MW00398027

LIPOSUCTION
& AESTHETIC
SURGERY

LIPOSUCTION & AESTHETIC SURGERY

Gerald H. Pitman, M.D.

Clinical Associate Professor of Surgery (Plastic Surgery),
Institute of Reconstructive Plastic Surgery, New York University
School of Medicine; Attending Surgeon, Manhattan Eye, Ear
and Throat Hospital, New York University–Bellevue Medical Center,
St. Luke's–Roosevelt Hospital Center, New York, N.Y.

ILLUSTRATOR

Virginia Cantarella

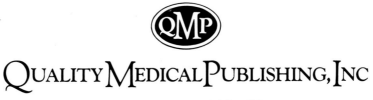

QUALITY MEDICAL PUBLISHING, INC

ST. LOUIS, MISSOURI
1993

Cover art:
PICASSO, Pablo
Les Demoiselles d'Avignon. Paris (begun May, reworked July 1907).
Oil on canvas, 8' × 7'8".
Collection, The Museum of Modern Art, New York. Acquired through the
Lillie P. Bliss Bequest.
Photograph © 1991 The Museum of Modern Art, New York.

Copyright © 1993 by Quality Medical Publishing, Inc.

All rights reserved. Reproduction of the material herein in any form
requires the written permission of the publisher.

Printed in the United States of America.

Credits are listed on p. 471.

PUBLISHER   Karen Berger

PROJECT MANAGER   Carolita Deter

PRODUCTION   Susan Trail, Billie Forshee, Judy Bamert

DESIGN   Diane M. Beasley

Quality Medical Publishing, Inc.
2086 Craigshire Drive
St. Louis, Missouri 63146

LIBRARY OF CONGRESS CATALOGING-IN-PUBLICATION DATA

Pitman, Gerald H., 1942-
    Liposuction & aesthetic surgery / Gerald H. Pitman.
      p.   cm.
    Includes bibliographical references and index.
    ISBN 0-942219-18-X (h)
    1. Liposuction. 2. Surgery, Plastic. I. Title. II. Title:
Liposuction and aesthetic surgery.
    [DNLM: 1. Esthetics. 2. Lipectomy—methods.   WO600 P685L]
RD119.5.L55P58   1993
617.9'5—dc20
DLC
for Library of Congress   92-532
                                           CIP

VT/WW/WW
5 4 3 2 1

To
Kay, Sam, and Max

Foreword

Some years ago when I first heard about liposuction from European colleagues I was not only skeptical but altogether unconvinced that a procedure that seemed so "unsurgical" had any long-term potential. Inserting a tube into the subcutaneous tissue space and literally suctioning excess fat without creating uncontrollable hemorrhage and unsightly secondary deformities was almost beyond comprehension.

Nonetheless, the concept of suction lipectomy was intriguing. Could the notoriously troublesome scars left by contouring the buttocks, thighs, and abdomen be avoided? Initially use of the technique was confined primarily to Europe. It was generally ill-regarded in the United States until over ten years ago a small group of surgeons commissioned by the American Society of Plastic and Reconstructive Surgeons visited Europe to observe the technique first hand. Their report sounded a note of cautious optimism.

Even after I began to grasp the advantages of the liposuction technique, I did not foresee the range of applications, nor did I appreciate the appeal of this procedure to young surgeons who were struggling to meet the requests of their patients for body contouring without extensive incisions.

Dr. Gerald Pitman was one of a small group of surgeons who transformed this rather gross procedure into one of finesse and control. He became interested in the field of liposuction early on. As Chairman of the Department of Plastic Surgery at Manhattan Eye, Ear and Throat Hospital I observed him work to hone his skills with this technique and eventually become a major contributor to our store of knowledge. His research helped to provide the necessary scientific validity. The study of the physiologic effects of liposuction, including fluid and electrolyte and blood replacement, as well as the possible effects of extracting body fat in large quantities was crucial to the well-being of the patient and obtaining good results. I remember well Dr. Pitman's first efforts to computerize the fat volume of a patient and to predict the consequences of liposuction based on computerized assessment.

Few of us could have conceived that liposuction would assume such an important role in plastic surgery. With technical refinements, the procedure has become at least as safe as any other plastic surgery operation. The results are quite predictable, and the complication rate is low. In many cases the extensive and objectionable scars of contour excisional surgery are eliminated by suction. The public demand for liposuction has made it one of the most common operations performed in the United States. Although the exact statistics are difficult to determine since many, if not most, of these procedures are performed as outpatient operations in surgeons' operating suites, it ranks among the top five surgical procedures performed over all.

In addition to its obvious advantage in treating body fat, liposuction has proved a major boon to those of us who confine our practice to the treatment of the head and neck. It has greatly facilitated face-lifting techniques and improved our results. The ability to suction fat from the neck and submental areas in particular is a tremendous advantage, especially as the cannulas became smaller and smaller, lending increasing precision to the technique. Direct suction of the buccal region has not been as rewarding in my experience, but some have reported interesting results.

Liposuction & Aesthetic Surgery is a testament to Dr. Pitman's knowledge and command of the subject. It should be read by everyone engaged in clinical practice of aesthetic surgery, even those performing few, if any, liposuction procedures. This book describes the state of the art and is thus essential to perfecting results in aesthetic surgery.

Thomas D. Rees

Preface

If any man wish to write a clear style, let him first be clear in his thoughts.
GOETHE

When I first became interested in liposuction in 1981, only a handful of people worldwide were performing the procedure. Little was known about its safety or efficacy, and most plastic surgeons were skeptical about such a radical departure from traditional surgical technique. Many looked at the procedure with disdain and even scorn. Nevertheless, I soon became convinced that liposuction could shape the body in a new and exciting way. I began to use it cautiously at first, but with increasing confidence as time passed.

Because the technique was novel and controversial, it demanded a rigorous, disciplined approach. For me, quantitative assessment was the key to good results and patient safety. Therefore, from the beginning, I measured weight, height, and pertinent body circumferences at every preoperative and postoperative examination. In the operating room, I recorded individual volumes removed from each area. Postoperative evaluation was conducted in light of preoperative measurements and knowledge of the precise volumes removed at surgery. Quantitative analysis of early cases refined clinical judgment and rapidly improved results. With time, use of small-diameter cannulas and an increasing sophistication in intraoperative evaluation of form and contour produced additional improvements. But it was the early insistence on meticulous quantitative assessment that set the stage for further refinements.

Quantitative assessment was also the foundation for safe management of fluid and blood loss. Meticulous record keeping helped define a linear relationship between suction volume and requirements for fluid and blood replacement. I believe that my record of safely treating large numbers of liposuction patients has been due in no small part to quantitative assessment.

My purpose in writing this book has been to share with my colleagues, particularly those just entering practice, my experience over the last 10 years. Although the work began as a treatise on liposuction, the broad application of this technique to multiple aesthetic and reconstructive operations encouraged me to enlarge the scope. I have interweaved related procedures when appropriate for a unified treatment approach. After all, patients come to the surgeon requesting improvement, not just a specific operation, and it is well to have the full range of surgical and nonsurgical options in mind during the initial consultation.

I have endeavored to present fairly my successes as well as some operations that did not turn out exactly as planned and disappointed either the patient or me. Sometimes I was able to improve the result with a secondary procedure, sometimes not. In all cases I have explained as clearly as possible what went wrong and how it might have been avoided.

The book is organized into two parts. The first section concerns fundamental clinical principles. The opening chapter is an overview of the surgeon's approach to the body contour patient and his or her unique needs. Enough information is provided in Chapter 2 on specialized instrumentation to help both the neophyte and more experienced surgeon in selection and purchase of equipment. Operative strategies providing a safe and inclusive framework for multiple body contouring procedures are the subject of Chapter 3. Chapter 4 covers fluid management. Mastery of this subject is key to avoiding major complications. In Chapter 5 I consider in some detail the tumescent technique, superficial suction, and syringe suction and the application of these recent refinements to the treatment of cellulite.

The second and larger section is organized into operations by anatomic area. For each area, I included a detailed consideration of the pertinent anatomy, not just the subcutaneous fat but also important underlying structures. Each chapter covers patient evaluation, technical operative details, avoidance of complications, and evaluation of results. Where appropriate, I describe related operations with or without adjunctive use of liposuction. Accordingly, the chapter on face and neck covers not just liposuction but significant segments on face and neck lift. Similarly, the chapter on the abdomen discusses liposuction and the various abdominoplasties as a continuum of treatment possibilities to be considered in evaluating and operating on patients. The chapter on thighs and buttocks logically includes thigh lifts.

One of the great pleasures in writing this book was that in seeking to educate others, I educated myself. Committing my thoughts to paper forced me to examine them not just in light of my own experience but also in light of the published experience of my colleagues and predecessors. As I reflected on issues concerning patient evaluation and operative technique and considered how best to express my ideas simply and clearly, the issues themselves became clearer. I developed a better understanding of my patients' needs and improved my skills in evaluation. As I simplified and refined the text, I also found myself doing the same in the operating room, and certain subtle variations in operating procedures evolved along with the book. In short, the writing process became a valuable adjunct to my surgical practice. It is my sincere wish that this record of my experience will be as helpful to the reader as it has been to the writer.

Gerald H. Pitman

Acknowledgments

More than five years have passed since the inception of this book to its birth. During this long gestation many people contributed their time, talents, and encouragement.

Dr. Tom Rees was Chairman of the Department of Plastic Surgery at Manhattan Eye, Ear and Throat Hospital when I performed the first liposuction procedure at that institution. By precept and example, he created an environment of innovation and excellence. He was generous in his support of a whole generation of young plastic surgeons. Dr. John M. Converse, Director of the Division of Plastic Surgery at New York University School of Medicine during my residency, was an inspirational leader, constantly challenging his residents to think critically and creatively. Dr. Joseph G. McCarthy, the current director, has continued to foster an academic atmosphere of inquiry and excitement. Other plastic surgery colleagues in New York whom I would like to thank for their interest and support include Dr. Sherrell J. Aston, Dr. William W. Shaw, and Dr. Nicholas Tabbal.

Dr. John Holzer, Chairman of the Department of Anesthesia at Manhattan Eye, Ear and Throat Hospital, was my original collaborator in working out the parameters and dynamics of fluid balance and blood replacement for liposuction. He also developed anesthetic techniques to make this operation as safe and pain-free as possible.

Dr. Bahman Teimourian introduced me to liposuction and was the father of this procedure in the United States. In 1987 I chaired the first of several annual symposia on liposuction in New York City sponsored by Manhattan Eye, Ear and Throat Hospital. Dr. Teimourian, Dr. Eugene H. Courtiss, and Dr. Frederick M. Grazer were among the initial faculty. Over the ensuing years we exchanged much useful information and continue to do so. I am grateful for their stimulating ideas and collegiality. More recently, Dr. Ted E. Lockwood of Kansas City and Dr. Luiz Toledo of São Paulo have shared their thoughts and techniques.

A book on plastic surgery depends as much on visual images as on the text. Virginia Cantarella provided most of the drawings, and her long effort and enthusiasm in interpreting operations and anatomic niceties are manifest throughout. Kevin Sommerville and Beth Willert also contributed drawings. Richard Imrie is a well-known fashion photographer and good friend. He produced several photographic personifications of ideal feminine beauty that can be easily recognized in this book.

Evaluation of results in liposuction, as in all plastic surgery, is dependent on skilled, honest photography. I was fortunate to have Wayne Pearson of Don Allen Studios take most of the clinical photographs. Early on, Wayne and I worked out appropriate views to show the sometimes subtle changes of body contouring. Wayne also provided extra prints and other photographic support, frequently on very short notice.

In the past 10 years I have worked with many surgical nurses, both in the office and at the hospital. My office scrub nurse, Jocelyn Choa, constantly seeks ways to improve efficiency and has provided expert assistance during our long-term association. At the Manhattan Eye, Ear and Throat Hospital Rafaella Diaz has worked to see that operations proceed smoothly and on time. Marilyn Ligouri was a superb organizer and much valued assistant in gathering clinical data for my initial studies on fluid balance and blood loss. Other nurses who have contributed their skills include Jeanie Bastone, Mary Jo Bertolino, Nancy Box, Dara Cantrell, Tracy Matthews, Debra Milbauer, Shirley Myers, and Linda Ramputti.

The support of my office staff has been much appreciated. Mrs. Helene Goodgold, my long-time assistant and patient coordinator, assumed numerous responsibilities to relieve me of tasks so that I could devote my energies to patient care and writing. Ms. Carolyn Morrow responded to a multitude of needs, typed much of the manuscript, and tirelessly filed and retrieved photographs. Vicki-Lee Wall also typed many pages of manuscript.

Ms. Rita Gams, reference librarian at The New York Academy of Medicine, and Ms. Dede Silverston, medical librarian at Manhattan Eye, Ear and Throat Hospital, provided bibliographic searches and tracked down obscure references with skill and dedication.

Several of the equipment vendors provided information and expertise. Robert Moffatt of Gast Manufacturing took the time to answer many questions on pump design and function. Gunter Grams of Grams Medical, Andy Halsey of M.D. Engineering Company, John Johnson of The Tulip Company, and John Wells of Wells-Johnson Company all contributed ideas and illustrations on short notice.

I would like to thank my publisher, Karen Berger, President of Quality Medical Publishing, Inc. Karen had the patience of Job and the strength of Samson. She coaxed, encouraged, cajoled, and when necessary threatened until this book finally emerged. Her organizational suggestions and editing skills added grace to the manuscript. She started as my publisher but ended as my friend. Special thanks are also due to the staff at Quality Medical Publishing.

My wife, Kay, provided unflagging support and encouragement. She endured my moods when things were going slowly and my weekend absences when they were going well. My sons, Sam and Max, were also ceaselessly supportive and understanding of my frequent need to be away.

Contents

Part I

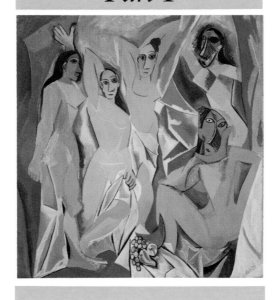

PRELIMINARY CONSIDERATIONS

Chapter 1

CONSULTATION AND PATIENT SELECTION

In the past decade liposuction has shed its status as a surgical curiosity to become a well-accepted procedure with clearly defined indications. Its increasing popularity and widespread appeal have made it the most frequently performed aesthetic operation in the United States. The majority of liposuction procedures involve primary cosmetic contouring to slim the torso and lower extremities. But liposuction is also used for reconstructive operations that reduce the debilitating effects of lymphedema and gynecomastia. Adjunctive applications increase the efficiency and refine the results of multiple aesthetic and reconstructive procedures.

CONSULTATION

The patient requesting liposuction is usually a woman (85% in my practice) desiring a slimmer, more sculpted face or body. The shapely, rounded proportions that characterize the abdomen, hips, and thighs are in many ways the essence of womanliness and have been a symbol of female sexuality throughout the ages. Yet these natural attributes are often seen as negatives in a society obsessed with youth, diet, and fitness.

Most patients fall into one of two categories. The larger group, more than 50%, is between the ages of 20 and 39 years (see p. 26). The typical patient in this group is not overweight but is very figure conscious and dissatisfied with figure faults that do not approach fashion's ideal. A second, smaller group is between 40 and 59 years of age. The typical woman in this older group may voice the same complaints as the younger patient with additional concerns related to changes brought on by weight gain and aging. The older patient's problems are attributable to gradual weight gain plus the inevitable age-related compaction, widening, and thickening of the midbody. Even the thin older woman may complain that her body has changed and her clothes do not fit.

The patient pursuing society's idealized standard of beauty often approaches the plastic surgeon's office with trepidation. During her encounter with the plastic surgeon she must subject to scrutiny areas of her body that she perceives to be imperfect and normally tries to camouflage. She may have feelings of insecurity, doubt, shame, and even revulsion. Certainly, she will be embarrassed. The surgeon conducting the consultation should be sensitive to the special needs and concerns of this patient.

FRAMEWORK FOR SURGEON-PATIENT DIALOGUE

Over the years I have developed a format for the body contour consultation that is sensitive to the patient's needs, puts her at ease as much as possible, and elicits essential information. The framework for this interaction is highly structured, but its very rigidity creates a neutral, professional atmosphere that calms and reassures the patient. The consultation consists of four parts: preliminary interview, metric examination, physical examination, and informed consent.

Interview

Before the interview the patient fills out a medical history form and reads a detailed letter on liposuction in the waiting room. If the patient indicates she is interested in abdominoplasty or thigh lift, the receptionist will give her letters on those procedures. The liposuction letter is reproduced on p. 5. The letters on abdominoplasty and thigh lift appear on pp. 244-245 and 362-365.

The initial meeting occurs in my private office. Time is allowed at the beginning of the conversation for an unstructured exchange of pleasantries and discussion of subjects other than surgery. The conversation may focus on the weather, the patient's profession, or any other appropriate subject. The object is not to extract medical information but to ease the patient's apprehension and afford an opportunity to observe her in a social situation.

I note the style and quality of her dress. Is she meticulously groomed and attentive to detail, or is she disheveled and unkempt? Obsessive attention to wardrobe may indicate a similar obsession with surgical results and a difficult-to-please patient. On the other hand, total inattention to dress may be symptomatic of psychosis.

INFORMATION LETTER

Liposuction

Liposuction is a surgical procedure for removing localized deposits of subcutaneous fat anywhere in the body. This technique uses small incisions and a high vacuum to remove fat cells in selected regions, thereby reducing contour in the treated areas.

A ⅛ to ¼ inch incision is made near the area from which the fat is to be removed, and a specially designed surgical cannula (tube) is placed through the incision into the fat. The cannula is attached by flexible tubing to a vacuum pump that removes the fat by suction as the cannula is manipulated beneath the skin.

Although the procedure was originally developed for the torso and thighs, it is now used on all areas of the body and has proved particularly helpful in contouring the area under the chin and as an adjunct to face lifting.

Fat distribution is determined by two factors, heredity and diet. Heredity determines the location and number of individual fat cells, which are fixed and unchanging after puberty. Diet can increase or decrease the amount of fat in each cell but will not affect the total number of cells or their distribution. For example, if you have inherited large numbers of fat cells on your thighs and small numbers of fat cells on your chest, you will always have more fat on the thighs than on the chest, and strenuous attempts at weight loss can leave you with a thin upper body and persistently bulky thighs.

Your appearance after liposuction will be influenced by your general state of health, the overall condition of your skin, age, weight, hormonal influences, and other factors. Each patient is unique, and during our consultation I will discuss with you in detail how these general factors apply to you in particular. Liposuction is not a substitute for a healthy diet nor is it useful for generalized weight reduction. While the foregoing may seem obvious, I mention it because some patients may expect localized fat removal to effect a dramatic weight loss. This is not possible.

Liposuction selectively removes fat only from those areas in which the patient desires reduction. Since the actual fat cells are removed, the procedure is permanent, and following liposuction the body will always have less fat in the treated areas.

Skin Elasticity   Good skin elasticity is a desirable attribute in all patients since it makes for a smooth surface contour. Tight skin is universally seen in the very young and is gradually lost as we age. Even through middle age, however, we retain some elasticity. The skin envelope always shrinks to adjust to the reduced contour following an appropriate liposuction.

Cellulite   The word "cellulite" has no precise medical meaning. Most people use the word to refer to dimpling and irregularities that occur on the surface of the skin. It is seen most frequently over the lower torso and thighs, worsens with age, and is frequently associated with loose skin (see below). Cellulite is due to protein degeneration in the skin and its supporting structures. While liposuction will not cure cellulite, it will remove fat and reduce contour.

In mild cases liposuction may lessen the intensity of cellulite. Severe cases, however, require abdominoplasty ("tummy tuck") or thigh lift for permanent improvement.

Loose Skin and Musculature   Some individuals have lax musculature and loose skin with or without excess fat. These patients require additional procedures such as abdominoplasty (tummy tuck) or thigh lifts. During your consultation I will evaluate your skin and musculature as well as localized fat deposition. If you require thigh lift or abdominoplasty for optimal results, I will so inform you.

Continued.

INFORMATION LETTER

Liposuction—cont'd

Permanency of Results The number of fat cells is fixed after puberty. Adults become thinner or fatter by reducing or increasing the amount of fat in each cell. Since liposuction reduces contour by removing fat cells, the procedure is permanent. Should you gain weight following liposuction, you will tend to deposit the fat in areas other than those treated.

Anesthesia When only one or two small areas are treated, particularly on the face and neck, the patient is given a local anesthetic. When multiple or large areas are treated, general or regional (spinal/epidural) anesthetics are administered by an anesthesiologist. The anesthesiologist's services are charged separately.

Duration of the Operation The operation lasts 30 minutes to 2 hours, depending on how many areas are treated.

Hospitalization vs. Office Surgery Patients having large amounts suctioned stay overnight in the hospital. Admission is the morning of operation, and discharge is at 10:00 A.M. 1 day after surgery. You may have a private room or semiprivate room shared with one other patient usually having a cosmetic procedure similar to yours. A private-duty nurse will add to your comfort following the operation but is not essential to your care. Please inform my office if you want a private room or private-duty nurse.

Patients having smaller amounts suctioned may have ambulatory surgery, reporting to the office the morning of surgery and remaining a few hours after the operation. If you live more than 1 hour away, you must stay overnight in Manhattan after surgery. If you desire, we will recommend a nearby hotel. You will need to have someone with you when you leave after the operation, remain with you overnight, and accompany you when you return to the office the next day for a postoperative check. If a relative or friend is not available, we will recommend a nurse.

After Surgery There are usually no bandages or dressings. Patients having larger amounts of fat removal may require a urinary catheter in the immediate postoperative period. If needed, this catheter is placed while the patient is asleep during surgery and is removed prior to discharge. Both placement and removal are painless.

Stitches are small surgical staples that are taken out the day after surgery. Removal is painless.

You will be placed in a support garment immediately after surgery, and you will wear the garment continuously for 2 to 3 weeks. You may remove the garment to shower starting 24 hours after surgery. If your calves and/or ankles are treated, you will wear support hose for up to 6 weeks.

You may experience some pain for an hour after surgery, for which you will be given as much medication as necessary. There is usually only mild discomfort thereafter, although you will have a prescription for light pain medication should you need it. All patients except those having very small volume removal (e.g., neck only or knees only) take an iron supplement for 1 month after surgery.

I will see you the first day after surgery and 1 week, 1 month, and 6 months after surgery. All patients may return to work in 1 week, although many return earlier. Vigorous sports are prohibited for 3 weeks. If skin tightening is done, recovery will be longer.

For the first week following surgery the treated areas will be swollen and will show no reduction in contour. In fact, you may appear larger than you did before surgery. Your clothes may fit more tightly, and you may weigh more. By the end of the first week, however, the swelling associated with surgery begins to subside, and sometime during the second week you will notice a diminution in contour and the treated areas will be smaller than they were before surgery. Resolution of swelling occurs rapidly after the first week, but your final improvement may not be apparent until as long as 3 months after surgery. If the calves and ankles have been treated, subtle additional improvements may take place even beyond 3 months.

Photographs Preoperative photographs will be taken. The body photographs do not show your face. They are important aids in planning and performing surgery and become a permanent part of your patient record. Postoperative photographs are taken 6 months after surgery.

Scars In the past, scars from body contouring were long and conspicuous. Liposuction scars are usually less than ¼ inch long and can be placed in natural body creases or in other areas where they are inconspicuous or easily hidden by clothing or bathing suits. In most patients the scars will be red or pigmented for 6 months and gradually fade thereafter until they are not noticeable by 12 months after surgery. The scars are rarely troublesome. Nevertheless, you should know that all scars are permanent and their height, width, and final color are not totally predictable.

Complications and Untoward Results
Serious complications are uncommon with this kind of surgery. All patients have bruising, which lasts 3 to 6 weeks, occasionally longer. A certain amount of numbness or reduced sensation in the treated area is also to be expected. As with any surgery, bleeding, infection, and other complications are possible.

Patients may experience contour irregularities in the treated areas following surgery. Usually this is temporary, but, in occasional patients, may be permanent. Perfect symmetry is the goal, although small side-to-side differences can occur. I will make every effort to give you as smooth and symmetric a result as possible.

Five percent of patients have secondary surgery or a "touch-up" after 6 months, most frequently for removal of additional fat. This is usually done in the office under local anesthesia but may require general anesthesia and/or hospitalization if the work is extensive.

Articles have appeared in the lay press publicizing and even sensationalizing disastrous consequences following liposuction. Fat embolization (small particles of fat traveling to the lungs or other parts of the body) has received particularly lurid coverage. I have investigated all serious complications and/or deaths associated with liposuction that have come to my attention either through reports in the medical literature or informally through my professional associations. I have found that almost all patients who had a disastrous consequence following liposuction had either been operated on by unqualified practitioners or had had additional simultaneous surgical procedures performed that were more likely to have caused the complication. I believe that fat embolization is a universal accompaniment of all surgery and is of no clinical significance in healthy patients. While no surgery can be totally safe, liposuction compares favorably with any cosmetic procedure.

I mention these problems because I want to give you full disclosure. I hasten to add, however, that the vast majority of patients are immensely satisfied with their results, and in my personal practice I have never seen a serious complication from this procedure.

Should you not understand any of the foregoing, or should you want further information, please ask. Occasional questions will arise after you have left the office. Feel free to call for additional information. If necessary, a second visit can be scheduled. Find out all you need to know. I wish all patients to be fully informed.

The nature of this interaction provides significant insights. Is the patient able to easily participate in a social, intellectual, and emotional interchange? Dr. Jack Sheen has quoted a psychiatrist as stating, "If you can't elicit a smile from a patient, don't operate." Although not every patient may smile during what may be a stressful interview, every person should be able to interact verbally with her surgeon at some mutually comfortable level. If I cannot establish some easy form of social intercourse in the first 5 minutes, I know that it portends trouble for the future doctor-patient relationship, and I do not offer surgery. Fortunately, such individuals are rare, and most patients are approachable and friendly.

After a few minutes' conversation I ask the patient, "Please tell me how may I help you?" or "Please tell me what brings you to the office?" I keep the question neutral and open; once the patient begins to respond, I allow her to speak freely without interruption. Even if she rambles somewhat, it is important to let her tell her story in her own way.

Patients sometimes respond to questions about their concerns by saying, "Doctor, you're the expert; I want you to tell me how I can look better." With this statement the patient may be voicing a legitimate wish to receive some expert guidance from her surgeon. But this plea for direction may also be a clue to generalized, emotional dissatisfaction having little to do with the body. A hostile, suspicious patient may also be wary of revealing the reasons for her visit. She may fear that the "avaricious" surgeon will seize on any complaint and offer to fix it for a fee. It is important to distinguish which type of patient is sitting across from me. I do so by first reassuring the patient that in due course I will perform a comprehensive examination and will not hesitate to recommend whatever surgery I feel appropriate. I go on to say, however, that the recommended procedure will depend not only on her physical characteristics but also on her personal needs and desires, and therefore I would like to know what concerns *her* the most so that I can properly focus my attention.

The depressed or suspicious patient will remain generalized, unfocused, and vague. Inability to articulate a specific concern raises a cautionary flag in my mind. If the patient has no specific dissatisfactions, surgery will not help, and if the patient is hostile now, she may be even more so after surgery, particularly if the result does not meet her expectations. Fortunately, most patients can be brought to the point and are reasonably articulate and specific in their desires with little coaching.

After establishing the patient's reasons for coming to the office, I move to questions concerning weight, diet, exercise, and fitting of clothes. The patient is asked for her lowest and highest weight since adolescence, the chronology of her weight change, her ideal weight, and the weight she is able to maintain. If the patient has complained about excess fullness in a particular body area, she is asked if the disproportion persisted at ideal or low weight. Patients who have "diet-resistant" fat will retain bulges in their thighs and buttocks even when at normal or near-normal weight. This group of patients responds well to liposuction. If the patient has demonstrated an inability to maintain normal weight by dieting and exercising, insisting on weight loss prior to surgery is futile. I have to decide, based on her current weight, whether or not the patient is a suitable candidate for surgery. I never ask the patient her present weight. She will be weighed by the nurse, and the actual weight recorded in the office may be embarrassingly more than the patient volunteers.

Major weight fluctuations and other history suggestive of eating disorders are noted. Actively anorectic or bulemic patients require psychiatric not surgical care. On the other hand, patients who have recovered from eating disorders can be helped by liposuction, and a past history of anorexia or bulemia is not a contraindication to body contour procedures.

The patient is asked about her exercise habits. Would she describe herself as sedentary, physically active, or somewhere in between? Although the level of exercise is not critical to making a decision about surgery, it does reflect on the patient's psychological makeup and body image orientation.

Questions concerning dress size and difficulty in fitting clothes yield important insights. It is not uncommon for patients to make a comment such as, "I am a size 8 on top and a 12 on bottom." Bra size is also a clue to general body proportions.

A brief gynecologic history includes the number of full-term pregnancies and menstrual history.

The general medical history is reviewed, eliciting further information and clarifying details as needed. Previous surgeries and serious illnesses are listed in chronologic order. Allergies are documented with specific information on the allergen involved and the exact nature of the reaction. Medications and dosages are also noted, including over-the-counter and illicit drugs, and inquiries are made about any systemic or psychological problems.

After the specific body contour history and the more generalized medical history, the patient is ready for a metric and physical examination.

Metric Examination

The nurse conducts the metric examination, recording height, weight, and blood pressure and measuring the circumferences of all pertinent body areas. This and other data are entered on a specially designed body contour consultation form.

Weight and circumferences are also recorded in the late postoperative period. If weight is constant at 6 months, then one can ascribe postoperative changes to surgery. If weight has changed, postoperative appearance is evaluated in light of the weight differential.

During the metric examination a skilled nurse is able to establish rapport and extract insights from the patient that extend beyond simple recording of data and may even include confidences not readily revealed to the surgeon. If the nurse has actually had body contour surgery, so much the better; she gains additional credibility with the patient and can more readily assure her and put her at ease. The nurse also previews for the patient what will occur during her examination by the surgeon. After seeing the patient, the nurse meets with me privately to review measurements and alert me to any additional information she has obtained.

Physical Examination

I examine the patient first from the back. Her general body habitus and posture are noted. The existence of any spinal curvature and the relative heights of right and left shoulders and right and left iliac crests are recorded on the intake sheet. Then the quality of the patient's skin is documented with comments on wrinkles or irregularities. I also estimate the approximate aspiration volumes of all areas. The patient is turned to the side to better assess buttocks and abdominal protuberances and finally examined from the front to observe the anterior abdomen and the presence and location of abdominal scars.

I test for thickness of the fatty layer to determine if bulges are caused by fat or are secondary to skin relaxation or bony prominences. Multiple tests have been developed for preoperative evaluation of the subcutaneous fat, but they all reduce to three maneuvers: pinching the skin, lifting the skin, and having the patient contract her muscles.

Body Contour Consultation

Name _____   Date _____/_____/_____
          (Last)   (First)   (Initial)

Areas of concern: _____
_____

G _____   P _____   A _____   _____
Dress size _____   Bra _____   Shoulder: R _____ L _____
Weight history _____ Hips: R _____ L _____
_____ Scoliosis: None Mild Mod Sev
Ht. _____   _____
BP _____/_____   _____
                                          _____
          Consult   _____
Date   ___/___/___ ___/___/___ ___/___/___   _____
Weight   _____ _____ _____   _____
Waist   _____ _____ _____   _____
Umbilicus _____ _____ _____   _____
Hip   _____ _____ _____   _____
Thigh   _____ _____ _____   _____
          R   L   R   L   R   L   _____
Knee   ___ ___ ___ ___ ___ ___   _____
Calf   ___ ___ ___ ___ ___ ___
Ankle   ___ ___ ___ ___ ___ ___
Arm   ___ ___ ___ ___ ___ ___   _____

Pinch Test

Pinching up the skin and underlying tissues verifies that the protuberance is composed of subcutaneous fat and not excess skin, intraperitoneal fat, or bone.

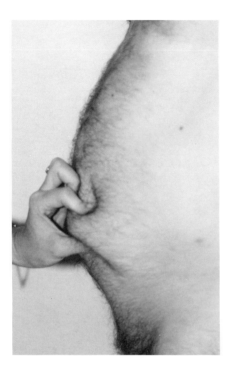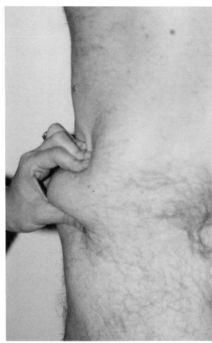

This man requested suction to reduce his abdomen. Most of his fat, however, was beneath the fascia, and pinching the skin revealed a relatively thin layer of subcutaneous fat, not enough to treat successfully. Pinching his flank area, however, revealed a substantial subcutaneous fat layer, and this area was treated.

Skin thickness in the area to be treated should be compared with thickness in adjacent areas. Although 3 cm (representing an actual skin and fat layer of 1.5 cm) has been suggested as a minimal pinch for areas to be suctioned, the minimum thickness of tissue that can be successfully suctioned is variable and depends on the peculiar and individual nature of each anatomic area.

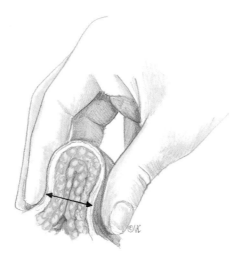

As shown in this schematic of the pinch test, when the skin is pinched it folds on itself, so that the actual thickness of the skin and subcutaneous fat layer is one-half the thickness of the tissue between the fingers.

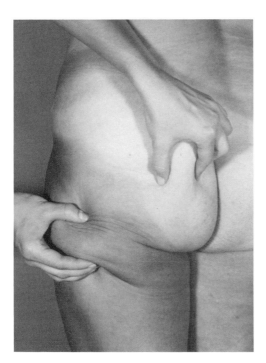 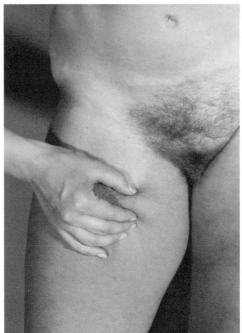

The pinch thickness over the buttocks and outer thigh is always greater than at the inner thigh. Over the buttocks, outer thighs, or abdomen a preoperative "pinch" thickness of at least 3 cm is desirable, but over the inner thighs or calves and ankles, preoperative pinch may be as little as 2 cm.

Lifting Test

The skin and subcutaneous tissues are elevated to note the effect on protuberant deformities. If most or all of the deformity is caused by loose skin, lifting the skin will significantly improve contour. This maneuver is particularly useful in identifying patients who require thigh lift.

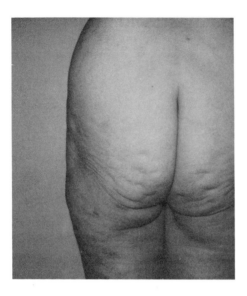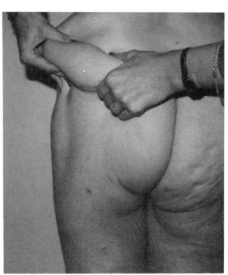

This patient has a small lateral thigh protuberance following liposuction. Her skin is lax and can be pulled up over the iliac crest, reducing the lateral thigh fullness; this suggests the need for thigh lift.

The lifting test can also be done on the abdomen with the patient standing to diagnose fullness due to skin laxity.

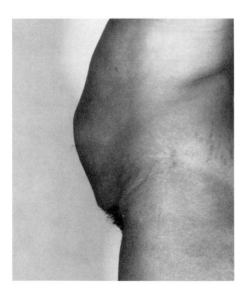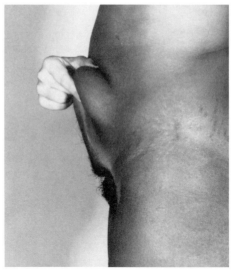

This woman's protuberant abdomen was due to excess skin, as demonstrated by the lift test.

If the patient is a candidate for abdominoplasty, she is examined supine so that the abdominal musculature can be tested for weakness or herniation. The abdomen should also be examined with the patient in a semisitting position so the surgeon can pinch up the skin of the lower abdomen to estimate if the entire skin segment between umbilicus and pubis can be excised.

Muscle Contraction

Having the patient tighten and pull in the abdominal musculature while the pinch test is performed can help distinguish between abdominal protuberance due to fat and protuberance from muscle laxity.

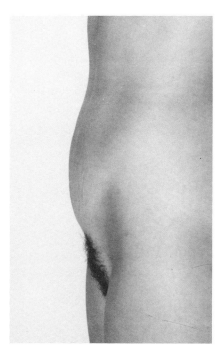 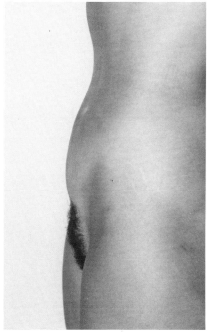 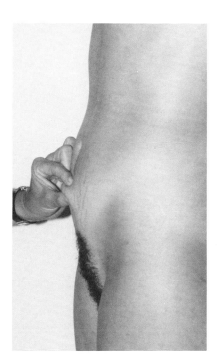

This patient's slight lower abdominal fullness was diminished when she contracted and pulled in the abdominal musculature. Pinching the skin while the muscles were contracted showed very little abdominal subcutaneous fat. This patient was not a candidate for liposuction. She was offered miniabdominoplasty (see Chapter 9).

Muscle contraction is also a useful technique for evaluating the lateral thighs.

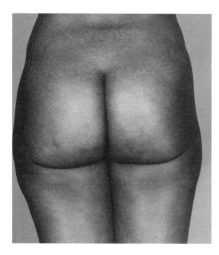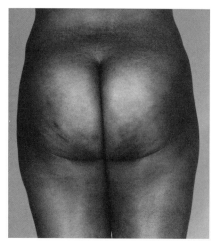

When the patient stands on her toes and tenses her buttocks, a reduction in the size of the lateral thigh bulk may sometimes be observed as the soft tissue mass of the buttocks is elevated by gluteal contraction. Note how this patient's full lateral thighs appear less full when the gluteal musculature is tensed, pulling her buttock mass in a superior direction and relieving pressure on her lateral thighs. When this happens, the lateral thighs should be treated not only by direct liposuction but also by removal of some of the buttock fat to reduce the mass transmitting pressure to the outer thighs.

Muscle contraction is also helpful in evaluating the calves and ankles.

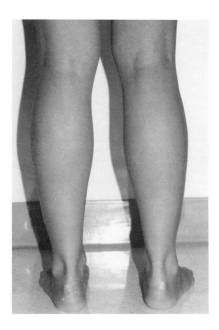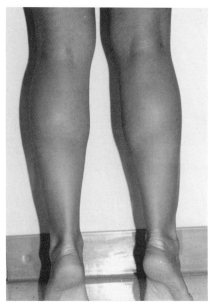

When the patient stands on her toes, the gastrocnemius muscles shorten and thicken, revealing their location and permitting the surgeon to plan fat removal so that the final result suggests the underlying presence of the muscle without undue accentuation.

Marking the Patient

When the examination is completed, I ask the patient for permission to mark her skin with a washable ink and mark all areas to be treated. The topographic outlines are the same as those used for preoperative markings; each access incision is also marked (see p. 46).

After the markings, the patient is given a hand mirror so that she can view each area to be treated and the planned incisions. I distinguish those areas I think will dramatically improve and those areas where only a subtle or limited change can be anticipated. I also point out skin irregularities and inform the patient that although it is unlikely she will have any new irregularities, old irregularities will probably persist.

I direct attention to asymmetries, telling the patient that I will compensate for these by removing more fat from fuller areas. Most asymmetries are skeletal in origin, however, and some persistent right-to-left differences are inevitable.

Informed Consent

I describe the nature of the procedure and recovery period in considerable detail. Much of this information is included in the letter that she has already read, but it is essential that this information be conveyed in a face-to-face conversation. During this conversation I mention alternatives to surgery. For the overweight patient, alternatives include weight loss. Of course, the patient always has the ultimate alternative of not having any surgery. I also outline the most common complications and untoward results.

The patient is asked if she has any questions concerning the procedure, and I take as long to answer them as necessary. Persistent questions on the same issues or repetitive review of possible complications are an indication that the patient is not emotionally ready for surgery.

Finally, I state my recommendation for treatment and the level of improvement that can be anticipated. After having spent a fair amount of time detailing alternatives, complications, and benefits, it is important to close with an unambiguous recommendation.

Before leaving the room I say, "Should any questions arise after you have left the office, please call. I will be happy to speak with you or return your call." The patient can also return for a reconsultation without charge. About 20% of patients ask for a second visit.

Special Consent for Operation or Other Procedures

Patient: _____

Date: _____ Time: _____

1. I hereby request and authorize Dr. Gerald H. Pitman and assistant(s) to perform a surgical operation(s) known as _____

   on _____.

   (Name of patient)

2. The procedure listed in paragraph 1 has been explained to me by Dr. Pitman, and I completely understand the procedure insofar as possible.

3. I have read Dr. Pitman's letter(s) entitled _____

   _____

   and dated _____. I understand the letter(s) and have had the opportunity to ask Dr. Pitman any questions concerning the letter(s).

4. I recognize that during the course of the operation unforeseen conditions may necessitate additional or different procedures than those set forth above. I therefore further authorize and request that Dr. Pitman, his assistants, or his designees perform such procedures as are, in his professional judgment, necessary and desirable, including, but not limited to, procedures involving pathology and radiology. The authority granted under this paragraph shall extend to remedying conditions that are not known to Dr. Pitman at the time the operation starts.

5. I consent to the administration of anesthetics to be applied by or under the direction and supervision of Dr. Pitman or such anesthesiologists as he shall select and to the use of such anesthetics as he may deem advisable.

6. I am aware that the practice of medicine and surgery is not an exact science, and that errors in judgment and implementation are possible in any surgery. Although good results are expected, I acknowledge that no guarantees have been made to me as to the results of the operation or procedure.

7. I consent to be photographed before, during, and after the treatment; these photographs shall be the property of Dr. Pitman and may be published in medical journals or books and/or shown for medical education. My name shall not be published.

8. I agree to keep Dr. Pitman informed of any change of address so that he can notify me of any late findings, and I agree to cooperate with him in my care after surgery until completely discharged.

9. I have read the above consent and fully understand the same and do authorize Dr. Pitman to perform this surgical procedure on me.

10. I am not known to be allergic to anything except: (list)

Dr. Gerald H. Pitman _____ Patient _____

Witness _____

Following her interview the patient meets with the patient administrator to discuss scheduling and fees. If she wishes to see "before and after" photographs, the administrator has a wide range of results to show. These pictures vary from thin, young women with small, localized deformities to middle-aged, overweight women with wrinkled skin. A selection of male photographs is also available.

The patient is provided with a copy of the consent for surgery at least 2 weeks before the operation so that she can study it in detail before signing. The consent is specific to the operation and makes reference to the information letter she has already read. The information letter is kept on permanent file in the office.

The signed document is not truly the informed consent; it is only evidence that the consent has taken place. The actual informed consent consists of the dialogue between patient and surgeon outlined above. This conversation gives the patient a full understanding of the risks and benefits as well as alternatives to the proposed surgery. It involves a sharing of responsibility and an acceptance by the patient of a level of risk. In this sense the informed consent is protective of the surgeon. More important, however, informed consent is simply good medical practice.

The patient consultation is focused and intense; distracting phone calls or interruptions are not permitted. The time varies depending on individual needs, but the quality of this exchange is more important than the actual quantity of time devoted. The patient is put at ease by the structure and orderly progression of the consultation. The form and content of this interaction are far more reassuring than elaborately decorated waiting rooms or glossy brochures.

PATIENT SELECTION
Health Status

Good health is a basic prerequisite for aesthetic body contouring procedures. Failure to screen out patients whose health is suboptimal is one of the important contributing factors to serious morbidity following liposuction. Obesity, hypertension, arteriosclerotic cardiovascular disease, diabetes mellitus, renal dysfunction, and other illnesses that compromise the patient's ability to recover from surgical trauma are all contraindications to liposuction and other forms of body contour surgery. Patients with minor medical problems may be suitable candidates for suction, depending on the severity of their disease and the magnitude of the planned procedure. Removal of small volumes of fat from limited areas under local anesthesia carries little risk, even for patients with minimally compromising conditions. As the volume of aspirate increases, however, or if multiple procedures are planned, medical contraindications become more absolute. Removal of 2000 cc under general anesthesia or performance of multiple simultaneous procedures carries significantly increased risk when general health is not optimal. All patients, whatever their medical status, deserve careful preoperative scrutiny and a prudent balancing of potential benefit vs. potential risk.

Localization of Fat

The most important criterion in patient selection is localization of excess fat. Patients with dramatically disproportionate, discrete, and localized fat deposits, whether large or small, can obtain correspondingly dramatic results. Patients with less well-localized excess fat or moderately overweight patients can still benefit from liposuction but with more limited results.

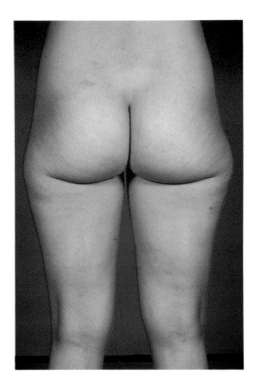 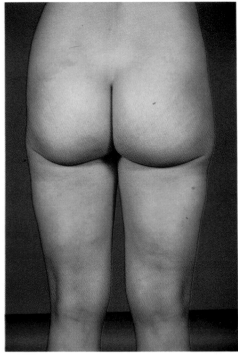

This rather petite woman (5 feet 3 inches, 108 pounds, dress size 3 on top, 5 on bottom) had small but very sharply localized excess fat. I was able to achieve a striking change in contour with removal of less than 150 cc of aspirate from each lateral thigh. Postoperatively, her weight remained constant, and she was able to fit a size 3 bottom as well as top.

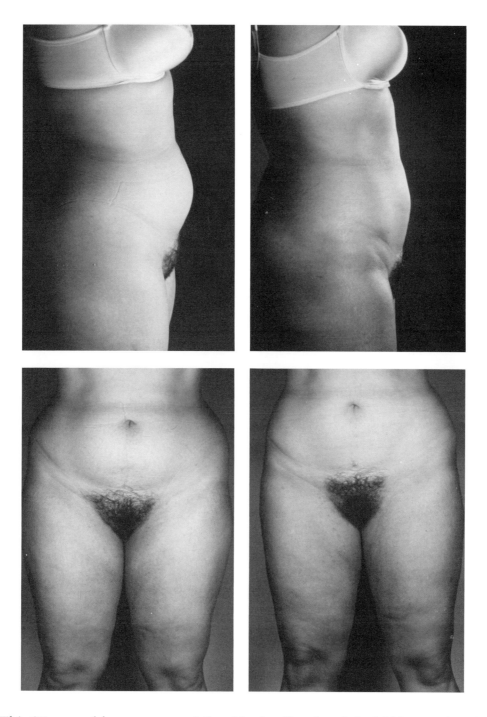

This 27-year-old woman was 6 feet 1 inch tall and weighed 200 pounds. Her three sisters and father were of similar build. Although she was moderately overweight, she still had enough localization of fat for successful treatment. I removed 500 cc from the abdomen, 500 cc from the left lateral thigh, 600 cc from the right lateral thigh, and 300 cc from each hip. Other areas were also treated. She shows a modest but definite improvement. Poor fat localization with or without obesity makes a pleasing result exceedingly difficult.

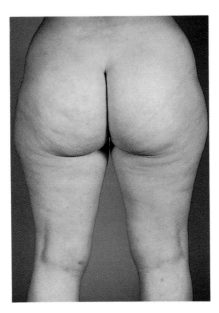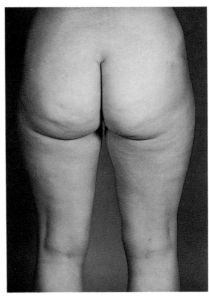

This patient had a very full figure (5 feet 3 inches, 140 pounds, dress size 12), but she still had pronounced localization of excess fat in her lateral thighs. I removed 425 cc from the left and 475 cc from the right outer thigh in one operation and 350 cc from the left and 450 cc from the right in a second operation 8 months later for a total of 775 cc from the left and 875 cc from the right outer thigh. I also treated her anterior thighs, medial thighs, buttocks, hips, and knees. When the second photograph was taken, she had lost 10 pounds by dieting and wore a size 8 dress, but the dramatic change in contour could not have been realized with weight loss alone. Localization of fat permitted an outstanding result.

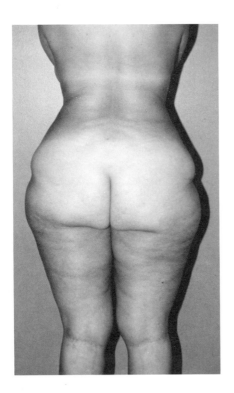

This 5-foot 2-inch patient weighed 145 pounds. Most important, her fat was diffusely distributed. Patients such as these are generally not offered surgery.

Weight

Weight is another factor to consider in patient selection. Patients seeking surgery can be divided into three weight groups: normal, moderately overweight, and severely overweight.

Normal Weight

Patients of normal weight may have disproportionate and excessive fat deposition, most frequently in the thighs and buttocks in women, but also in the hips and abdomen in both sexes. Attempts to reduce contour by dieting and exercise are unsuccessful because these patients are genetically programmed to retain fat in the affected areas. These regions are the last to lose fat during weight loss, retaining fullness even as the patient approaches cachexia. The common denominator for these patients is that they are more successfully treated by surgery than by weight loss and exercise.

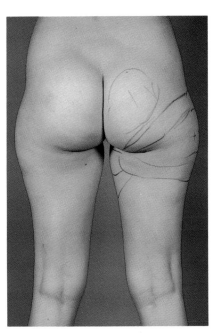 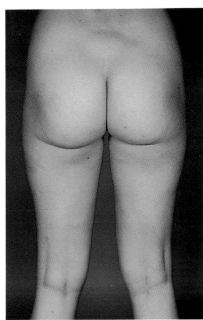

This 5-foot 2-inch woman weighed 100 pounds; she had persistent and disproportionate lateral thigh and buttock fullness despite an exercise program and normal weight. Note preoperative markings of area to be treated. She is shown 6 months after removal of 500 cc from each lateral thigh. The buttocks and medial thighs were also treated.

Moderately Overweight

Despite being moderately overweight this group of patients may have disproportionate fat deposition in the torso and extremities, but the common denominator for these patients is that at least a portion of the desired reduction in contour can be achieved with diet and exercise.

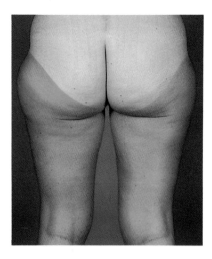 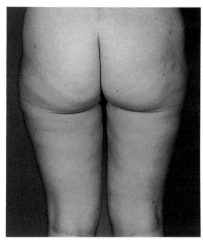

This woman was 5 feet 8 inches tall and weighed 146 pounds. She had lost 10 or 15 pounds on many occasions, always returning to about 145 pounds. At lower weights her outer thigh contour was partially reduced but always remained disproportionately full. Suction of 500 cc from each lateral thigh produced a significant and permanent contour reduction at a constant weight of 146 pounds. I also treated the hips, medial thighs, and medial knees.

Some of these patients can be convinced to undergo a trial of weight loss, but most, having already failed, perhaps several times, will want a surgical solution to an intractable problem. Patients 10 to 20 pounds above ideal weight can have satisfactory results and benefit from surgery as long as they have good fat localization. Nevertheless it is still the surgeon's responsibility to present the alternatives of diet and exercise for even the slightly overweight patient. Patient evaluation always includes an assessment of nonsurgical solutions. Anterior abdominal fat is extremely labile in most persons and is lost quickly with weight reduction. Buttock and lateral thigh fat is usually more resistant to dieting and exercise, particularly in women. If the patient still elects surgery, the surgeon has not only followed good medical practice but has also provided one of the essential components of an informed consent, namely, an alternative to the surgical procedure.

If the patient is accepted for surgery, she is not encouraged to diet preoperatively. It is technically easier to remove fat from patients with slightly distended fat deposits. Weight loss tends to make the fat more fibrous and difficult to extract.

Severely Overweight

For severely overweight patients, removal of even large volumes of tissue will make little discernible difference in their appearance. Moreover, surgery will be fraught with complications and untoward results such as wrinkled, hanging skin or pseudobursae. These patients should be rejected for surgery.

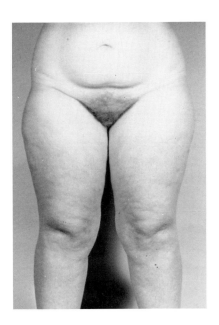

This 5-foot 1-inch woman weighed 165 pounds; she had been unsuccessful in her repeated efforts to lose weight; I judged her to be a poor candidate for liposuction because of her obesity combined with poor skin quality and absence of fat localization. She was referred to a weight-loss program, which she was unable to complete.

Skin Elasticity and Cellulite*

Although smooth, tight skin is a desirable attribute, it has been overrated as a criterion for patient selection in liposuction. Patients with skin wrinkling or multiple fine and coarse irregularities, so-called cellulite, can still benefit from liposuction as long as they have disproportionate fullness secondary to fat.

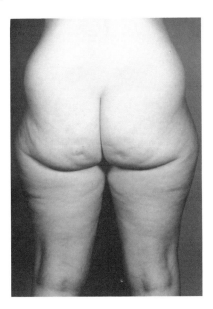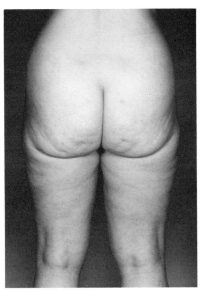

This patient exhibited poor-quality skin with "cellulite," but she also had large, disproportionate lateral thigh fat excess that was improved by removal of 650 cc from each outer thigh in two operations: 400 cc from each thigh at the first operation and 250 cc from each thigh at the second operation. Her hips, medial thighs, and medial knees were also treated.

*See also pp. 101-107.

Although cellulite is seen most frequently in women over 35 years of age, it can occur in genetically predisposed women and men in their late teens and twenties. Patients with cellulite who request liposuction should be evaluated with particular care since frequently the wrinkled skin disturbs them more than the fullness of contour. It is well to take extra time in the initial consultation to emphasize that cellulite is not totally correctable by liposuction, and some skin irregularity will persist. Patients who accept these limitations will usually be satisfied with their improved contour, and those who primarily want improvement in the appearance of their skin will be spared an operation. The surgeon is also spared the difficulty of dealing with a disappointed postoperative patient.

Patients who have poor skin elasticity or generalized soft tissue laxity *without* disproportionate localization of excess fat will not benefit from liposuction but may be candidates for skin excision and tightening procedures whether on the arms, torso, or thighs (see Chapters 7, 9, and 11).

Age

The majority of patients are in their thirties or forties, but I have operated on patients as young as 14 and as old as 79. In a personal series of 200 consecutive patients, the median age was 38 years, with more than 75% of patients between 30 and 49 years old.

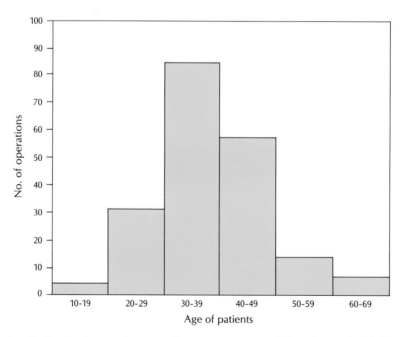

Patients in their sixties and seventies are not too old to benefit if they are in good medical condition. The patient's chronologic age is less important than her intrinsic skin elasticity and the presence of localized fat deposits. So long as the patient has excess fat, liposuction can reduce contour.

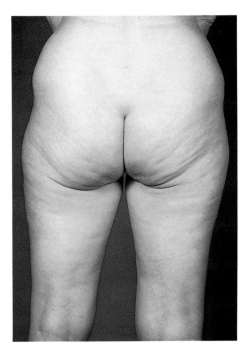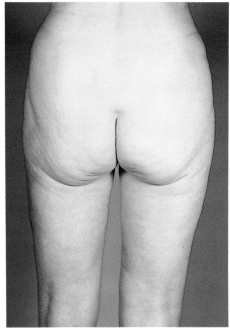

This 60-year-old, 5-foot 5-inch woman noted that she could not fit into her existing wardrobe despite a constant weight of 119 pounds. A total of 1450 cc was removed: 200 cc from each hip, 375 cc from each lateral thigh, 100 cc from the left medial thigh, 50 cc from the right medial thigh, and 50 cc from each medial knee. She was pleased with her appearance and the improved fit of her clothes.

SPECIAL ANATOMIC CONSIDERATIONS

Localized fat excess is more common in certain anatomic areas; the lateral thighs (trochanteric area), the hips in women (area adjacent to the iliac crest), the flanks in men (area superior to the iliac crest and extending posteriorly—the so-called spare tire), the medial knees, and the lower abdomen. These areas can generally be treated in a straightforward manner to reduce unwanted protuberances and achieve the most consistently satisfactory results.

Treatment of the hips and medial knees usually produces a favorable result, even for the surgeon with minimal experience. Although results in the abdomen are generally good, irregularities of the anterior abdominal skin surface are more likely if the skin has lost elasticity or if the surgeon tries to achieve a totally flat contour in patients with relatively small fat deposits.

Although the buttocks frequently have large amounts of localized excess fat, they are more difficult to treat because their intrinsic roundness must be maintained for a pleasing result.

The calves and ankles require meticulous circumferential sculpting with fine cannulas. It is best to treat these areas only after experience is gained in sculpting other more forgiving regions.

The posterior aspect of the arms can be treated effectively with suction, but only limited amounts can be removed without creating noticeable wrinkling. The patient must be advised in advance of the limited nature of the results she may expect.

The medial thighs are difficult to treat because of the paucity of fat, the relatively thin skin, and the frequent presence of skin laxity. The sparse subcutaneous layer in this area more readily shows irregularities and hyperpigmentation. The anterior thighs are even more difficult to treat because fat localization is not discrete.

Circumferential treatment of the thighs is possible, but it is difficult to maintain a smooth, rounded skin surface. Irregularities and depressions, particularly on the anterior thighs, are common in patients who undergo circumferential liposuction.

—————————— SUGGESTED READINGS ——————————

Baker JC, Kolin IS, Barlette ES. Psychosexual dynamics of patients undergoing mammary augmentation. Plast Reconstr Surg 53:652-659, 1974.

Bennett AE. Communication Between Doctors and Patients. New York: Oxford University Press, 1976.

Bersheid E, Walster E, Bohrnstedt G. Body image. Psychology Today 14:119-131, 1973.

Bird B. Talking With Patients, 2nd ed. Philadelphia: WB Saunders, 1973.

Blumgart HL. Caring for the patient. N Engl J Med 270:449-456, 1964.

Bostwick J III. Plastic and Reconstructive Breast Surgery. St. Louis: Quality Medical Publishing, 1990, pp 3-55.

Campion FX. Ground Rounds on Medical Malpractice, chap 3. Milwaukee: American Medical Association and The Risk Management Foundation of the Seward Medical Distributors, 1990, pp 109-125.

Curray WJ. Informed consent in malpractice cases: A turn toward reality. N Engl J Med 314:429-431, 1986.

Edgerton MT, Webb WL, Slaughter R, Meyer E. Surgical results and psychosocial changes following rhytidectomy. Plast Reconstr Surg 33:503-521, 1964.

Edgerton MT, McClory AR. Augmentation mammoplasty. Psychiatric implications and surgical indications. Plast Reconstr Surg 21:279-305, 1958.

Edgerton MT, Jacobson WE, Meyer E. Surgical psychiatric study of patients seeking plastic (cosmetic) surgery: 90 consecutive patients with minimal deformity. Br J Plast Surg 13:136-145, 1960.

Edgerton MT, Meyer E, Jacobson WE. Augmentation mammoplasty II. Fuller surgical and psychiatric evaluation. Plast Reconstr Surg 27:270-302, 1961.

Fletcher C. Listening and talking to patients. III. The exposition. Br Med J 2:21-24, 1980.

Goin MK, Bergoyne RW, Goin JM. Face lift operation: The patient's secret motivations and reactions to "informed consent." Plast Reconstr Surg 58:273-279, 1976.

Goldwyn RM. The woman and aesthetic surgery. In Notman MT, Nadelson CC, eds. The Woman Patient: Medical & Psychological Interfaces, vol I. Sexual and Reproductive Aspects of Women's Health Care. New York: Plenum Press, 1978, pp 271-278.

Goldwyn RM. Patient selection: The importance of being cautious. In Courtiss EH, ed. Aesthetic Surgery: Trouble, How to Avoid It and How to Treat It. St. Louis: CV Mosby, 1978, pp 14-16.

Goldwyn RM. Aesthetic surgery: Basic principles. In Regnault P, Daniel RK, eds. Aesthetic Plastic Surgery. Boston: Little, Brown, 1984, pp 31-44.

Goldwyn RM. The Patient and the Plastic Surgeon, 2nd ed. Boston: Little, Brown, 1991.

Gorney M. Malpractice. In Courtiss EH, ed. Aesthetic Surgery: Trouble, How to Avoid It and How to Treat It. St. Louis: CV Mosby, 1978, pp 1-13.

Grunder TM. On the readability of surgical consent forms. N Engl J Med 302:900-902, 1980.

deGutheisl TG, Gurgatjn H, Brodsky A. Malpractice prevention through the sharing of uncertainty. N Engl J Med 311:49-51, 1978.

Gifford S. Cosmetic surgery and personality change: A review of some clinical observations. In Goldwyn RM, ed. The Unfavorable Result in Plastic Surgery: Avoidance and Treatment. Boston: Little, Brown, 1972, pp 11-33.

Hecht MC. Setting up a cosmetic surgery office (from a lawyer's point of view). Part I: Printed Forms. Am J Cosmetic Surg 5(2):113-116, 1988.

Holzer JF. The process of informed consent. Bull Am Coll Surg 74:10-14, 1989.

Illouz Y-G, de Villers YT. Body Sculpturing by Lipoplasty. New York: Churchill Livingstone, 1989, pp 72-93.

Katz J. Informed consent: Are "miracle, mystery, and authority" better medicine? Conn Med 50:457-600, 1982.

Leeb D, Bowers DG, Lynch JB. Observations on the myth of "informed consent." Plast Reconstr Surg 58:280-282, 1976.

Lewis CM. Patient selection: Psychological aspects. In Hetter GP, ed. Lipoplasty: The Theory and Practice of Blunt Suction Lipectomy. Boston: Little, Brown, 1990, pp 113-117.

MacGregor FC. Social and psychologic considerations in aesthetic plastic surgery: Old trends and new. In Rees TD. Aesthetic Plastic Surgery. Philadelphia: WB Saunders, 1980, pp 29-39.

Millard DR. Principalization of Plastic Surgery. Boston: Little, Brown, 1986, pp 51-71.

Myerscough PR. Talking With Patients: A Basic Clinical Skill. New York: Oxford University Press, 1989.

Parsons T. The silk robe and the role of the physician considered. Mibank Mem Fund Q 53:257- 278, 1975.

Redden E, Baker DC, Meisel A. The patient, the plastic surgeon and informed consent: New insights into old problems. Plast Reconstr Surg 75:270-276, 1985.

Rees TD. Selection of patients. In Rees TD, ed. Aesthetic Plastic Surgery, vol 1. Philadelphia: WB Saunders, 1980, pp 19-28.

Reich J. The surgery of appearance: Psychological and related aspects. Med J Aust 2:5-13, 1969.

Sheen J, Sheen AP. Aesthetic Rhinoplasty. 2nd ed, vol 1. St. Louis: CV Mosby, 1987, pp 129-140.

Sherlock R. Reasonable men and sick human beings. Am J Med 80:2-4, 1986.

Trieger M. Practical guidelines to informed consent for the cosmetic surgeon. Am J Cosmetic Surg 1(4):36-37, 1984.

Wright MR, Wright UK. A psychological study of patients undergoing cosmetic surgery. Arch Otolaryngol 101:145-151, 1975.

Chapter 2

INSTRUMENTATION

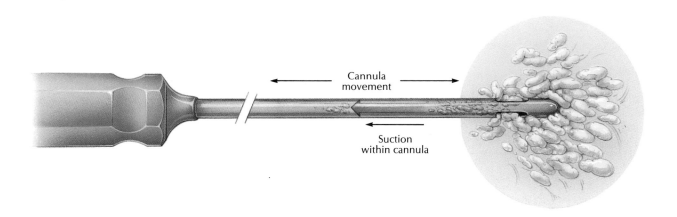

Cannula
movement

Suction
within cannula

Liposuction is a simple, two-stage mechanical process for dislodging and evacuating subcutaneous fat. A stiff, hollow tube (cannula) is directed into the subcutaneous fat through a small skin incision. The proximal end of the cannula is connected to a vacuum source, and the cannula is thrust back and forth through the fat. Suction causes the fat to adhere to one or more apertures at the distal end of the cannula, and the piston-like motion avulses the fat from its bed. The suction draws the fat through the cannula into a receptacle.

Despite this conceptual simplicity, equipment manufacturers have produced a bewildering array of instruments and suction machines. Selection of equipment, nevertheless, is really quite straightforward. This chapter is a practical review of the various instrumentation options for cannulas, suction pumps, syringe systems, and associated devices. Although I will discuss most of the commonly used instruments, I can only recommend the few systems that I have selected for my practice.

31

I hasten to add that I have no commercial relationships with any manufacturer or purveyor of instruments or pumps. These recommendations are based solely on personal clinical experience.

CANNULAS

Three important features determine the efficiency of a cannula: tip configuration, diameter, and length.

Tip Configuration

The shape of the distal end of the cannula and the number, configuration, and position of the apertures are critical in determining the safety and efficiency of liposuction.

The tip should be gently rounded and tapered. A sharp, pointed tip is more likely to penetrate the fascia or skin, whereas a rounded tip permits easy movement through the tissues with less danger of penetration.

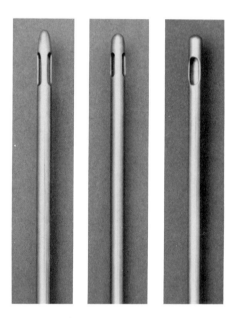

The tip shape of these three cannula varies from tapered on the left to blunt on the right. I prefer the more tapered tip on the left since it requires the least effort to maneuver through the tissues yet is still rounded so that it is less likely to penetrate fascia or skin.

The distal aperture should be set back from the tip. The advantage of rapid suction with the aperture at the tip is more than offset by the increased likelihood of extracting fat from close to the skin surface and creating a depression as the cannula tip inevitably hits the undersurface of the skin. With the aperture set back from the tip, pressing the tip against the skin is less likely to result in removal of fat close to the skin surface.

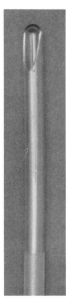

This plastic cannula has a single large opening at the tip and extracts fat rapidly. I do not use it because of the risk of overresecting the undersurface of the skin.

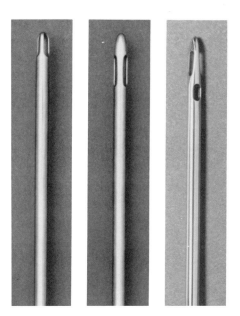

Multiple openings near the cannula tip increase the cross-sectional area to which the fat can adhere and thus the efficiency of fat removal. Multiple apertures also increase the shearing and rasping action of the edges of the aperture and therefore increase the speed of fat evacuation. Increased efficiency of extraction correlates to fewer passes of the cannula and reduced tissue trauma.

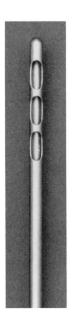

Some arrangements of multiple openings can, however, cause excessive rasping and increase rather than decrease trauma. For example, cannulas designed with three apertures oriented longitudinally along the axis and separated by narrow bars are likely to act like sharp curettes and cause bleeding.

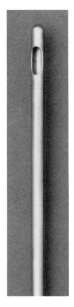

A single, side-facing aperture set back from the tip is relatively safe because the aperture can be directed away from the surface of the skin. The single aperture, however, makes for a slower rate of fat extraction. The cannula requires more passes through the tissue to extract a given amount of fat. Therefore tissue trauma is increased.

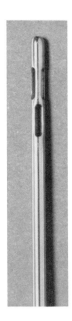

This cannula is designed so that it can be used with all three apertures facing away from the skin surface.

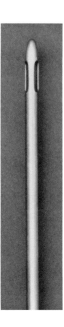

My personal preference is a Mercedes Type cannula that has three apertures set back from the tip and oriented at 120 degrees to each other around the long axis of the cannula. I find these cannulas more rapid and efficient than those with single side-facing apertures. The flow rate of Mercedes Type cannulas is not quite as rapid as cannulas with the apertures set at the very tip, but I find this negligible difference does not justify the possible risk of excessive fat removal close to the skin surface such as might occur with use of cannulas with apertures at the tip.

The Mercedes Type cannulas have been criticized because one of the openings always faces the surface of the skin and theoretically could remove fat from close to the undersurface and create surface irregularities. I have used Mercedes Type cannulas exclusively for more than 7 years; so long as the tip is directed to the appropriate fat layer I have not found surface irregularities to be a problem. The relatively small size of each of the three holes and use of narrow-diameter cannulas (see below) make a noticeable depression less likely if one of the holes is placed near the surface of the skin.

Diameter

The cannulas should be as narrow as possible to permit smoother resection and refinement of results. Small-diameter cannulas also slide back and forth through the tissues more easily, thereby reducing operator fatigue.

Narrow-diameter cannulas diminish flow rates. To compensate for this reduction the surgeon needs to take additional steps to increase the efficiency of fat extraction. Cannulas with multiple apertures at the tip have already been discussed as one means of maximizing the speed of fat dislodgment and evacuation. Powerful suction pumps that vaporize water under operating room conditions are another means of improving flow rate when narrow-diameter cannulas are used. These pumps are discussed in the next section. Finally, distention of the tissues with large volumes of injected solutions also facilitates use of narrow-diameter cannulas (see Chapter 5, pp. 88-93).

No single cannula diameter is suitable for all anatomic areas under all conditions. As a general rule, large, deep fat deposits should be treated with large-diameter cannulas, and small, superficial fat deposits should be treated with small-diameter cannulas. A range of Mercedes Type cannulas 2 to 6 cm in diameter suffices to treat all areas of the neck and body. Facial suction requires cannulas 1.5 to 2.4 cm in diameter.

Length

Shorter cannulas afford better control since the tip can be directed more easily and accurately. Longer cannulas provide access to distant areas and diminish the number of incisions, but since incisions are small and generally inconspicuous, I prefer to use short instruments. I work with cannulas 18 to 20 cm long for most areas of the body. In the smaller areas of the face and neck I use cannulas 10 to 14 cm long.

A minimal set consists of five Mercedes Type cannulas, each 20 cm long with diameters of 2.4, 3.0, 3.7, 4.6, and 6.0 cm. The 2.4 and 3.0 cm cannulas may be used for the neck. If the face is to be suctioned, the surgeon should also have a 1.8 cm diameter cannula that is 14 cm in length. All cannulas should be constructed of high-quality stainless steel and should be capable of being bent and straightened by the surgeon. The handle should be ergonomic and fit comfortably into the hand. I find the hexagonal handles easiest to grip.

ASPIRATORS

Fat can be aspirated through a cannula attached to a syringe by drawing back on the plunger, but the most efficient and rapid method involves a high-powered, medical-grade suction pump. A set of cannulas that can be used with a Toomey-type syringe can be purchased as a backup system. If the surgeon performs liposuction on an occasional basis, the syringe system can be used exclusively, avoiding the expenditure for a suction machine. If liposuction is performed frequently, an efficient pump speeds the operation considerably and is well worth the investment.

The primary requirement for a pump is the ability to vaporize water under operating room conditions. A second important and related feature is a high flow rate so that vapor pressure is reached quickly and fat is evacuated rapidly. Other technical considerations in choosing a pump are noise level, reliability, ease of maintenance, size of collection bottle, and mobility in the operating room. A vacuum gauge is convenient but not essential. The reputation of the vendor and efficient, rapid service for the equipment are important additional factors.

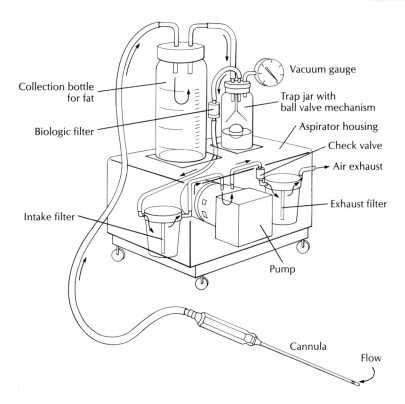

Collection bottle for fat

Biologic filter

Intake filter

Vacuum gauge

Trap jar with ball valve mechanism

Aspirator housing

Check valve

Air exhaust

Exhaust filter

Pump

Cannula

Flow

The component parts of an aspirator for liposuction are:

1. A collection bottle for the fat
2. An additional vacuum trap to protect the pump from overflow
3. A biologic filter to protect the pump and operating room personnel from microbes
4. An intake filter to protect the pump from other contaminants
5. The pump
6. An exhaust filter to protect the operating room environment from oil or other vaporized substances.

VAPORIZATION OF WATER

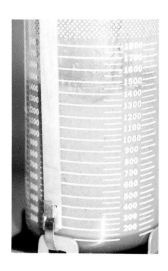

Water vapor in the aspirate (note the bubbles in the fat) significantly increases the rapidity of fat evacuation and is a crucial adjunct when fine cannulas are used. Vaporization improves efficiency by reducing the viscosity of the mixture of fat, blood, and other substances traveling through the cannula and tubing. Much of the aspirate is water, either in the form of tissue water, serum, or solutions injected into the fat prior to suction. Water that has been vaporized to its gaseous phase flows 100 times more rapidly than water in its liquid phase. By reducing viscosity and increasing flow rate, vaporization of water compensates for the reduction in flow rate when using fine cannulas.

The same decrease in viscosity can be achieved by periodically withdrawing the cannula from the access incision so that air from the atmosphere enters the cannula. This method is, however, inconvenient and can lead to excessive suctioning of tissue from the area around the access incision. A sump-type cannula has been designed that permits the operator to bring air into the system by periodically removing his thumb from an intake port, but this is unnecessary if the machine generates vapor pressure.

To boil water a suction pump must be able to evacuate enough air so that pressure in the system falls to the vapor pressure of the water in the aspirate. Vapor pressure of water at body temperature (37° C) is 47 mm Hg. Vapor pressure of water at room temperature (20° C) is 17 mm Hg. Although the aspirate is initially at body temperature, it loses heat rapidly once it is in the cooler operating room environment. It never quite reaches room temperature, however, and if a pump is capable of reaching a pressure of 20 mm Hg, it will suffice to vaporize the water in the aspirate under operating room conditions. Oil-sealed rotary vane vacuum pumps can easily evacuate enough air to achieve vapor pressure at room temperature. These pumps, commonly called high-vacuum pumps, can produce very low ultimate pressures at low sound levels. Two-staged oil-less rotary vane pumps do not achieve as deep a vacuum as the oil-lubricated pumps but will reach vapor pressure.

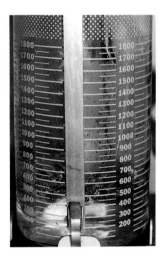

An aspirator can be easily tested to determine if it is suitable for liposuction. Put water in the collection bottle to a height of 1 inch. Occlude the intake port on the collection bottle and turn on the pump. The water should boil in under 20 seconds, preferably under 10 seconds. The fact that the water boils at all is evidence that the pump is powerful enough to reach vapor pressure. The length of time it takes for the water to boil depends on the flow rate of the pump (how rapidly it can move air) and the size of the collection bottle (a pump takes longer to empty the air from a bigger collection bottle). Most pumps in use today have flow rates of 50 to 100 L/min, which is adequate to achieve vapor pressure in 10 to 20 seconds.

OTHER CONSIDERATIONS

Oil-lubricated pumps require more maintenance: the oil must be changed periodically as must the exhaust filter, which is needed to prevent oil droplet contamination of the operating room. A reliable vendor will service the machine at appropriate intervals, although the oil can be changed by a member of the office staff. Oil-less pumps require less maintenance but are noisier. The noise level of an aspirator can be checked by simply turning it on prior to purchase.

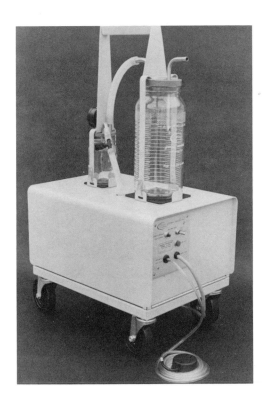
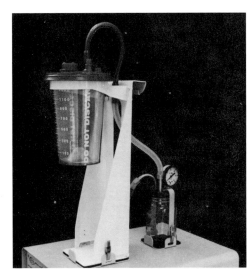

Most aspirators come with appropriate-sized bottles with markings. A 1500 to 2000 cc bottle is convenient. Smaller bottles must be changed too frequently during procedures, whereas larger bottles require inordinately long waits to achieve vapor pressure and are awkward to deal with. Most machines have mounts that can accommodate disposable hard plastic receptacles. These should be implosion-proof.

The aspirator should be mounted on wheels for mobility. All machines come with gauges that in the United States are usually marked in inches of mercury (29.9 being the maximum) or millimeters of mercury (760 being the maximum). The gauges are frequently inaccurate and usually not very helpful. If the machine is working properly, you can observe the aspirate boiling.

Several reliable vendors supply aspirators that will reach vapor pressure. Some of them are listed at the end of the chapter.

Computerized Scale for Recording Aspirate Weight and Composition

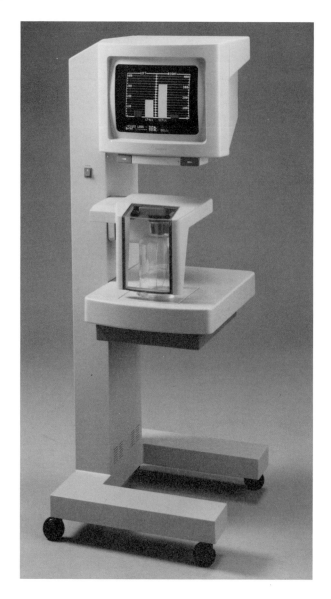

The M.D. Engineering Company manufactures a computerized scale that can be used in conjunction with any pump. The scale accurately measures the weight of the aspirate and projects it on a monitor that has the capacity to display amounts removed from five different areas simultaneously. This device is convenient for measuring small volumes of aspirate removed from multiple areas. A printout is also available.

The collection bottle on the computerized scale is equipped with a device that uses the electrical impedance of the aspirate to determine the percent solid vs. liquid. This can be used to estimate the amount of blood vs. fat in the aspirate.

Tubing

Tubing connects the cannula to the pump and connects the various parts of the pump. A 7-foot length of tubing is enough to reach from the pump to all areas of the body. Longer tubing is unnecessary and can be awkward.

The internal diameter of the tubing can range from ¼, ⅜, to ½ inch. The internal diameter should be appropriate to the size of the cannula handle.

Disposable tubing is generally made of clear vinyl. If disposable tubing is preferred, the walls must be strong enough to resist collapse under conditions of vapor pressure.

I prefer reusable silicone rubber tubing. The tubing is strong and will not collapse. It can be rinsed out and steam autoclaved. Although it is initially clear, there is some discoloration with time, but this does not affect function.

Filters

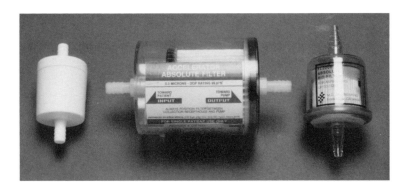

Biologic filters capable of removing particles up to 0.3 μm in size are readily available. These should be placed in the system between the overflow bottle and the pump mechanism to prevent bacterial contamination of the pump and oil. These filters do not protect against viral transmission. There is, however, no reported instance of viral transmission to operating room personnel from aerosolization of aspirate.

Syringe Systems

Liposuction can be performed without suction pumps using 60 or 10 ml syringes with wide necks fitted to specially designed cannulas. Although this method does not achieve vapor pressure, it can be used for removal of small and large amounts of fat. Although less efficient than liposuction with a pump aspirator, it is used by some plastic surgeons as their exclusive method of liposuction because of its perceived advantages (see Chapter 5, pp. 96–101).

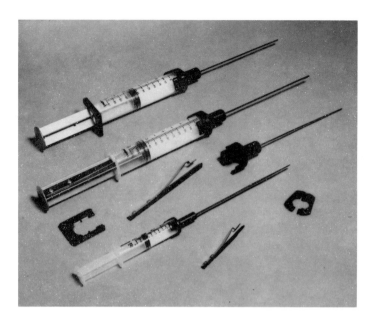

The systems consist of a Toomey-type syringe and a set of cannulas fitted with receptacle ends for the syringe instead of handles. A locking device fits over the barrel of the syringe. The cannula with attached syringe is inserted into the fat and the plunger of the syringe withdrawn to create a vacuum. The plunger is locked in the withdrawn position using the locking device.

Syringe systems are marketed by several manufacturers; some are listed at the end of this chapter.

■   ■   ■

Although it is helpful to have state of the art devices, ultimately it is the skill of the surgeon that determines the surgical result.

─────────────── SUGGESTED READINGS ───────────────

Chajchir A, Wexler EA. New model of liposuction cannula. Aesthetic Plast Surg 9:101-106, 1985.

Cukier J. Filter update. Lipoplasty Newsletter 5:73, 1988.

D'Assumpcao EA. Cannula for liposuction. Plast Reconstr Surg 74:731-732, 1984.

Gast Manufacturing Corporation. Vacuum and Pressure Systems Handbook. Benton Harbor, Mich.: Gast, 1986.

Grazer FM. Atlas of Suction Assisted Lipectomy in Body Contouring. New York: Churchill Livingstone, 1992, pp 15-29.

Hetter GP. Physics and equipment. In Hetter GP, ed. Lipoplasty: The Theory and Practice of Blunt Suction Lipectomy. Boston: Little, Brown, 1990, pp 147-162.

Hetter GP. Optimum vacuum pressures for lipolysis. Aesthetic Plast Surg 8:23-26, 1983.

Illouz Y-G, de Villers YT. Body Sculpturing by Lipoplasty. New York: Churchill Livingstone, 1989, pp 97-107.

Kesselring UK. Suction curette for removal of subcutaneous fat [letter]. Plast Reconstr Surg 63:560, 1979.

Teimourian B. Suction Lipectomy & Body Sculpturing. St. Louis: CV Mosby, 1987, pp 45-64.

VENDORS OF INSTRUMENTS AND MACHINES

This selective list of manufacturers represents those with whom I have worked and have personal knowledge. There are many other fine manufacturers and vendors not listed here.

PUMPS

Byron Medical Corporation
3280 East Hemisphere Loop
Tucson, AZ 85706
#800-777-3434

Grams Medical
2443 Norse Avenue
Costa Mesa, CA 92627
#714-548-7337

Robbins Instruments, Inc.
2 North Passaic
P.O. Box 441
Chatham, NJ 07928
#201-635-8972

Unitech Corporation
P.O. Box 9989
Fountain Valley, CA 92728
#714-963-3525

Wells-Johnson Company
P.O. Box 30395
Tucson, AZ 85751-0395
#800-528-1597

CANNULAS AND SYRINGE SYSTEMS

Byron Medical Corporation
3280 East Hemisphere Loop
Tucson, AZ 85706
#800-777-3434

Grams Medical
2443 Norse Avenue
Costa Mesa, CA 92627
#714-548-7337

The Tulip Company
2535 Kettner Boulevard
Suite 3B1
San Diego, CA 92101
#800-325-6526

Wells-Johnson Company
P.O. Box 30395
Tucson, AZ 85751-0395
#800-528-1597

COMPUTERIZED SCALE

M.D. Engineering Company
2536 Barrington Court
Hayward, CA 94545
#800-633-8423

Chapter 3

OPERATIVE PLANNING AND SURGICAL STRATEGIES

All liposuction operations share common elements: marking, anesthesia, positioning, and fat evacuation. Individual technical details change constantly, and the surgeon devises new refinements over time or incorporates those of his colleagues. Over the years I have evolved a routine for operative treatment that works well for most patients. It provides a constant, fixed framework yet permits multiple variations to encompass individual needs. Most important, it facilitates consistent achievement of satisfying aesthetic results in a safe environment.

PREOPERATIVE CONSIDERATIONS
Markings

Patient markings for liposuction should be made before the patient is brought to the operating room. If delayed until the patient is in the surgical suite, the lack of privacy and the cooler temperature make for patient discomfort and impede accurate marking. Areas to be treated should be outlined with the patient standing since this is the position in which contour excesses are most noticeable. When the patient is recumbent, subcutaneous fat assumes a different shape and location, making accurate assessment of the amount to aspirate from each site more difficult.

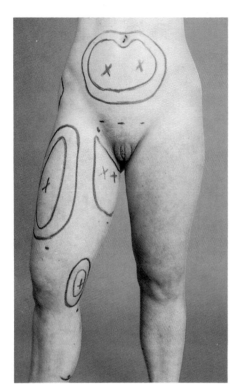 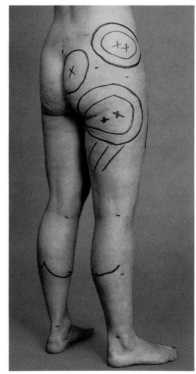

Topographic markings denote each area to be treated, with the innermost ring showing the maximal fat deposition and protuberance. Straight lines emanating from the periphery indicate areas to be feathered to ensure a smooth transition from treated to untreated areas. Sites for access incisions are designated by short lines in the direction of minimal skin tension.

When the markings are completed, I review the areas to be suctioned with the patient to ensure that she fully understands the scope of the operation and to afford her an opportunity to ask last-minute questions.

Anesthesia

If only a few areas are to be treated, local anesthesia is adequate. I use 0.05% lidocaine in a 1:1,000,000 epinephrine solution. Large volumes of this dilute injectate (at least 1 ml for each cubic centimeter of planned aspirate) can achieve profound and long-lasting anesthesia (see Chapter 5, pp. 88-93). Local anesthesia can also be used for secondary operations on very limited areas, but injection through the unyielding scar tissue is more painful, and diffusion may be incomplete. Most secondary operations and all operations on multiple areas are performed under general endotracheal or epidural anesthesia. The patient has total and complete analgesia, and the surgeon operates in a tranquil field without being distracted by patient discomfort or motion.

Positioning, Prepping, and Draping

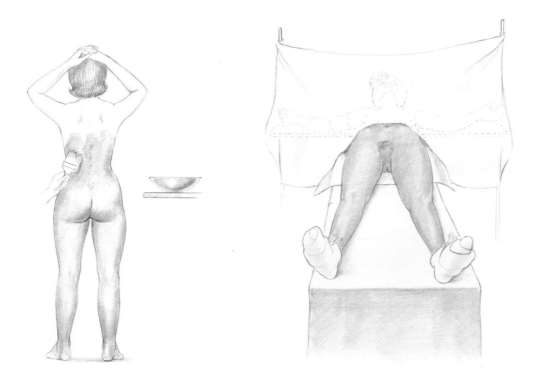

No preoperative narcotics or sedatives are administered since the patient must stand while she is painted circumferentially from chest to feet with warm povidone-iodine (Betadine) solution. After the prep the patient lies supine on a sterile-draped operating table with her arms extended on arm boards at a 90-degree angle. Her feet are wrapped in sterile towels. A Mayo stand cover placed under the midsection serves as a sterile drawsheet and facilitates positioning. The patient is covered with another sterile sheet while the anesthesiologist performs induction and intubation. Following intubation the covering sheet is lifted and suspended between two poles to separate the anesthesiologist from the sterile field. All areas of the torso and lower extremities are now accessible for suctioning, either from the supine position or by turning the patient side to side.

When epidural anesthesia is used, the epidural catheter is introduced before the patient is prepped. Once the catheter is positioned and secured, it is covered with a sterile adhesive drape (Steri-Drape; 3M Corporation, St. Paul, Minn.). The patient then stands for circumferential prepping that includes the Steri-Drape covering the catheter. After prepping, she is placed supine on the sterile-draped operating table, the regional anesthetic is administered through the epidural catheter, and the operation proceeds. Of course, the same prepping and draping procedures may be used with local anesthesia.

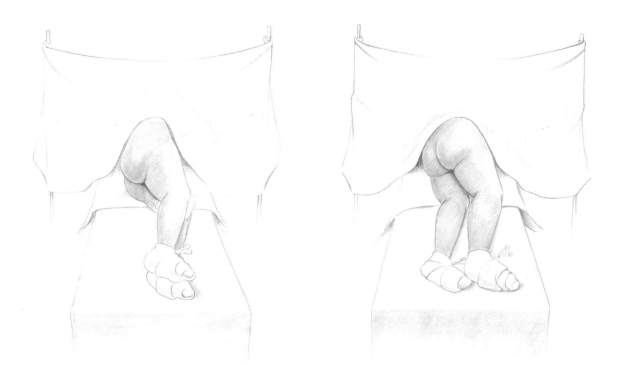

The sterile drawsheet is used to help move the patient to her side for access to lateral areas. Note that the patient is completely in the decubitus position. The hip is kept extended to a neutral position to help maintain laxity of the subtrochanteric skin. Folded towels between the knees keep the thighs slightly abducted and also maintain laxity in the subtrochanteric area. If the skin is stretched tight in this area, accurate palpation is inhibited. More posterior areas are reached by turning the patient slightly more prone, as shown.

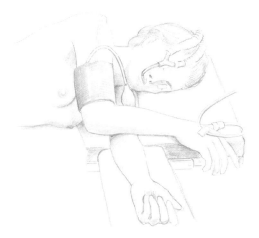

The anesthesiologist actively participates in moving the patient from side to side, protecting her upper body from positional injury. A roll can be placed under the chest adjacent to the axilla to protect the brachial plexus, but since the patient is on her side for a relatively short period of time (usually 15 to 30 minutes), we have not found this maneuver necessary. Because there is no restraining strap and the lateral decubitus position is inherently unstable, surgeon and assistant must take care to maintain patient position.

This method of prepping, induction, and positioning takes less than 10 minutes from the time the patient is brought into the operating room until she is ready for surgery. Furthermore, because all areas of the body below the breast are prepped, the patient does not have to be reprepped and redraped for treatment of anterior and posterior surfaces. The unrestricted patient mobility afforded by this approach permits ready access to all areas. The patient is never fully prone; therefore respiratory exchange is not inhibited, and the anesthesiologist has unrestricted access to the airway.

The few disadvantages of this method are easily overcome. Prepping in the standing position can be embarrassing to the patient and awkward for the operating room staff. Once the staff has become accustomed to the routine, however, their comfort level improves, and they readily reassure the patient and minimize her embarrassment. Operating on a patient in the lateral decubitus position does not permit simultaneous visual or palpatory comparison of opposite sides of the body. The surgeon therefore must compare the feel and appearance of the two sides of the body from memory and rely more on volumetric control measures to ensure side-to-side symmetry (pp. 52-55). This technique requires continual communication between the anesthesiologist and surgeon with regard to patient positioning. I find this interaction advantageous since the anesthesiologist becomes a more active participant in the procedure.

Alternative Positioning

If only the anterior chest or abdomen is to be treated, the patient is placed supine on the operating table and then prepped.

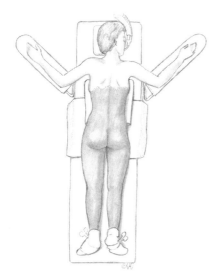

If only posterolateral areas are to be treated (back, hips/flanks, lateral thighs), the patient may be intubated supine on a stretcher next to the operating table, turned prone onto the operating table, and prepped and draped. Rolls are positioned under the lateral torso to leave the central chest and abdomen free for respiratory excursion.

Position of Operating Room Personnel and Instruments

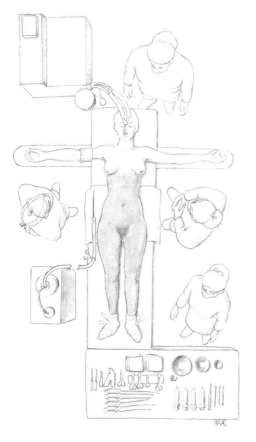

The assistant stands directly opposite the surgeon to help position and stabilize the patient. The scrub nurse stands to the left of the assistant. If an assistant is not available, the nurse stands opposite the surgeon. All instruments are kept on a case cart at the foot of the table. The aspirator is to the right of the surgeon.

Minimizing Heat Loss

Liposuction patients tend to lose heat during surgery. Operating rooms are frequently cool, most of the patient's body may be exposed, and her skin is washed with solutions causing heat loss by vaporization. Core temperatures may easily reach 93° F or less.

Heat loss cannot be totally eliminated, but it can be lessened. The operating room should be kept at 72° F, and as much of the body as possible should be kept covered. An aluminum-shielded heat reflective cap (Thermadrape; O.R. Concepts, Inc., Roanoke, Tex.) will reduce heat loss from the scalp. Intravenous solutions and local injections should be warmed, as should all preps and washes.

PRINCIPLES OF TREATMENT

The goals of liposuction are predictable, smooth contour reduction achieved in a consistent, reproducible manner. The operation should be efficient and safe. Adherence to the following principles makes these goals attainable:

- Use quantitative assessment of volume removal to plan fluid and blood replacement and to achieve symmetry.
- Inject large volumes of dilute lidocaine and epinephrine solution to achieve local anesthesia, create vasoconstriction, distend treated areas, and reduce postoperative pain.
- When treating multiple sites, have a plan for systematic progression of treatment from area to area so that the patient is manipulated as little as possible and treatment proceeds efficiently.
- Use small cannulas for small volumes and large cannulas for large volumes.
- Use two access incisions for most areas to avoid "waviness."
- Keep the tip of the cannula in the deep central fat for large-volume removal and suction with small cannulas at a more superficial level for fine contour adjustments. Do not injure the dermis above or the musculofascia below.
- Use a piston motion to slide the cannula back and forth. Do not move the cannula side to side in an arc.
- Be gentle.
- Note the color of the aspirate as tunneling proceeds.
- Judge the end point by tactile and visual assessment of contour supplemented by quantitative assessment of volume removed.
- Be conservative. If insufficient volume is removed, more can be suctioned, but it is virtually impossible to correct an overresection. As a corollary, it is sometimes better to correct very large deformities in two stages, both to prevent possible overresection and to permit skin to adjust more gradually and smoothly to a reduced volume.

Quantitative Assessment

Quantitative assessment of fat removal is critical to obtaining consistently satisfying aesthetic results and to calculating fluid and blood loss for safe operative conduct (see Chapter 4).

At the initial consultation I estimate volume of tissue extraction necessary to produce the desired contour reduction in every area to be treated. These volumes are recorded on the patient intake sheet and brought to the operating room for reference during surgery. Preoperative pinch thicknesses are also noted.

The quantitative estimate of volume removal is supplemented in the operating room by high-quality photographs of the patient in the standing position. Small slides are not suitable for this purpose, and I use 5 × 7 black and white prints that include the patient's front, back, and both profiles. The photographs and preoperative volume assessments provide important information on the patient's fat distribution and side-to-side symmetry. I refer to them constantly during the procedure.

Since I treat most of my patients in the lateral decubitus position, a direct visual comparison of the two sides is not possible. To ensure symmetry I take equal volumes from right and left areas (of course, if the areas are asymmetric to start, I will compensate by taking more from the fuller side).

Quantitative volume estimates also help in treating individual areas. When using two access incisions, about half the planned volume is taken from one access incision and the remaining volume from the second access incision. Taking approximately equal volumes from each access incision helps create a smooth grid pattern of subcutaneous tunnels and minimizes postoperative waviness.

Quantitative assessment of volume is central to obtaining consistent, reproducible, and symmetric contour reduction. Nevertheless, final suction volume may be more or less than preoperative estimates both in individual areas and for total volume. Although preoperative estimates are important initial guides to treatment, appearance of the area and intraoperative palpation remain the benchmark parameters for determining final suction volume.

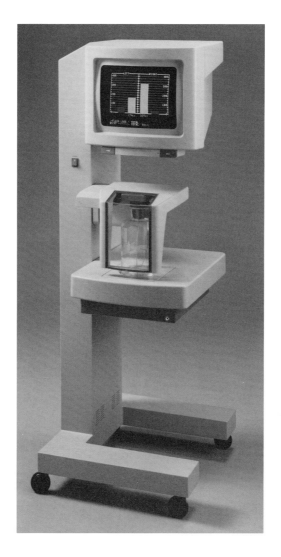

Assessment of the exact amount of volume removed from each area is facilitated by use of an aspirator connected to a computerized scale and monitor (LS 1000 power aspirator; M.D. Engineering Company, Hayward, Calif.). This device permits precise measurement of even small amounts of fat and allows accurate simultaneous comparison of right and left sides for up to five areas. While I have found the computerized scale convenient and useful, a simple pencil and paper tally can serve as well. Use of syringes for aspiration also allows measurement of small volumes.

A preprinted operative report with spaces to fill in volumes of aspirate permits quantification and comparison of tissue removal from left and right sides of multiple areas. Filling in the report as the operation proceeds keeps all operating room personnel apprised of volume removal. At the end of the procedure I review the report and add any significant additional notes before signing.

Injection Regimen*

Injection of the fat with a solution of dilute lidocaine and epinephrine diminishes bleeding by producing vasoconstriction[1-3] and smoothes emergence from anesthesia by reducing postoperative pain. Despite a recent report[4] advocating abandonment of epinephrine injection to reduce blood loss in liposuction, I continue to find it useful for this purpose.[5] Large volumes of injectate also distend the tissues and facilitate passage of the cannula. Whether using general, epidural, or local anesthesia, I inject 0.05% lidocaine in 1:1,000,000 epinephrine. The solution is conveniently made as follows:

1:1000 epinephrine	1 ml
8.4% sodium bicarbonate (1 mEq/ml)	5 ml
1% lidocaine	50 ml
Physiologic saline solution	1000 ml
0.05% lidocaine with 1:1,000,000 epinephrine	1056 ml

Volumes of injectate are generally equal to or more than volumes of planned aspirate. The total injection may reach 4000 cc. All areas are injected 10 minutes before suctioning begins. Although the amount of injected lidocaine is well in excess of the manufacturer's recommended maximal dose of 7 mg/kg or 500 mg total,[6] I have never had a patient experience an untoward effect. Systemic absorption of dilute lidocaine and epinephrine is slow, and serum lidocaine does not reach toxic levels.[7]

Toledo[3] uses a slightly lower concentration of lidocaine (0.04%) and increases the concentration of epinephrine to approximately 1:500,000. He claims his solution is effective for local anesthesia if the volume suctioned from all areas totals less than 1000 cc. For larger extractions he uses general or regional anesthesia and injects 2 to 3 L, suctioning as much as 4000 cc without transfusion.

*See also Chapter 5, pp. 88-93.

Operative Report

Date: _____/_____/_____   Name: _____

Attending surgeon: _Pitman_____   Assisting surgeon: _____

Anesthesia: _____   Attending anesthesiologist: _____

Procedure performed: _Liposuction_____

Preoperative diagnosis: _Localized adiposity, ICD #278.1_____

Postoperative diagnosis: _Same_____

Pathology: _There was excess fat in the areas listed below:_____

Volumes

	Left	Right
Face	_____	
Neck	_____	
Abdomen	_____	
Hips/flanks	_____	_____
Buttocks	_____	_____
Med. thigh	_____	_____
Ant. thigh	_____	_____
Lat. thigh	_____	_____
Post. thigh	_____	_____
Knee	_____	_____
Calf/ankle	_____	_____
_____	_____	_____
_____	_____	_____
_____	_____	_____

TOTAL   _____ + _____ = _____

Procedure   The patient was prepped in the standing position, placed on a sterile-draped operating room table, induced, and intubated. Areas to be treated were infiltrated with 0.05 lidocaine with 1:1,000,000 epinephrine. Transverse stab incisions were made at appropriate places. Liposuction was carried out through the incisions. Incisions were closed with staples. The patient was then extubated and taken from the operating room in good condition. *Cannulas:* _____

Addendum: _____
_____
_____
_____
_____
_____

_____

Gerald H. Pitman, M.D.

Progression of Treatment

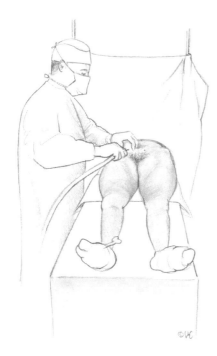

When treating multiple sites, I start on the right side of the table with the patient supine and treat the abdomen first followed by the right anterior thigh.

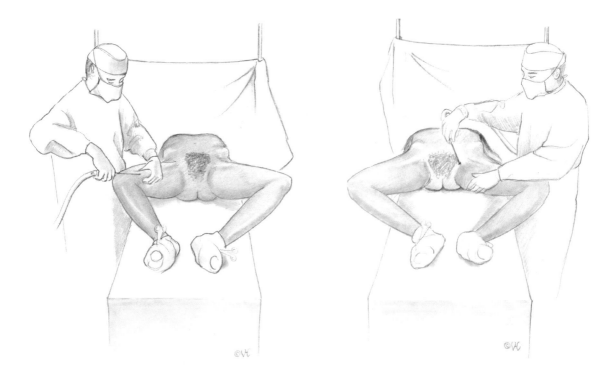

I then place the patient in a frog-leg position and suction the right medial thigh and right medial knee. Next, I move to the left side of the table to treat the left medial thigh and left medial knee. The legs are taken out of the frog-leg position to treat the left anterior thigh.

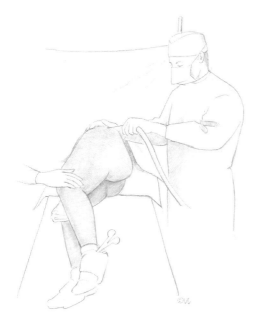

Turning the patient to the right lateral decubitus position, I proceed to suction the left hip, left flank, and left trochanteric area. Placing the patient into a slightly more prone position makes the buttocks and posterior thighs accessible. The left lateral leg and right medial leg and knee can also be suctioned with the patient in the right lateral decubitus position.

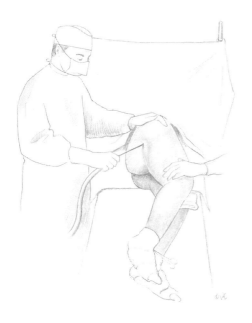

Finally, the patient is turned to the left lateral decubitus position so that the right hip, flank, buttock, and trochanteric areas can be treated. Again, if the calves and ankles are suctioned, the right lateral leg and left medial leg are treated from this position.

Cannula Selection

Small-diameter cannulas penetrate the fat more easily than large ones, causing less tissue trauma and creating fewer irregularities. Small-diameter cannulas can also be used nearer to the skin than large-diameter cannulas, which will leave visible irregularities. Fat removal is slowed, however, as cannula diameter decreases. The surgeon must strike a balance between finesse and speed. Multiple ports at the tip of the cannula increase the rate of extraction and partially compensate for the decreased efficiency of the smaller diameter cannulas. A suction pump powerful enough to vaporize body water is mandatory for successful use of small cannulas. My personal preference is a Mercedes Type cannula for almost all areas, using different cannula diameters based on the size of the fat deposit and how close I want to work to the skin surface. The cannulas I use most frequently are:

6 mm	Large deep fat deposits
4-5 mm	Medium fat deposits
3-4 mm	Small superficial fat deposits

Cannula length varies from 15 to 20 cm, with narrow-diameter cannulas being shorter than large-diameter instruments. Use of longer cannulas permits fewer access incisions, but I find the shorter cannulas easier to control. They permit more precise contouring.

Access Incisions

Access incisions are placed adjacent to but not within the treated area. Placement of the incision within the treated area can easily result in over-resection around the incision.

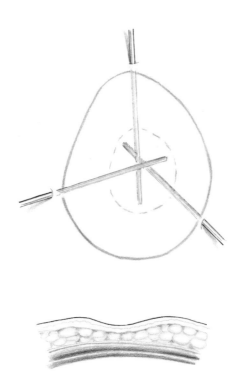

More than two access incisions are unnecessary and unwise since multiple access incisions may cause excessive resection in the central zone of maximum overlap, resulting in a permanent depression.

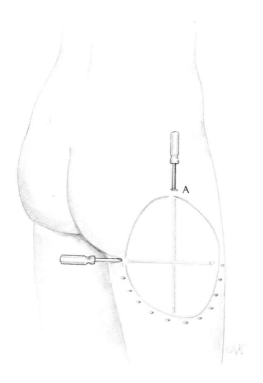

The incisions are located so that tunnels intersect as much as possible at or near 90 degrees. If the first access incision is at point *A,* the second access incision is ideally made somewhere on the opposite circumference of the treated area to create the maximum number of tunnel intersections in a grid pattern. The desirability of inconspicuous scars, however, sometimes dictates other locations. Two access incisions are used for most areas, but a very small area (medial knee, for example) may require only one incision for adequate treatment.

Access incisions should be slightly longer than the diameter of the cannula. Incisions that are too small grip the cannula barrel tightly, impeding free motion of the cannula and causing excessive trauma to the sides of the wound. Edge necrosis and a wide, depressed scar are the ultimate result. Larger incisions permit easier movement of the cannula and less trauma to the skin.

Access incisions are always less than 10 mm in length, with the majority becoming inconspicuous 6 to 12 months after surgery. As a general rule, the surgeon should place incisions for optimal ease of contouring, use as many as necessary, and make them large enough to easily accommodate the cannula. They are rarely problematic.

Suctioning Techniques

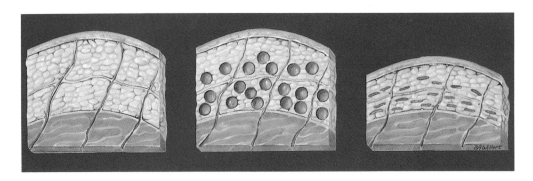

Liposuction removes the subcutaneous fat while leaving the supporting fascial framework containing neurovascular and lymphatic elements. Reduction of fat volume produces a "collapsing" action and diminution of surface contour. Preservation of sensory nerves and nutrient vessels between the muscle fascia and skin permits treatment of large areas without vascular compromise or permanent numbness. Maintenance of the fascial connections also prevents skin shifting, discourages seroma formation, and promotes early healing.

Liposuction creates a discontinuous cavity or multiple small cavities as opposed to the single, large, continuous cavity created by fat removal using traditional flap dissection. Liposuction is often described as creating a series of "tunnels," a useful visual construct that I will refer to frequently in this chapter and elsewhere. More accurately, however, the treated area is characterized by a fascial-neurovascular-lymphatic framework from which the fatty stroma has been evacuated.

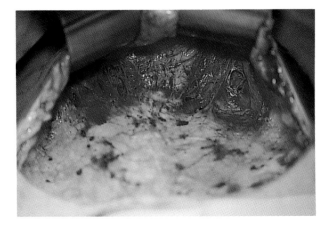

Multiple intact cords can be observed between investing fascia and skin after fat has been suctioned from beneath an abdominoplasty flap. Some fat remains in place around the umbilical stalk near the center of the flap. Cords contain nerves, perforating vessels, and lymphatics.

Cannula Insertion

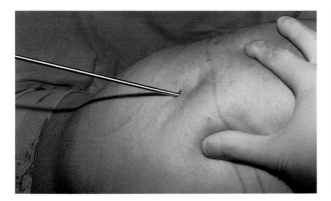 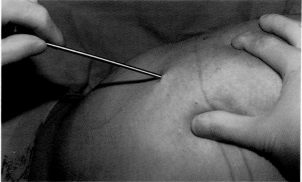

Insertion is facilitated if the surgeon grasps the skin and subcutaneous fat surrounding the access incision and stabilizes the tissue mass. The tip of the cannula is then inserted into the superficial tissue until it encounters the fascia separating the superficial and deep fat layers. The skin is slightly depressed around the cannula as fascial connections transmit the pressure of the tip to the skin surface (left). An additional thrust penetrates the fascia and places the cannula at the correct level; the surgeon feels the tissues "give" as the cannula penetrates the deep fat. The skin is released and is no longer depressed (right).

Maintaining Correct Cannula Depth

Keeping the tip of the cannula in the deep fat, the surgeon turns on the suction and moves the cannula back and forth in a gentle, piston-like motion. Although there are times when the surgeon will wish to selectively suction fat near the dermis,* for most anatomic areas and most patients the tip of the cannula should remain in the deep central fat.

Unintended repenetration of the tip through the fascia to the superficial fat is felt as a "catching" as the cannula slides back and forth. Movement becomes more arduous, the outline of the cannula may be seen through the skin, and the skin is transiently depressed as the fascia transmits the pull of the cannula. If this occurs, the surgeon should withdraw the cannula completely and reestablish the correct plane of dissection before proceeding.

If the tip remains superficial and fat close to the dermis is evacuated, noticeable irregularities may be created on the skin surface and the subdermal plexus may be injured, resulting in pigmentary changes in the skin. If the tip is too deep, it may injure the vascular plexus lying on the investing fascia and cause excessive bleeding. Maintenance of the tip in the central deep fat permits contour reduction, yet leaves the superficial fat undisturbed to provide a smooth, soft cover above the treated area.

*See Chapter 5, pp. 94-95.

Keeping the cannula tip in the deep, central fat is always desirable, but some anatomic areas may only have a single, thin fat layer (e.g., calves, ankles, neck superficial to the platysma); the surgeon will, of necessity, direct the tip closer to the skin surface in these areas. On other occasions the surgeon will smooth out surface irregularities by removing small amounts of fat near the skin surface.

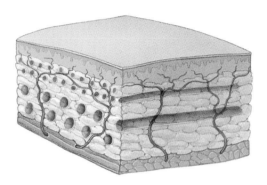

Suctioning may be performed close to the skin surface if the surgeon uses fine cannulas and removes only small amounts of fat. In general, removal of large volumes from thick fat deposits is performed with large-diameter cannulas kept at deep levels. Removal of small volumes from thin fat deposits is performed with small-diameter cannulas, and removal may be done closer to the skin surface. Even in areas of thick fat deposition with well-defined deep layers, however, the surgeon will unavoidably remove some superficial fat. The goal remains, nonetheless, to avoid large-volume fat removal close to the skin surface.

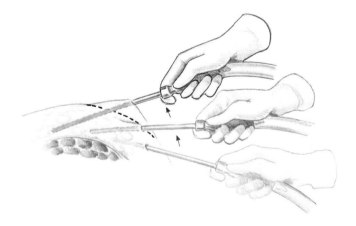

In suctioning a convex area the surgeon should elevate the handle of the cannula as he moves forward. Upward motion at the handle lowers the tip and keeps it in a deep plane as it moves over a convex surface.

Since the cannula removes fat by mechanically avulsing it from its bed, a certain vigor of motion is essential. Nevertheless, a rough, thrusting technique is unnecessary and should be avoided.

Crisscross Tunneling (Creating a Grid Meshwork)

If all of the fat in an anatomic area is evacuated through tunnels radiating from a single access incision, there will be a tendency for surface waviness since the extraction is carried out through radiating, near parallel lines. Therefore the plan for most areas (except for very small ones) is to create a series of tunnels radiating from one access incision and then a second intersecting series of tunnels radiating from a different access incision (crisscross tunneling).

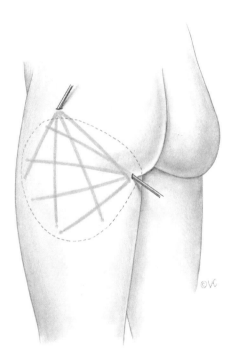

About half the expected volume is removed from the entire area using tunnels from the first access incision. A second access incision is then used to remove the remainder of the fat, creating a modified grid pattern.

Treatment from both access incisions is performed systematically and precisely. I begin by suctioning along one edge of the treatment area. After creating the first tunnel, I partially withdraw the cannula and redirect it to an adjacent radiating line, creating a second tunnel. The process is repeated to create as many tunnels as necessary to treat the entire area.

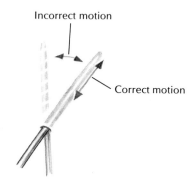

The direction of the cannula must not be changed until it is almost completely withdrawn. Attempts to change direction while the cannula is still deeply inserted cause a rough sideways motion (similar to a windshield wiper) and disrupt neurovascular connections between the deep fascia and skin. Excessive sideways motion will create a single large cavity between skin and fascia rather than the desired discontinuous cavity or grid undermining.

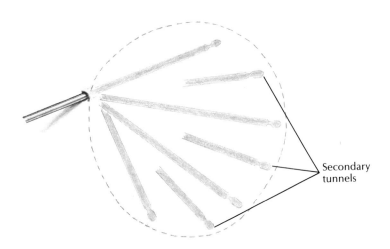

The distance between each tunnel increases with increasing distance from the access incision. Therefore I redirect the cannula to create additional shorter tunnels between the distal parts of the initial tunnels. The secondary tunnels fill in between primary tunnels as distance from the access incision increases. I spend more time and make more passes in the central portion of the treated area since this is the area of maximum fat deposition.

Evaluating Blood in the Aspirate

Initially the aspirate from any one area is pure yellow, indicating a high fat content. As suction continues in the same tunnel, the aspirate becomes progressively more red, indicating more blood and less fat content. Some surgeons advise cessation of suctioning as soon as the extract turns bloody.[8] Although surgeons inexperienced in performing liposuction procedures will avoid overresection by following this advice, they may also frequently underresect. It is often necessary and desirable to continue working in an area from which the aspirate is relatively bloody. Removal of this last bit of bloody tissue may transform an ordinary into a superior result.

Some areas (notably the anterior abdomen) are bloodier than others, and some patients bleed more readily than others. It is imperative that the surgeon and anesthesiologist be alert to the amount of blood in the tubing. An experienced surgeon will have little difficulty in assessing whether a patient is bleeding more or less than usual.

I clearly recall the case of a 35-year-old woman in whom I planned to remove 1800 cc of aspirate. While treating the left hip and thigh, I noticed the color of the aspirate was excessively red, and bleeding was profuse. I aborted the procedure after removing 900 cc from the left side and did not treat the right side.

On awakening, the patient admitted that she had taken aspirin prior to surgery. Her hematocrit fell to 23 postoperatively. She was not transfused but was started on supplemental iron. Aside from feeling fatigued for 3 days, the patient had no untoward sequelae. She returned to work in a week, abstained from aspirin, and underwent uneventful liposuction of her right side 8 weeks later. There was no excessive bleeding at the second procedure. Had I not observed the color of the aspirate and stopped the operation, the patient would almost certainly have required an unplanned homologous transfusion.

When to Stop—The Pinch Test

The end point of liposuction is optimal contour reduction with a smooth skin surface. At the initial consultation and, again, just before surgery I examine the patient in the standing position to assess the thickness and tone of the skin and subcutaneous tissues. Skin thickness is estimated in centimeters and recorded on the consultation sheet along with the estimated volumes.

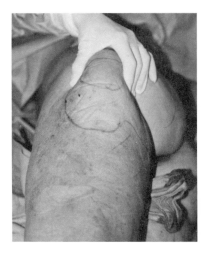 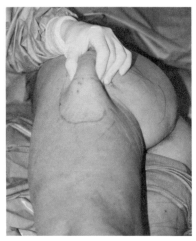 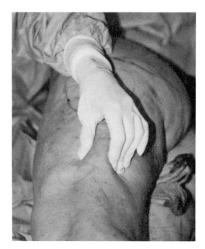

When the patient is anesthetized and after injection of lidocaine and epinephrine, I again inspect and pinch the soft tissues, as is being done on this patient's lateral thigh. I note contour and pinch thickness just before suctioning is started.

After removing half of the expected volume, I repeat the pinch test. I also visually check for surface irregularities and run my hand over the treated area to feel for bumps and depressions. I then work from the second access incision, creating a series of tunnels intersecting with those from the first access incision and paying particular attention to smoothing out irregularities until the area looks and feels correct.

The final thickness should be approximately the same as that of an adjacent nontreated area (the distal lateral thigh in this example). I find comparative thicknesses of treated areas vs. untreated areas of more help than absolute measurements since normal skin thickness varies considerably from patient to patient.

Feathering

Before concluding the procedure I palpate the edge of the treated area looking for bumps and abrupt steps from treated to untreated areas. If present, I smooth them by removing small amounts of fat in the transition zone using a fine-diameter cannula.

Conservatism: The Key to Avoiding Overresections

When the pinch test demonstrates a satisfactory thickness, when the treated area looks and feels smooth, and when equal volumes have been removed from bilaterally symmetric areas, suctioning is terminated. If in doubt, it is better to underresect than to overresect. Underresections are correctable, but overresections are not retrievable. Although I have had considerable experience with liposuction, I find that I still perform secondary procedures on about 5% of my patients, most frequently because they wish additional tissue removed. I prefer to perform secondary surgery for additional fat removal on a few patients rather than have a group of patients with uncorrectable overresections.

WOUND CLOSURE AND DRESSINGS

Access incisions are closed with surgical staples, which are removed 1 or 2 days after surgery and do not leave marks. Some surgeons leave the wounds open to drain, reasoning that egress of blood reduces swelling and bruising.[9] Although this method has the virtue of simplicity, profuse drainage is alarming to the patient and necessitates increased nursing care. I prefer a closed wound with minimal drainage and a comfortable patient.

After wound closure the patient is sent to the recovery room without a wound dressing or support garment. Recovery room staff check for bleeding from the access incisions, place additional staples as necessary, and put an elastic support garment on the patient.

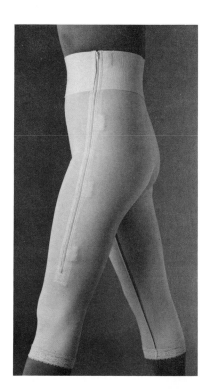

The Polli garment (Caromed International, Inc., Raleigh, N.C.) has zippered sides reinforced by hook and eye closures. Side openings facilitate putting the garment on the unconscious patient, and an open crotch permits voiding without having to remove the garment. Use of this stocking in the immediate postoperative period limits swelling and bruising.

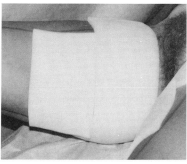

In some patients I support the treated areas with ¼-inch thick self-adherent foam sponge (Reston; 3M Corporation, St. Paul, Minn.) to limit bruising. It can be used as the sole or supplemental dressing underneath an elastic garment.

POSTOPERATIVE CARE AND RECOVERY

Economic considerations dictate that most liposuction procedures be performed in an ambulatory setting where their safety has been documented.[10,11] Nevertheless, if large volumes are to be removed, I keep the patient overnight if feasible. The patient always feels more comfortable and able to care for herself 24 hours rather than 4 hours after surgery.

Warming the Patient

Despite efforts to reduce heat loss during surgery (see p. 51), some patients will feel cold and shiver when they awaken in the recovery room. In the past, radiant heat lamps were used to provide warmth and reduce shivering.

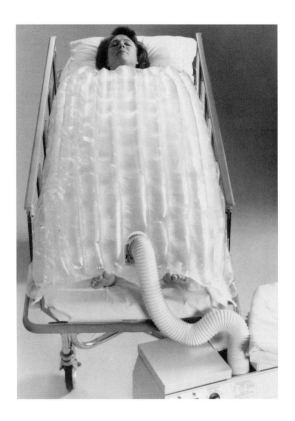

More recently, I have used a specially designed patient-warming device (Bair-Hugger; Augustine Medical, Inc., Eden Prairie, Minn.) that produces extremely fast warming and makes recovery much more pleasant and rapid for patients undergoing large-volume liposuction or multiple procedures. Heated air at a controlled temperature is forced through a disposable paper and plastic blanket. The heated air enters the blanket via the large corrugated tube at the foot of the bed and exits via microperforations in the blanket's paper underlayer, flowing over the patient and resulting in rapid convective warming.

Pain

Patients may experience transient burning in treated areas as the local anesthetic wears off. Small, frequent doses of intravenous narcotics provide rapid and effective relief. Patients usually need an oral narcotic the afternoon or evening following surgery but rarely require pain relief medication after the first 24 hours. Use of the tumescent technique sometimes eliminates the need for narcotics altogether.

Gradually decreasing levels of discomfort and soreness persist for several days. Generally there is no discomfort when lying or standing still, but changes of position will cause pain in treated areas until approximately 1 week after surgery. Occasional patients experience sharp, fleeting pain as late as 6 weeks after surgery. This pain is usually precipitated by vigorous motion and muscle contracture under the treated area. The anterior abdomen is most commonly the site of this problem, although any area may be affected. Such episodes usually occur only once or twice before disappearing.

Compression Garments

One or two days after surgery the treated areas are inspected and staples removed. A fresh compression garment is put on before the patient returns home. Patients wear the garment continuously (even when sleeping) for as long as 3 weeks (4 to 6 weeks for calves and ankles). They are given two sets of garments so that they can put on fresh garments while the soiled ones are washed. The garments limit swelling and bruising and help reduce late edema. Nevertheless, except in the calves and ankles, their use is not critical to obtaining a good final result. Some patients enjoy the support and security afforded by the garments and prefer to wear them longer than 3 weeks. Others find them uncomfortable and discard them in less than a week.

If Reston foam sponge has been used, it is removed 3 to 4 days after surgery. Over the past year I have seen no difference in final result between patients who have worn a Reston sponge and those who have had surgical support garments. I do recommend that after removal of the Reston sponge patients wear an inexpensive commercial elastic garment they can purchase at any department store. Patients having calf and ankle suction always wear medical-grade support hose for at least 4 to 6 weeks.

Swelling and Bruising

Swelling reaches a plateau at 48 to 72 hours and persists at peak levels for several days. During the first postoperative week patients will notice that their clothing fits more tightly and that they have gained weight due to fluid retention. Their enlarged body is covered with unsightly bruises. While these sequelae are routine and expected by the surgeon, they come as a depressing surprise to the unprepared patient. It will save considerable emotional discomfort to the patient and multiple telephone calls to the office if patients are told about their postoperative appearance before surgery and the information is reinforced at the first postoperative visit.

Patients frequently cannot see any contour improvement until the end of the first week. About 50% of the expected reduction occurs within 30 days, another 25% at 2 months, and most of the final 25% by 3 months. Occasional patients, particularly those who undergo calf and ankle suction, have significant additional diminution in contour up to 6 months after surgery. Bruising usually lasts 3 to 6 weeks. The intensity and duration of bruising are less severe when the tumescent technique is used (see pp. 88-93).

Resumption of Normal Activities

Patients may shower 24 hours after surgery. Tub baths are permitted at 5 days. Although patients are told to allow a week off from work, many feel well enough to return to part-time or even full-time sedentary activities in 48 hours. By 96 hours after surgery 80% of patients are able to return to work, and by 1 week 100% are back at work if they want to be. The patient's motivation is the single most important factor in determining return to full activity. Sports are resumed gradually starting the second week after surgery. By 3 to 4 weeks most patients can enjoy unlimited sports activity.

SECONDARY SURGERY

If a noticeable asymmetry or underresection is apparent 6 weeks after surgery, it is advisable to talk frankly to the worried patient. I tell the patient that if no significant improvement is seen by 6 months I will offer her a secondary procedure if I believe it will help. To dismiss the patient's complaints with the comment that she is "still swollen" and will improve with time can only be regarded as self-serving by the disappointed, anxious patient and will reflect adversely on the surgeon. It is reassuring to the patient for the surgeon to sympathetically acknowledge that a problem may exist, that he is aware of it, and that he is ready to take corrective steps if necessary.

———————————————— REFERENCES ————————————————

1. Hetter GP. The effect of low-dose epinephrine on the hematocrit drop following lipolysis. Aesthetic Plast Surg 8:19-21, 1984.
2. Klein JA. The tumescent technique: Anesthesia and modified liposuction technique. Dermatol Clin 8:425-437, 1990.
3. Toledo LS. Syringe liposculpture: A two-year experience. Aesthetic Plast Surg 15: 321-326, 1991.
4. Courtiss EH, Kanter MK, Kanter WR, Ransil BJ. The effect of epinephrine on blood loss during suction lipectomy. Plast Reconstr Surg 88:801-803, 1991.
5. Pitman GH. Discussion of Courtiss EH, Choucair RJ, Donelan MB. Large-volume suction lipectomy: An analysis of 108 patients. Plast Reconstr Surg 89:1080-1082, 1992.
6. Xylocaine package insert. Astra Pharmaceutical Products, Inc., Westborough, Mass., 1990.
7. Klein JA. Tumescent technique permits lidocaine doses of 35 ml/kg for liposuction: Peak plasma lidocaine levels are diminished and delayed 12 hours. J Dermatol Surg Oncol 16:248-263, 1990.
8. Illouz Y-G, de Villers YT. Body Sculpturing by Lipoplasty. New York: Churchill Livingstone, 1989.
9. Courtiss EH. Personal communication, 1990.
10. Clayton DN, Clayton JN, Lindley TS, Clayton JL. Large volume lipoplasty. Clin Plast Surg 16:305-312, 1989.
11. Ersek RA. Serial suction lipectomy. Clin Plast Surg 16:313-317, 1989.

Chapter 4

MANAGEMENT OF FLUID AND BLOOD LOSS

The cornerstone of safe liposuction is skillful management of fluid and blood loss; management is guided by the same physiologic principles that apply to any surgical procedure: (1) circulating volume is maintained by infusion of appropriate levels of asanguineous fluid and (2) oxygen-carrying capacity is supported with red cell transfusions. Although these principles are basic to surgeons, their application to liposuction needs to be examined, particularly in light of the fact that many of the catastrophic complications associated with liposuction have involved inadequate or inappropriate fluid and blood replacement.[1,2] The guidelines I use for calculating fluid and blood replacement are keyed to volume of fat removal and have evolved from my clinical experience since 1982.

FLUID REPLACEMENT
Early Experiences

Initially the anesthesiologist and I assumed fluid losses would be similar to those associated with major general surgery. Therefore all patients were given 500 ml of crystalloid in the perioperative-induction period. At first, additional crystalloid was given at a rate of 6 to 10 ml/kg/hr.[3] Subsequent rate and volume of replacement were determined by clinical evaluation of the patient, relying especially on neck vein filling[4] and urine output. It soon became apparent that as suction volume increased, so did fluid requirements. This observation prompted me to quantify the relationship between fluid replacement and volume of aspirate.

Development of Fluid Replacement Guidelines

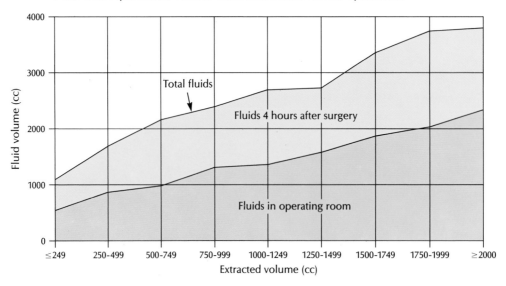

Mean fluid replacement volume vs. suction volume in 200 operations.

Detailed retrospective analysis of a personal series of 200 operations showed that average fluid replacement had a linear relationship to volume of aspirate.[5-7]

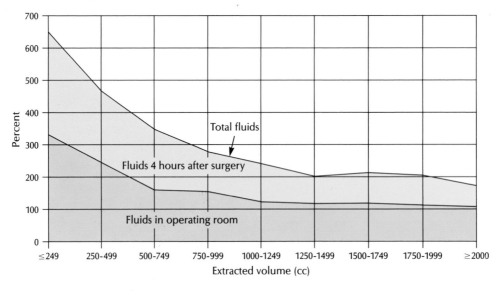

Mean fluid replacement volume as percentage of suction volume vs. suction volume in 200 operations.

When suction volume was 1000 to 2500 cc, the average volume of crystalloid replacement in the operating room slightly exceeded 100% of suction volume. Additional fluids in the first 4 hours after surgery brought total average volume of fluid replacement to approximately 200% of aspirate.

The following formulation fluid guidelines were developed for use when aspirating 1000 to 2500 cc of fat.[7]

Intraoperative	1.0 ml crystalloid/cc aspirate
First 4 hours postoperatively	1.0 ml crystalloid/cc aspirate
Total	2.0 ml crystalloid/cc aspirate

If more than 2500 cc of aspirate is suctioned, or if other procedures are performed simultaneously, a Foley catheter is inserted and hourly measurements of urinary output are used as an additional clinical determinant of fluid replacement. Most liposuction operations take 1 to 2 hours, but when large volumes of fat are removed quickly (e.g., more than 2500 cc in less than 1 hour), volume for volume replacement in a short period can result in fluid overload. In such instances the protocol is modified so that less fluid is administered in the operating room and more fluid postoperatively.

These general guidelines were developed when I was injecting relatively small amounts into the subcutaneous space. I now inject larger volumes of dilute lidocaine and epinephrine (tumescent technique). Subcutaneous injection may reach 4000 ml (see pp. 88-93), and intravenous fluid requirements are reduced.

Mobilization of fluid from the subcutaneous space occurs most impressively in the early postoperative period and is usually reflected in diuresis beginning 4 to 6 hours after surgery. Intraoperative diuresis does not occur unless the patient is given significant volumes of intravenous fluid during surgery.

Quantitative guidelines for the tumescent technique are being developed. My current practice is to give approximately 500 ml of intravenous crystalloid during induction followed by administration of 6 to 10 ml/kg/hr during surgery. Postoperative intravenous replacement is based on clinical observation, with urinary output of 0.5 to 1.0 ml/kg/hr being the most reliable indicator of adequate fluid replacement.

Preliminary experiences with large-volume subcutaneous injections indicate that postoperative intravenous fluid requirements are substantially reduced, and patients can be discharged soon after surgery.

If the patient stays overnight in the hospital, the intravenous solution is continued at a rate of about 100 ml/hr until discharge the next day. Oral fluids are also given. If the patient goes home the day of surgery, she is instructed to drink 8 ounces (250 ml) of fluid every hour until bedtime. Sodium-rich fluids such as V_8 juice and chicken broth are encouraged.

Crystalloid vs. Colloid

Some surgeons use commercially available colloids (Dextran, Hespan, etc.) and/or albumin to replace fluid losses as suction volumes exceed 1000 cc.[8-11] I avoid these preparations since they can cause allergic reactions, increase bleeding, and impair renal function.[12]

Crystalloid alone provides adequate volume replacement for most operations. If suction volume is large and red cell mass is depleted, I transfuse autologous blood (see below). Although the purpose of red cell transfusion is to increase oxygen-carrying capacity, it also restores intravascular oncotic pressure. Compared with commercially available products, the patient's own blood is a more effective, safer, and longer lasting plasma expander.

BLOOD LOSS AND TRANSFUSION

Large-volume aspirations result in significant loss of red cell mass and may require transfusion. The surgeon will want to avoid transfusions when possible; however, if transfusions are necessary, plans must be made in advance to have autologous blood available. A rational approach to minimize blood loss and facilitate planning for autologous transfusion involves four steps, as described below.

Preoperative Identification of Patients Likely to Require Transfusion

Despite ongoing efforts to purify the blood supply, a recipient of a single unit of homologous blood has a 1:100 chance of contracting hepatitis[13] and a 1:40,000 chance of acquiring AIDS.[14,15] Patients who are likely to require transfusion should be identified at the initial consultation so that preparations can be made for predeposit of autologous blood.

Which patients will require transfusion? Various existing guidelines advocate preparation for transfusion when planned aspiration exceeds 1000 cc,[16] 1300 cc,[17] 1500 cc,[10,18-23] 1750 cc,[24] or 2000 cc.[21,25,26] These recommendations, while based on clinical experience, are wide ranging and arbitrary. In my experience, patients having aspirations of less than 1500 cc do not need to be prepared for autologous transfusion. Patients having aspirations of more than 2500 cc and/or multiple simultaneous procedures will frequently require blood. A middle group of patients having aspirations of 1500 to 2500 cc suctioned may or may not require transfusion. If all patients in this middle group are prepared for transfusion, homologous transfusions may be avoided, but many patients will be needlessly subjected to the inconvenience, expense, and risks of phlebotomy and autologous transfusions. Unfortunately, some patients will be rendered so anemic by preoperative phlebotomy that they will require transfusions after surgery simply because they donated blood.[27]

The ideal goal is to identify those patients likely to require transfusion at the initial consultation by predicting expected volume of blood loss from liposuction and deciding if the predicted volume of blood loss necessitates transfusion.

Predicting Blood Loss From Liposuction

Blood loss from liposuction is always proportionate to suction volume.[5-7] Measurements of the average amount of blood in suction aspirates have ranged from 15% to 35%.[2,11,18,19,23,24,28-30] Blood in the aspirate, however, is less than total blood loss since it does not include loss into the tissues evidenced by swelling and bruising.

One can use fractional changes in preoperative and postoperative hematocrits to estimate total blood loss. Average blood loss increases with suction volume.[5-7]

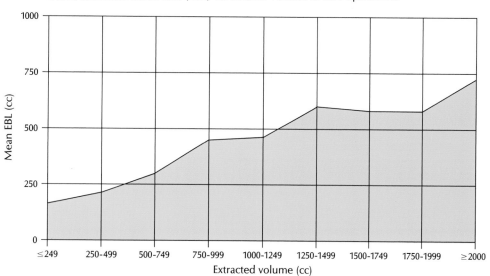

Mean estimated blood loss (EBL) vs. suction volume in 200 operations.

Average blood loss is a relatively constant percent of suction volume.[5-7]

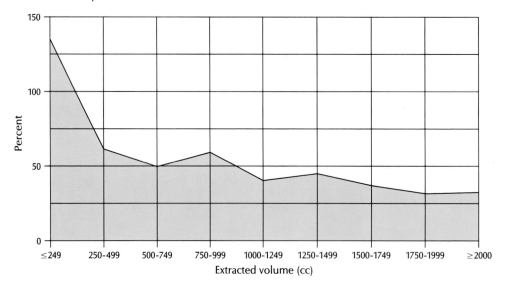

Mean estimated blood loss (EBL) as a percentage of suction volume vs. suction volume in 200 operations.

In my patients the average blood loss prior to use of the tumescent technique was 44% (±2.5%) of suction volume.[5-7] My clinical impression is that the tumescent technique has reduced blood loss still further, particularly during large-volume liposuction.

I am, therefore, comfortable in predicting that for most of my patients, blood loss will be less than 50% of suction volume. For example, patients undergoing liposuction of 1000 cc could be expected to lose less than 500 ml of blood, and patients undergoing liposuction of 2000 cc could be expected to lose less than 1000 ml of blood.

Guidelines for Deciding When to Prepare for Autologous Transfusions

Two concepts have emerged.

Maximal safe blood loss   Maximal predicted volume of blood loss acceptable without having autologous blood available

Maximal safe suction   Maximal volume of aspirate without having autologous blood available

Since volume of blood loss is less than one-half the volume of aspirate in my patients,

$$\text{Maximal safe suction} = 2 \times \text{Maximal safe blood loss}$$

Most healthy young adults will easily tolerate a loss of 25% of blood volume without transfusion.[31-33] For a person with a preoperative hematocrit of 40, 25% loss of blood volume will produce a post-equilibration hematocrit of 30. As acute blood loss exceeds 25% of blood volume (hematocrit <30), the desirability of transfusion increases in proportion to the loss.[33] Unreplaced acute blood loss of 50% of blood volume (hematocrit <21) is usually lethal.[31]

Given these considerations, I have autologous blood available for all operations in which predicted blood loss exceeds 25% of estimated blood volume.

LIPOSUCTION VOLUME AND PREDICTED BLOOD LOSS				
	Patient Weight (kg)	Blood Volume (ml)*	Maximal Safe Blood Loss (ml)†	Maximal Safe Suction Without Transfusion (cc)‡
Women	40	2600	650	1300
	50	3250	812	1625
	60	3900	975	1950
	70	4550	1138	2275
	80	5200	1300	2600
Men	40	2800	700	1400
	50	3500	875	1750
	60	4200	1050	2100
	70	4900	1225	2450
	80	5600	1400	2800

*65 ml/kg for women and 70 ml/kg for men.
†25% of estimated blood volume.
‡Twice the maximal safe blood loss.

The figures in the chart can be expressed as a simple graph that permits selection of "trigger points" at which to prepare patients for autologous transfusion.

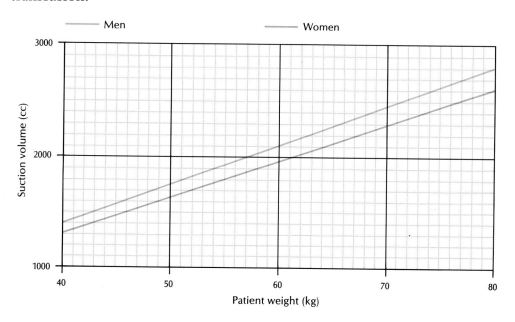

I prepare patients for autologous transfusion when the line intersecting patient weight and predicted suction volume lies above the diagonal line appropriate to gender (black for men, red for women). Depending on the clinical circumstances (e.g., older patient, performance of simultaneous additional operations), I also ask some patients whose weight and predicted suction volume intersect below the diagonal line to predonate blood. Patients may donate more than 1 unit of blood, depending on planned suction volume and other factors.

Early Autologous Blood Donation*

When a patient has been selected for possible autologous transfusion, blood donation should be completed 3 to 4 weeks before surgery to minimize anemia and maximize reticulocytosis.[34] Several factors influence planning.[27]

1. Following withdrawal of a single unit it takes 10 days for a maximal erythropoietic response[32] and more than a month to completely restore red cell mass.[35]
2. Iron stores are the rate-limiting factor in erythropoiesis,[32,36-38] and oral iron supplements will permit red cell production at a rate three times normal.[32,38]
3. Modern blood bank techniques permit storage of unfrozen packed red cells for up to 42 days.[39-41]
4. Removing 1 unit of blood at weekly intervals from patients who are given supplemental iron permits a steady state to develop with a drop in hematocrit averaging 3 to 6 points in many series.[36,42-43]
5. Although units can be withdrawn up to 3 days prior to surgery,[44] there is only minimal compensatory erythrocytosis in this time. Plasma protein and blood volume are fully restored in 72 hours.[45,46]

I have patients begin donations as early as 40 days prior to surgery. They start taking ferrous sulfate, 325 mg PO tid, 5 days before withdrawal of the first unit and continue for 30 days after the operation. They can donate 3 units at weekly intervals, with the last unit drawn almost 4 weeks before surgery. When appropriate, the interval between phlebotomies can be reduced, or the first unit can be drawn more than 42 days in advance and then infused at the same time that the patient donates 2 units.

*Reprinted with minor changes from Pitman GH. Discussion of Courtiss EH, Choucair RJ, Donelan MB. Large-volume suction lipectomy: An analysis of 108 patients. Plast Reconstr Surg 89:1080-1082, 1992.

Intraoperative Use of Dilute Epinephrine to Reduce Blood Loss

There is near universal agreement among plastic surgeons that injection of epinephrine into the subcutaneous tissues reduces blood loss during procedures involving the skin and subcutaneous tissues. I[27] as well as others[18,37,48] have observed that blood loss during liposuction is also reduced by this maneuver. Although one study challenges this practice,[49] I find the results unconvincing.[27] My current practice is to inject large volumes of the following solution into the subcutaneous tissues 10 minutes prior to starting liposuction:

1:1000 epinephrine	1 ml
8.4% sodium bicarbonate (1 mEq/ml)	5 ml
1% lidocaine	50 ml
Physiologic saline solution	1000 ml
0.05% lidocaine with 1:1,000,000 epinephrine	1056 ml

See pp. 88-93 for additional details.

Intraoperative and Postoperative Evaluation to Determine When Transfusion Is Necessary

Having autologous blood available does not necessarily mean it should be transfused. Although safer than homologous blood, autologous transfusions are not without risk.[50,51] Clerical error can result in a mismatch and fatal hemolytic transfusion reaction. Sepsis may occur from bacterial contamination during phlebotomy or storage. In addition, transfusions can cause pulmonary dysfunction from circulating cell fragments or fluid overload.

In the absence of large, unexpected blood loss or hemodynamic instability, the decision to transfuse is usually made after surgery based on postoperative hematocrit and other clinical considerations such as age and probability of ongoing blood loss.

The minimal acceptable hematocrit level for surgical patients is a moot issue.[31,52,53] A hemoglobin level of 10 or hematocrit level of 30 has traditionally been regarded as the minimum value for elective surgery,[54] but treatment of patients with chronic anemia and use of normovolemic hemodilution[55-58] have shown that patients with hematocrit levels in the low twenties can tolerate surgery.

Given a demonstrated ability to manage patients with low hematocrits, plastic surgeons have been advised to avoid transfusion until the hematocrit falls to 21.[59] Such advice is inappropriate for elective cosmetic operations for several reasons.

We do not know with certainty that it is safe to permit the hematocrit to drift into the low twenties without full monitoring just because this policy has worked well in some groups of patients.[31] Moreover, although no proof exists that mild or even moderate anemia contributes to perioperative morbidity,[53] my clinical impression, which is supported by others who are experienced in liposuction,[2,17,60] is that use of autologous transfusion in appropriately selected patients does hasten recovery.

The risks associated with autologous transfusion are less than those of homologous transfusion, and what seems reasonable in a nonelective or emergency situation in which only homologous blood is available is not reasonable in elective cosmetic surgery when autologous blood can be readily banked. In short, indications for autologous transfusions can be more liberal than indications for use of homologous blood.

It is my practice to use autologous transfusions to maintain the postoperative hematocrit near 30. This level provides a comfortable cushion of functional reserve and oxygen-carrying capacity. Should the hematocrit drift into the mid- or even low twenties in an otherwise healthy young patient, I do not use homologous transfusions to restore the hematocrit. I do, however, use autologous blood for this purpose when it is available.

Note: The presence of autologous blood does not mean that homologous units will not have to be used should there be unexpected blood loss. It is prudent, therefore, to so inform the patient in advance.

CONCLUSION

Safe liposuction demands attention to fluid flux and blood loss. The guidelines set forth in this chapter have been helpful in calculating fluid replacement, estimating blood loss, and planning transfusion in my personal practice. These recommendations are subject to modification by the unique requirements of each patient and the unique circumstances of each individual surgeon's approach. They are a starting point, but, in the end, the surgeon's informed clinical judgment determines detailed management of fluid and blood replacement.

REFERENCES

1. Mladick RA. Panel discussion: Catastrophic complications of lipoplasty. Presented at the Fifty-ninth Annual Scientific Meeting of the American Society of Plastic and Reconstructive Surgeons. Boston: October 25, 1990.
2. Teimourian B. Suction Lipectomy and Body Sculpturing. St. Louis: CV Mosby, 1987.
3. Tonneson AS. Crystalloids and colloids. In Miller RD, ed. Anesthesia. New York: Churchill Livingstone, 1990, pp 1443-1446.
4. Holcroft JW. Shock. In Wilmore DW, Brennan MF, Harken AH, Holcroft JW, Meakins JL, eds. The American College of Surgeons Manual on Care of the Surgical Patient, vol 1. New York: Scientific American, 1989.
5. Pitman GH, Holzer J. Anesthetic management for suction lipectomy of the torso and extremities. Presented at the Twentieth Annual Meeting of The American Society for Aesthetic Plastic Surgery. Los Angeles: March 23, 1987.
6. Pitman GH, Holzer J. Safe suction: Fluid replacement and blood loss parameters. Presented at the Fifty-eighth Annual Scientific Meeting of the American Society of Plastic and Reconstructive Surgeons. San Francisco: October 30, 1989.
7. Pitman GH, Holzer J. Safe suction: Fluid replacement and blood loss parameters. Perspect Plast Surg 5(1):79-89, 1991.
8. Cohen S. Lipolysis: Pitfalls and problems in a series of 1246 procedures. Aesthetic Plast Surg 9:207-214, 1985.
9. Fournier PF, Otteni FM. Lipodissection in body sculpturing: The dry procedure. Plast Reconstr Surg 72:598-609, 1983.
10. Hetter GP. Blood and fluid replacement for lipoplasty procedures. Clin Plast Surg 16:245-248, 1989.
11. Mladick RA, Morris RL. Sixteen months' experience with the Illouz technique of lipolysis. Ann Plast Surg 16:220-223, 1986.
12. Miller RD. Transfusion therapy. In Miller RD, ed. Anesthesia. New York: Churchill Livingstone, 1990, pp 1467-1499.
13. FDA Drug Bulletin, July 1989.
14. Bove JR. Transfusion-associated hepatitis and AIDS: What is the risk? N Engl J Med 317:242-245, 1987.
15. Ward JW, Holmberg SD, Allen JR, Cohn DL, Critchley SE, et al. Transmission of human immunodeficiency virus (HIV) by blood transfusions screened as negative for HIV antibody. N Engl J Med 318:473-478, 1988.
16. Courtiss EH. Invited comment. Mladick RA, Morris RL. Sixteen months' experience with the Illouz technique of lipolysis. Ann Plast Surg 16:233-234, 1986.
17. Mandel MA. Blood and fluid replacement in major liposuction procedures. Aesthetic Plast Surg 14:187-191, 1990.
18. Clayton DN, Clayton JN, Lindley TS, Clayton JL. Large volume lipoplasty. Clin Plast Surg 16:305-312, 1989.
19. Illouz Y-G, de Villers YT. Body Sculpturing by Lipoplasty. New York: Churchill Livingstone, 1989.
20. Gargan TJ, Courtiss EH. The risks of suction lipectomy: Their prevention and treatment. Clin Plast Surg 11:457-463, 1984.
21. Shirakabe T. Japanese suction-assisted lipectomy. Clin Plast Surg 11:549-565, 1984.
22. Teimourian B, Fisher JB. Suction curettage to remove excess fat for body contouring. Plast Reconstr Surg 68:50-58, 1981.
23. Courtiss EH, Choucair RJ, Donelan MB. Large-volume suction lipectomy: An analysis of 108 patients. Plast Reconstr Surg 89:1068-1079, 1992.
24. Goodpasture JC, Bunkis J. Quantitative analysis of blood and fat in suction lipectomy aspirates. Plast Reconstr Surg 78:765-769, 1986.

25. Ersek RA, Zambrano J, Surak GS, Denton DR. Suction-assisted lipectomy for correction of 202 figure faults in 101 patients: Indications, limitations, and applications. Plast Reconstr Surg 78:615–624, 1986.
26. Hetter GP. Closed suction lipoplasty on 1,078 patients: Illouz told the truth. Aesthetic Plast Surg 12:183–185, 1988.
27. Pitman GH. Discussion of Courtiss EH, Choucair RJ, Donelan MB. Large-volume suction lipectomy: An analysis of 108 patients. Plast Reconstr Surg 89:1080–1082, 1992.
28. Grazer FM. Discussion of Goodpasture JC, Bunkis J. Quantitative analysis of blood and fat in suction lipectomy aspirates. Plast Reconstr Surg 78:770–772, 1986.
29. Apfelberg DB, Lash H, Maser MR, White DN. Computerized suction lipectomy aspirator monitor for improved results in suction lipectomy. Plast Reconstr Surg 82:896–903, 1988.
30. Courtiss EH. Suction lipectomy: A retrospective analysis of one hundred patients. Plast Reconstr Surg 73:780–794, 1984.
31. Greenburg AG. Indications for transfusion. In Wilmore DW, Brennan MF, Harken AH, Holcroft JW, Meakins JL, eds. The American College of Surgeons Manual on Care of the Surgical Patient, vol 1. New York: Scientific American, 1989.
32. Hillman RS. Acute blood loss anemia. In Williams WJ, Bentler E, Erslev AJ, Lichtman MA, eds. Hematology, 4th ed. New York: McGraw-Hill, 1990, pp 700–704.
33. Schwartz SI. Hemostasis, surgical bleeding, and transfusion. In Schwartz SI, ed. Principles of Surgery. New York: McGraw-Hill, 1989, p 128.
34. Kruskall MS, Glaser EE, Leonard SS, Wilson SC, Pacini DG, Donovan LM, Ransil BJ. Utilization and effectiveness of a hospital autologous preoperative blood donor program. Transfusion 26:335–340, 1986.
35. Walsh RJ, Sewell AK. Some effects of blood loss on healthy males. Med J Aust 1:73–75, 1946.
36. Finch S, Haskins DM, Finch CA. Iron metabolism: Hematopoiesis following phlebotomy: Iron as a limiting factor. J Clin Invest 29:1078–1086, 1950.
37. Hamstra RD, Block MH. Erythropoiesis in response to blood loss in man. J Appl Physiol 27:503–507, 1969.
38. Hillman RS, Henderson PA. Control of marrow production by the level of iron supply. J Clin Invest 48:454–460, 1969.
39. Valeri CR. Measurement of viable Adsol-preserved human red cells [letter]. N Engl J Med 312:377–378, 1985.
40. Vovric VA, Archer GT, Wisdom L, Robson J, Raftog J, Coulits N, Ribeifora A, Stewart M, Jindra J, Schiller M. Thirty-five day modified red cells and 7-day stored platelet concentrates from triple bags of identical PVC formulation. Vox Sang 49:181–186, 1985.
41. Nasouredis SP. Preservation and clinical use of erythrocytes and whole blood. In Williams WJ, Bentler E, Erslev AJ, Lichtman MA, eds. Hematology, 4th ed. New York: McGraw-Hill, 1990, pp 1628–1647.
42. Gilcher RO, Belcher L. Predeposit programs. In Sandler SG, Silvergleid AJ, eds. Autologous Transfusion. Arlington, Va.: American Association of Blood Banks, 1983, p 18.
43. Haugen RK, Hill GE. A large-scale autologous blood program in a community hospital. JAMA 257:1211–1214, 1987.
44. Holland PV, ed. Standards for Blood Banks and Transfusion Services, 13th ed. Arlington, Va.: American Association of Blood Banks, 1989, pp 20, 40.
45. Ebert RV, Stead EA, Gibson JG. Response of normal subjects to acute blood loss. Arch Intern Med 68:578–590, 1941.
46. Adamson J, Hillman RS. Blood volume and plasma protein replacement following acute blood loss in normal man. JAMA 205:609–612, 1968.

47. Hetter GP. The effect of low-dose epinephrine on the hematocrit drop following lipolysis. Aesthetic Plast Surg 8:19-21, 1984.
48. Toledo LS. Syringe liposculpture: A 2-year experience. Aesthetic Plast Surg 15:321-326, 1991.
49. Courtiss EH, Kanter MA, Kanter WR, Ransil BJ. The effect of epinephrine on blood loss during suction lipectomy. Plast Reconstr Surg 88:801-803, 1991.
50. Toy PT, Strauss RG, Stehling LC, Sears R, Price TH, et al. Predeposited autologous blood for elective surgery. A national multicenter study. N Engl J Med 316:517-520, 1987.
51. Bell W. The hematology of autotransfusion. Surgery 84:695-699, 1987.
52. Allen JB, Allen FB. The minimum acceptable level of hemoglobin. Int Anesthesiol Clin 20:1-22, 1982.
53. Perioperative red blood cell transfusion. National Heart, Lung, and Blood Institute Consensus Development Panel. JAMA 260:2700-2703, 1988.
54. Messmer KF. Acceptable hematocrit levels in surgical patients. World J Surg 11:41-46, 1987.
55. Fahmy NR, Chandler HP, Patel DG, Lappas D. Hemodynamics and oxygen availability during acute hemodilution in conscious man [abst.]. Anesthesiology 53:S84, 1980.
56. Jobes DR, Gallagher J. Acute normovolemic hemodilution. Int Anesthesiol Clin 20:77-95, 1982.
57. Laks H, Pilon RN, Klovekorn WP, Anderson W, MacCallum JR, O'Conner NE. Acute hemodilution. Ann Surg 180:103-109, 1974.
58. Rose D, Forest R, Coutsoftides T. Acute hormovolemic hemodilution [abst.]. Anesthesiology 51:S91, 1979.
59. Kruskall MS. Autologous blood transfusions and plastic surgery. Plast Reconstr Surg 84:662-663, 1989.
60. Courtiss EH. Personal communication, 1991.

Chapter 5

REFINEMENTS IN LIPOSUCTION
TUMESCENT TECHNIQUE, SUPERFICIAL SUCTION, SYRINGE SUCTION, AND TREATMENT OF CELLULITE

Three recent technical refinements (the tumescent technique, superficial suction, and syringe suction) have been touted together and separately as effective treatment for cellulite and flaccid skin.[1-5]

The tumescent technique and superficial suction are major technical improvements that enhance our ability to contour the subcutaneous fat, particularly in patients with suboptimal skin conditions and/or small fat deposits. Both modalities offer individual and unique advantages. In combination, they are superadditive, interacting and building on one another to permit a more sophisticated level of treatment with improved results in many areas.

Syringe suction has become increasingly popular as a convenient alternative to utilization of a mechanical aspirator. It is particularly efficient for fat transfer and is used to reinject fat for filling isolated depressions and smoothing generalized surface irregularities (cellulite). Unfortunately, results of fat injection remain unreliable and inconsistent. Occasional patients do benefit from long-lasting correction of solitary surface depressions. Cellulite, however, is characterized by multiple fine and coarse skin irregularities, and I have seen no convincing evidence that fat transfer is an effective remedy.

Despite my skepticism about treatment of cellulite, the tumescent technique, superficial suction, and syringe suction have a broad range of clinical applications that merit consideration.

TUMESCENT TECHNIQUE

The tumescent technique involves injecting very large volumes of dilute lidocaine with epinephrine into the subcutaneous fat. Enough fluid is infiltrated so that the tissues become swollen and firm (hence the name "tumescent"). Although the technique was initially developed as a method to achieve local anesthesia, it also offers several technical advantages that help achieve a smoother skin surface.

Early practitioners of liposuction injected a variety of substances into the fat. Illouz[6] and Fournier and Otteni[7] used a hypotonic solution containing hyaluronidase ("wet technique") to speed adipocyte dissolution and evacuation, but hypotonicity did not improve liposuction, and hyaluronidase caused allergic reactions. These solutions were subsequently abandoned.[7]

Teimourian and Fisher[8] preinjected 1:200,000 epinephrine to limit bleeding. Use of epinephrine in even more dilute concentrations (1:500,000) produced a quantifiable reduction in blood loss.[9-11] Although Courtiss et al.[12] reported no decrease in blood loss with the use of epinephrine, almost all clinicians agreed that preinjection of epinephrine significantly reduced bleeding. Addition of lidocaine to the injectate permitted liposuction of limited areas under local anesthesia.

Although most surgeons did not report or even note the volume of injection, the customary amount was less than 500 ml.[9] Klein[13] and Toledo,[1] however, advocated injection of very large volumes of highly dilute solutions to achieve local anesthesia in multiple areas and to further decrease blood loss. Toledo reported that 0.04% lidocaine with 1:500,000 epinephrine was effective for this purpose. Klein[14] recommended 0.05% lidocaine with 1:1,000,000 epinephrine to reduce blood loss in all patients and to achieve local anesthesia in patients undergoing removal of up to 3000 cc of fat.

The tumescent technique has four major advantages: enhanced local anesthesia, reduced blood loss, reduction of intravenous fluid requirements, and enlargement of the subcutaneous space.
1. *Enhanced local anesthesia.* Large volumes of dilute lidocaine provide profound anesthesia in the entire operative area during surgery and well into the postoperative period. Anesthesia may be maintained for as long as 12 hours. The need for postoperative narcotics is significantly reduced or eliminated in all patients. Patients frequently are able to leave the recovery area and return home without pain medication.

2. *Reduced blood loss.* Blood loss is diminished if the surgeon stops suctioning before blood appears in the aspirate. If, however, suctioning continues after the aspirate turns red, blood loss will increase. Nevertheless, overall blood loss is reduced.[1,13] I documented that combined blood loss into the aspirate and third space averaged 44% of suction volume in earlier publications,[10,11] but my clinical experience with the tumescent technique indicates that blood loss is even lower. Postoperative bruising is significantly decreased in many patients.

3. *Reduction of intravenous fluid requirements.* Intravenous fluid requirements are reduced as some of the large volume of injectate is absorbed into the circulation by hypodermoclysis. In the past, I have replaced suction volume with crystalloid in a ratio of 1:2. That is, the patient received 2 ml of crystalloid in the perioperative period for each 1 cc of aspirate.[10] Klein[14,15] believes that intravenous fluid replacement is altogether unnecessary when the tumescent technique is used. I have noted a diminution in fluid requirements with the tumescent technique, but the magnitude of the reduction has not been quantified. Suffice it to say that fluid requirements are reduced but should be determined on a clinical basis for the individual patient.

4. *Enlargement of the subcutaneous space.* Distention of the tissues by the large volume of injectate results in a hydrodissection that amplifies the volume of the subcutaneous space, permitting suction closer to the surface of the skin, facilitating more precise removal of small fat collections, and minimizing skin surface irregularities.

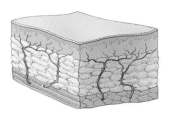 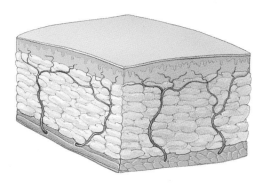

The volume enlargement of the fat compartment is analogous to the visual enlargement of the operative field produced when using loupe or microscopic magnification. The distention produced by hydrodissection also enlarges the space between fibrous elements, eases passage of the cannula, decreases tissue trauma, and reduces work effort.

Solutions for Injection

I use 0.05% lidocaine with 1:1,000,000 epinephrine. The addition of sodium bicarbonate (1 mEq for each 10 ml of 1% lidocaine) neutralizes the pH and decreases the pain of injection.[16] The solution is conveniently made as follows:

1:1000 epinephrine	1 ml
8.4% sodium bicarbonate (1 mEq/ml)	5 ml
1% lidocaine	50 ml
Physiologic saline solution	1000 ml
0.05% lidocaine with 1:1,000,000 epinephrine	1056 ml

The volume injected into each area is at least equal to and frequently double or triple the volume of planned tissue removal. Injected volumes may reach 4000 ml.

Klein's formula is identical to the above except that he uses 12.5 ml of bicarbonate.[14] Toledo[1] uses a slightly weaker solution of lidocaine with lactated Ringer's solution as his diluent.

The manufacturer's recommended maximum dose for subcutaneous injection of lidocaine with epinephrine is 7 mg/kg or 500 mg total. Recent studies have shown, however, that much larger doses can be used safely.[14,17] Klein[14] has suggested a maximum safe lidocaine dose of 35 mg/kg *if* the lidocaine is in dilute solution, *if* it is injected over 45 minutes, and *if* the solution contains epinephrine. Under these conditions, he has shown that lidocaine is absorbed very slowly into the circulation and that serum lidocaine concentrations do not reach toxic levels. I have injected as much as 2000 mg of dilute lidocaine with epinephrine over 10 minutes without untoward effect.

Equipment

Infiltrating cannulas come in varying diameters and lengths. A 3 mm cannula is narrow enough to pass through the tissues with minimal pain but strong enough so that it does not bend easily. The cannulas should be slightly longer than those used for suction since the local solution has to be injected beyond the treatment area. I use 25 cm infiltrating cannulas, which are 5 cm longer than my longest suction cannulas.

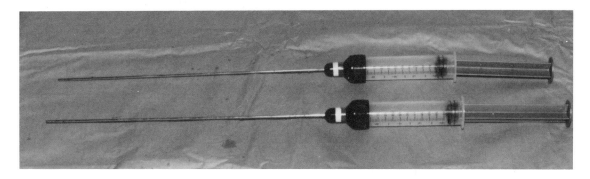

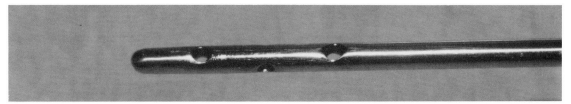

The infiltrating cannulas are mounted to 60 ml Toomey syringes filled with injectate. A close-up view of the tip of the cannula shows the multiple fenestrations for rapid delivery of fluid.

Operative Technique

A small amount of local anesthesia is injected into the access incisions, and a stab wound is made in the anesthetized skin. The 3 mm cannula is passed through the stab wound into the deep subcutaneous fat 5 cm beyond the area to be treated. Passage of the cannula causes surprisingly little discomfort. The local anesthetic is injected as the cannula is withdrawn. Keeping the tip of the cannula in the deep fat and away from the more richly innervated subcuticular tissues minimizes the pain of injection, as does slow, gradual injection. The soft tissues will visibly swell as the injection proceeds. The object is to produce a uniform swelling and firmness. If the patient is being treated under local anesthesia, intravenous sedation may be used during the injection period.

Two access incisions are used to create a grid pattern of injection so that the fluid is uniformly distributed in the entire fat compartment. Two syringes and two injection cannulas should be available so that the nurse or assistant can keep the surgeon continually supplied with a full syringe.

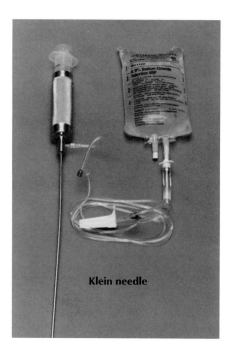

Klein needle

Injection devices are available that permit use of a single syringe and cannula attached by tubing to a container filled with the injectate. These devices require the surgeon to draw back on the syringe plunger to continually refill the syringe as the injection proceeds. I find having an assistant perform this task with a separate syringe faster and more efficient, but this is a matter of individual preference; others find the self-filling devices convenient.

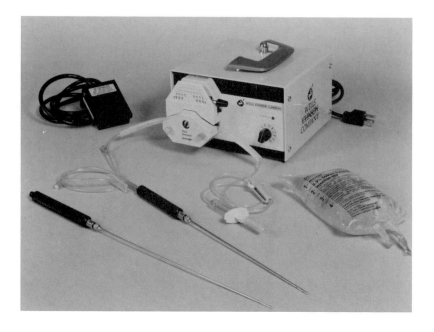

Injection pumps used with specially designed infiltrating cannulas permit continuous foot-pedal–controlled infusion.

I infiltrate a volume of solution equal to or greater than the expected volume of aspirate. If the injection is into the deep fat, the awake patient tolerates it easily. Flow through the cannulas is very rapid, and large volumes can be infused quickly; the only limiting factor is the pain due to rapid distention. Suction should not be started until at least 10 minutes after injection.

When suction begins, the aspirate is pure yellow or white and remains so until the surgeon has been working in the area for a while. Eventually, some blood appears, the amount depending on how long and how vigorously one works. Suction volumes are larger because the aspirate contains more water.

Using visual cues and the pinch test to determine the end point is similar to standard liposuction procedures except that the superficial subcutaneous tissues may initially feel somewhat stiffer because of the large volume of injectate.

Results

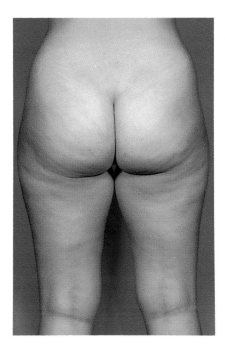 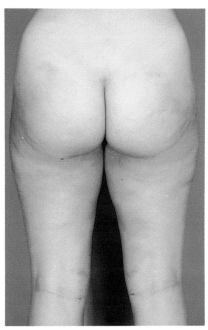 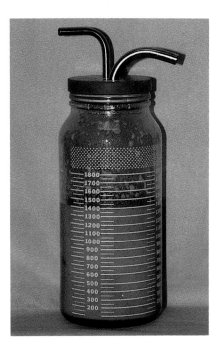

This 19-year-old woman is shown before and 3 days after liposuction of 2000 cc from her thighs, buttocks, and knees using the tumescent technique. There is almost no bruising in the postoperative view. Because swelling is also decreased when the tumescent technique is used, some improvement in contour is already evident. The fullness at the top of the medial thighs is the result of swelling above the top of the compressive garment. The aspirate is shown on the right.

SUPERFICIAL SUCTION

Liposuction was originally performed with cannulas 10 mm in diameter[6] and larger.[8,18] Early practitioners emphasized keeping the cannulas in the deep fat since removal of fat close to the skin resulted in unsightly surface irregularities. The advent of more efficient multiport cannulas (see pp. 32-36) permitted use of instruments as small as 1.5 mm in diameter. Cannulas 2 to 3 mm in diameter allow the surgeon to work closer to the undersurface of the skin without creating noticeable irregularities[19] and permit liposuction of areas of sparse fat deposit such as the calves and ankles.

Even with the use of fine cannulas, however, liposuction of areas containing minimal amounts of fat is technically challenging. Treatment of single or multiple small surface irregularities, as seen in secondary procedures or in patients being treated for cellulite, is also problematic. The surgeon sometimes has to suction minute amounts of fat from areas surrounding a depression to create a smooth effect. The goal is to reduce contour without creating irregularities. The margin for error is small because of the small size of the fat deposit, and inexpert treatment can exacerbate rather than ameliorate the condition for which treatment was sought. The tumescent technique combined with the use of fine cannulas is an important technical aid in performing superficial liposuction.

Operative Technique

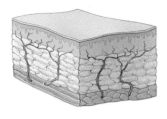 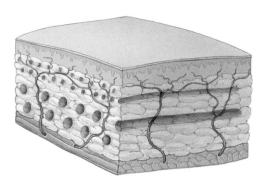

Injection of large volumes of solution into the fatty space expands the volume of the fat compartment and temporarily converts small fat compartments into large ones. The practical effect is that fine cannulas can be moved more easily in the expanded compartment. Moreover, instead of having to work directly adjacent to the dermal layer, the surgeon can place the fine cannulas at a slightly deeper level but still close to the skin surface. Expansion of the fat compartment increases the margin of safety and reduces the likelihood of creating surface irregularities.

Results

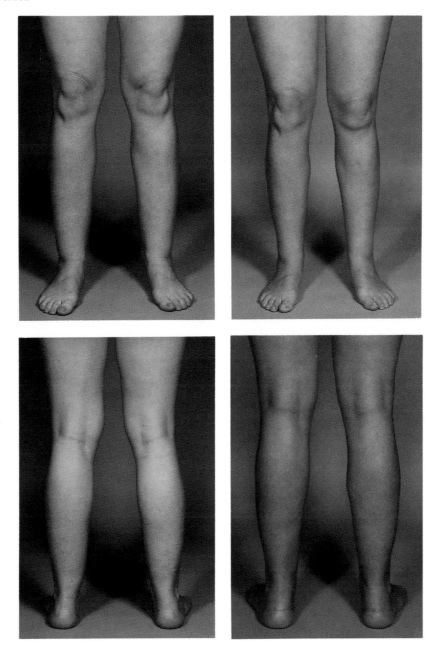

The calves and ankles have a narrow fat compartment that allows little margin for error. Treatment of this area can easily result in surface irregularities despite the use of fine cannulas. Expansion of the fat compartment by injecting large volumes of infiltrate into the knees, calves, and ankles of this 30-year-old woman permitted removal of a relatively small amount of fat without creating irregularities. She is shown before and 6 months after liposuction of 300 cc from each calf and ankle. Approximately 400 ml of dilute lidocaine with epinephrine was injected into each lower extremity before beginning suction. A 3.0 mm Mercedes Type cannula was used.

Syringe Suction

In 1985 Pierre Fournier[4] began to use a syringe for liposuction. Others adopted his techniques, at first only to harvest small amounts of fat for grafting or to treat limited areas. A few surgeons abandoned mechanical aspirators altogether and performed even large-volume liposuction with syringes.[1,4] The recent interest in syringes has prompted manufacturers to produce a wide range of new instrumentation. Videotapes are available to demonstrate the technique.[20,21]

Syringe liposuction is performed by manually creating a vacuum with a syringe. A wide-neck Toomey syringe is inserted into the tight-fitting proximal end of a specially designed cannula. The cannula is introduced beneath the surface of the skin, and the plunger of the syringe is pulled back to produce a vacuum. The vacuum is not strong enough to create vapor pressure (see pp. 37-38) but will, nevertheless, draw fat into the syringe as the cannula is thrust back and forth.

The syringe system has several advantages. The surgeon is not tethered by tubing leading from the cannula handle to the aspirator. Since there is no suction pump, the operating room is quiet. There is no aerosolization of either tissue or oil from an oil-lubricated machine. Small volumes are easily measured with increased accuracy. Finally, syringe suction is relatively inexpensive since it can be used without a suction pump. If the surgeon eventually purchases a suction pump, investment in the syringe system is not wasted since adapters permit the syringes to be attached to suction machines.

The syringe system is also said to minimize blood loss, but efficient use of the syringe system requires injection of large volumes of dilute epinephrine solution into the fat prior to suction (tumescent technique). Reduction in bleeding is attributable to the injection rather than any inherent advantage of the syringe.

A major convenience of syringe systems is that fat can be reinjected with ease. The fat is transferred from one syringe to another through available connecting devices and can be quickly rinsed of blood and oil. Since the same syringes that collect fat can inject fat, reinjection becomes very efficient. Although the syringe system facilitates fat transfer, unfortunately there is no evidence that it improves efficacy. Most grafted fat is resorbed (see pp. 460-464), and fat reinjection remains an unpredictable technique.

The syringe system has two disadvantages. It is slower than using a vacuum pump so that operations with the syringe take one-third to one-half again as long as operations using an aspirator. The syringe system is also labor intensive, requiring the full-time attention of an assistant to repeatedly empty, clean, and prepare the syringe-cannulas for use.

Equipment

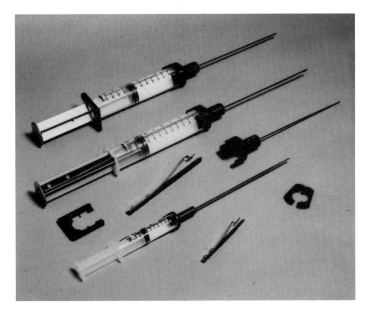

Toomey syringes come in 10 and 60 ml sizes with wide necks that can be fitted to specially designed cannulas. To relieve the surgeon of the physical effort of constantly pulling back on the barrel to maintain the vacuum, a locking device is fitted to the hub of the barrel and used to fix the plunger in the withdrawn position.

ASPIRATION TECHNIQUE

The cannula attached to a syringe is inserted into the subcutaneous tissue through an access incision.

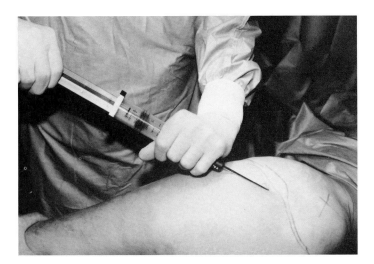

The surgeon pulls back on the plunger as far as possible to create a vacuum within the syringe.

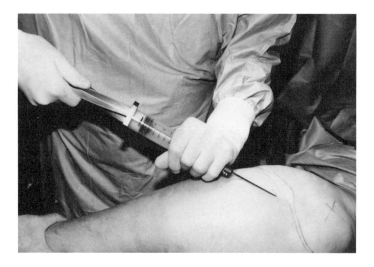

Twisting the plunger locks it into position. The vacuum is maintained as long as the cannula remains in the tissues.

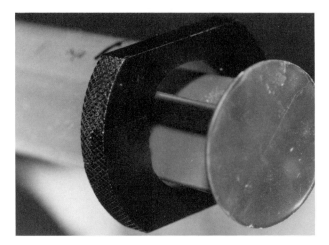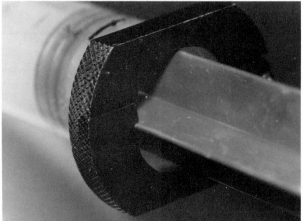

A close-up view of the barrel of the cannula and locking device is shown on the left. The barrel has been twisted and is locked into position on the right.

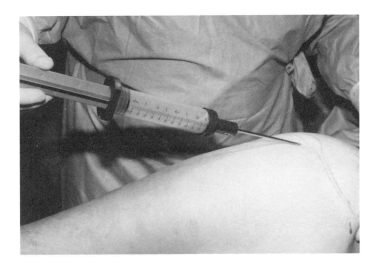

The cannula is then thrust back and forth through the tissues, and the syringe fills with aspirate. In patients with large fat compartments the fat flows quite readily into the syringe. In patients with smaller fat compartments or when aspirating from more fibrous areas, fat does not flow readily into the syringe unless the tissues have been overdistended with local anesthetic (tumescent technique).

Several technical features of this method are important to maximize efficiency. The syringe should remain attached to the cannula throughout the procedure. When the surgeon has filled the syringe with fat, he hands the assembled syringe and cannula to the assistant, who gives the surgeon another empty syringe with cannula attached. The surgeon then reinserts the cannula into the subcutaneous fat and repeats the process. While the surgeon is aspirating with the second syringe, the assistant expels the fat from the first syringe and readies it for reuse. A small amount of saline or lactated Ringer's solution should always be in the syringe when the assistant hands it to the surgeon so that the vacuum will be maintained. The assistant ejects the fat from the syringe without detaching the cannula. Detaching and reattaching the cannula is time consuming and messy. A basin of saline or lactated Ringer's solution should be used to rinse out the cannula and syringe each time. With some rehearsal and practice, the surgeon and assistant can work in smooth coordination. Nevertheless, the technique is labor intensive.

Results

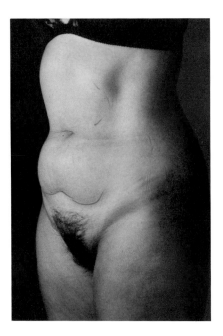 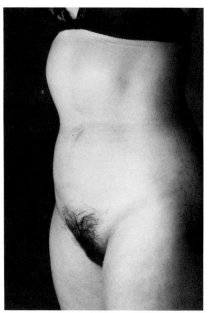

A 46-year-old woman is shown before and 6 months after removal of 400 cc of anterior abdominal fat using syringe aspiration. Results are satisfactory but not significantly different from results in other patients when a mechanical suction pump was used (see pp. 250-256).

FAT TRANSFER TECHNIQUE

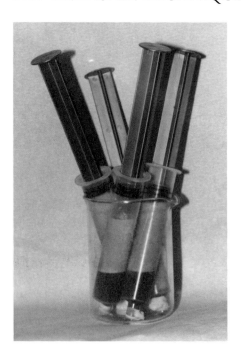

After the fat has been drawn into the Toomey syringe, the syringe is placed upright and the fat allowed to layer out. The excess fluid is then ejected from the syringe, and the fat can be reinjected with the same cannulas used for harvesting or transferred to smaller syringes and cannulas to use on the face.

Although occasional patients will have long-lasting isolated contour improvement, injection of fat has not resulted in generalized smoothing of the surface of the skin. See pp. 460-464 for further discussion of fat grafting.

TREATMENT OF CELLULITE

The term "cellulite" originated in nineteenth-century French medical literature.[22] It refers to a generalized and irregular pattern of fine and sometimes coarse irregularities usually occurring on the skin of the buttock and thigh, but also seen in the abdomen, nape of the neck, and upper arms. A defining characteristic is the "mattress phenomenon,"[22] a surface motif of alternating discoid protrusions and linear depressions. The protrusions are filled with fat. All women and some men will develop cellulite with age. In those with a genetic predisposition or in the obese, cellulite may occur before the third decade of life.

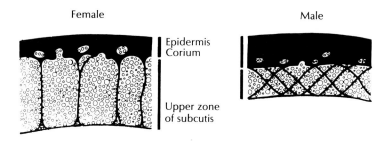

Nürnberger and Müller[23] biopsied the subcutaneous fat of the thighs and found two patterns of fascial architecture in the subdermis. In women, vertically oriented fascial bands divide the superficial fat into small cuboid compartments or "standing fat-cell chambers" averaging 0.5 × 1.5 cm in cross section. The fascial bands (retinacula cutis) anchor the dermis to the deeper fascia. Small protrusions from the fat-cell chambers (papillae adiposae) project into the dermis. In men the subdermal fat layer is thinner, and the fascial architecture is composed of a lattice-like network of crisscrossing connective tissue that creates multiple small polygonal units of fat instead of the cuboidal fat chambers seen in women. The dermal layer is thicker in men.

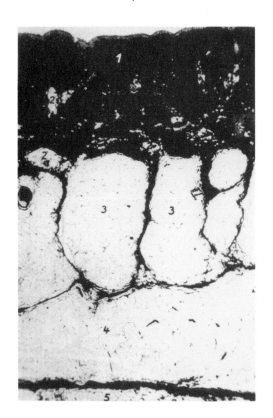

Nürnberger and Müller[23] also divided the subcutaneous fat into three layers. The most superficial layer *(3)* lies just beneath the skin *(1)* and corresponds to the standing fat-cell chambers above. Papillae adiposa *(2)* protrude from the superficial layer of fat into the undersurface of the dermis. The second layer *(4)* lies just deep to the standing fat-cell chambers but is superficial to the deep layer of subcutaneous fat *(5)*.

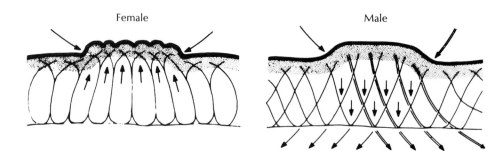

According to Nürnberger and Müller, the discrete vertical anchoring of fascia into the dermis in women as well as hypertrophy of the papillae adiposa are responsible for the expression of cellulite in the skin of women. Cellulite does not normally occur in men because of the more diffuse attachments of the superficial fascia to the dermis. The thicker skin of men is also less likely to show irregularities secondary to underlying fascial attachments. The pinch test in women (left) produces fine deformation and pitting of the skin while the pinch test in men (right) creates larger folds and furrows.

Cellulite results from tethering of the skin to the underlying fascial framework by the retinacula cutis in combination with hypertrophy of fat. The tethering fascial bands are responsible for the alternating areas of depression and protrusion.

Although cellulite is a demonstrably normal anatomic finding,[22-24] most women consider it an unsightly affliction, and there is a long history of attempts to treat the condition with a wide variety of techniques, including topical agents, enzymes injected into the subcutaneous tissues, suppositories, electrical stimulation, massage, and diathermy.[22] The profusion of therapies attests to their inefficacy.

It was recognized early on that liposuction had little if any beneficial effect on the quality of the skin surface; in fact, the best results were obtained in patients with smooth, tight skin prior to surgery.[7] Nevertheless, our increasing ability to work close to the surface of the skin with fine cannulas, an interest in selective surgical division of restraining fascial bands, and a renewed attention to and facility in fat grafting all combined to focus interest on surgical therapy for cellulite.[1,3,5]

Theoretically, releasing fascial bands should ameliorate cellulite by permitting the depressed areas to elevate to the level of the surrounding raised areas. Simultaneous removal of some of the fat from the protruding areas should also contribute to a smoother effect. Obviously, a combination of both modalities could be used. These thoughts form the theoretical basis for recent attempts to treat cellulite.[1-5]

Markings

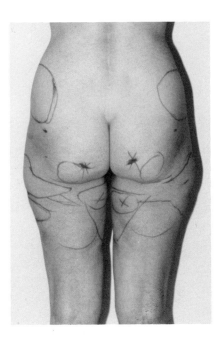

The patient is marked in the standing position. Individual depressed areas requiring surgical release are marked on the lower medial buttocks in this patient. Use of a strong side light during marking is helpful to emphasize fine skin irregularities.

Operative Technique

Treatment of cellulite combines elements of the tumescent technique and superficial suction. The area to be treated is infiltrated with large volumes of dilute lidocaine with epinephrine to distend the tissues. Tethered areas will remain relatively flat or depressed, whereas areas of fat protrusion are more easily expanded and will be emphasized. In any case, the tethered areas will have been marked preoperatively.

Fine Cannula Suction

Ten minutes after infiltration areas containing excess fat are aspirated. The deep fat is treated first, after which the superficial layers are suctioned with fine cannulas (2 to 3 mm in diameter). The superficial aspiration of necessity breaks some of the tethering bands.

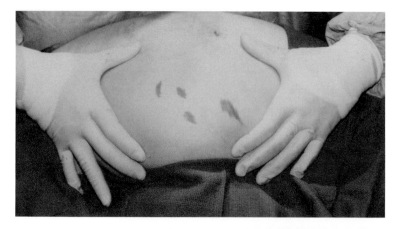

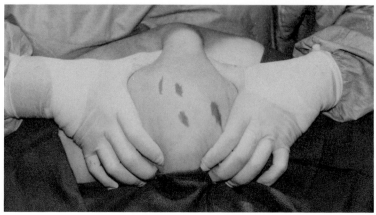

Gently pressing the skin between the hands mimics the effect of gravity and emphasizes the contrast between depressed and protuberant areas.

Cutting Constricting Bands

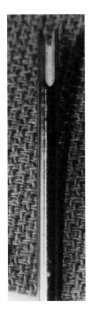

A specially designed instrument that has a distal end consisting of a sharpened concave edge is used by some to release constricting bands. This instrument is inserted through the access incision and directed to areas where the skin is tethered to the fascia. When a band is encountered, the tip of the instrument meets resistance. Pulling up on the surface of the skin with one hand while carefully advancing the instrument close to the skin undersurface severs the constricting band(s).

Fat Injection

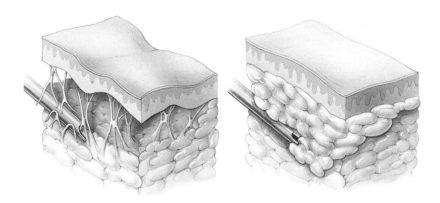

Several authors have suggested that if sharp lysis of tethering bands is followed by injection of fat into the areas of depression, adhesions and recurrence of depressions are less likely.[1-5]

In my personal experience, use of sharpened cellulite lysing instruments and injection of fat into the subcutaneous space *have not improved results beyond those achieved with superficial suction and the tumescent technique.*

Results

These patients range in age from 25 to 60 years. Preoperative skin texture varies from smooth and tight with minimal irregularities to generalized alternating protrusions and depressions with and without laxity.

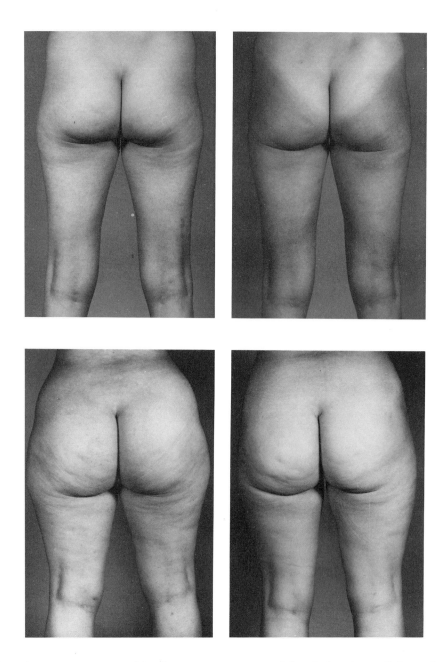

All patients were treated in the same manner. After injection of the subcutaneous space with large volumes of dilute lidocaine with epinephrine, varying amounts of fat were aspirated at deep and superficial levels. Small-diameter cannulas (maximum 3.7 mm) were used in the superficial levels. No patient underwent sharp division of constricting bands, and fat was not reinjected. Some patients were treated more than once.

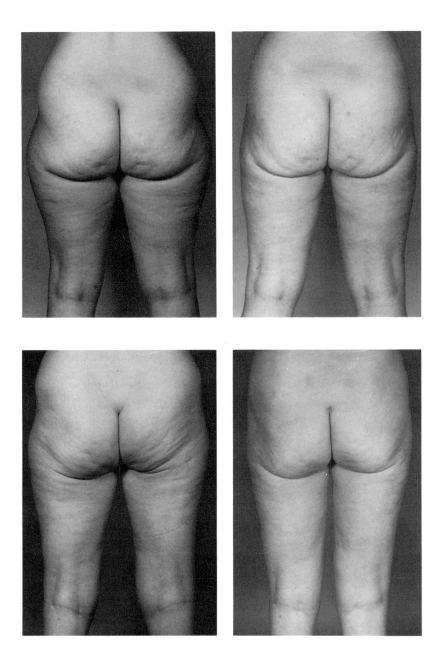

The postoperative photographs were taken at least 6 months after the last surgery. Although the photographer took great care to keep pre- and post-operative photographic conditions identical, there are subtle changes in light and exposure. Nevertheless, most patients demonstrate a contour change *plus* an overall smoothing of the skin. I believe the smoothing of the skin results from fine-cannula fat removal in the superficial plane.

REFERENCES

1. Toledo LS. Syringe liposculpture: A 2-year experience. Aesthetic Plast Surg 15:321-326, 1991.
2. Grazer FM. Atlas of Suction Assisted Lipectomy in Body Contouring. New York: Churchill Livingstone, 1992, pp 217-218, 400-401.
3. Grazer FM. Cellulite lysing. Aesthetic Surg 11:11, 1991.
4. Fournier PF. Liposculpture: The Syringe Technique. Paris: Arnette, 1991.
5. Gasprotti M. Superficial liposuction: A new application of the technique for aged and flaccid skin. Aesthetic Plast Surg 16:141-153, 1992.
6. Illouz Y-G. Body contouring by lipolysis: A 5-year experience with over 3,000 cases. Plast Reconstr Surg 72:591-597, 1983.
7. Fournier PF, Otteni F. Lipodissection in body sculpturing: The dry procedure. Plast Reconstr Surg 72:598-609, 1983.
8. Teimourian B, Fisher JB. Suction curettage to remove excess fat for body contouring. Plast Reconstr Surg 68:50-58, 1981.
9. Hetter GP. The effect of low-dose epinephrine on the hematocrit drop following lipolysis. Aesthetic Plast Surg 8:19-21, 1984.
10. Pitman GH, Holzer J. Safe suction: Fluid replacement and blood loss parameters. Perspect Plast Surg 5(1):79-89, 1991.
11. Pitman GH. Discussion of Courtiss EH, Choucair RJ, Donelan MB. Large-volume suction lipectomy: An analysis of 108 patients. Plast Reconstr Surg 89:1080-1082, 1992.
12. Courtiss EH, Kanter MA, Kanter WR, Ransil BJ. The effect of epinephrine on blood loss during suction lipectomy. Plast Reconstr Surg 88:801-803, 1992.
13. Klein JA. The tumescent technique for liposuction surgery. Am J Cosmetic Surg 4:263-267, 1987.
14. Klein JA. Tumescent technique permits lidocaine doses of 35 mg/kg for liposuction: Peak plasma lidocaine levels are diminished and delayed 12 hr. J Dermatol Surg Oncol 16:248-263, 1990.
15. Klein JA. The tumescent technique: Anesthesia and modified liposuction technique. Dermatol Clin 8:425-437, 1990.
16. McKay W, Morris R, Mushlin P. Sodium bicarbonate attenuates pain on skin infiltration with lidocaine with or without epinephrine. Anesth Analg 66:572-574, 1987.
17. Lewis CM, Hepper T. The use of high dose lidocaine in wetting solutions for lipoplasty. Aesthetic Plast Surg 22:307-309, 1989.
18. Kesselring UK, Meyer R. A suction curette for removal of excessive local deposits of subcutaneous fat. Plast Reconstr Surg 62:305-306, 1978.
19. Pitman GH. Suction lipectomy of the face and body: Precision and refinement. In Riley WB Jr, ed. Plastic Surgery Educational Foundation Instructional Courses, vol 1. St. Louis: CV Mosby, 1988, pp 71-106.
20. The Tulip technique. Videotape from The Tulip Company, San Diego, Calif., 1991.
21. Wells-Johnson videotape, Phoenix, Ariz., 1991.
22. Scherwitz S, Braun-Fazco O. So-called cellulite. J Dermatol Surg Oncol 4:230-234, 1978.
23. Nürnberger F, Müller SG. So-called cellulite: An invented disease. J Dermatol Surg Oncol 4:221-229, 1978.
24. Rose EH, Vistnes LM, Ksander GA. A microarchitectural model of regional variations in hypodermal mobility in porcine and human skin. Ann Plast Surg 1:252-266, 1978.

Part II

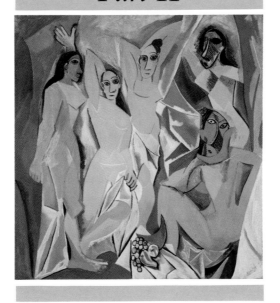

OPERATIONS BY ANATOMIC AREA

Chapter 6

FACE AND NECK

Liposuction offers singular benefits for face and neck contouring. In the younger patient, it can be used as a single modality or combined with an open surgical approach through limited incisions to remove deep fat and modify the platysma. In the older patient, liposuction can be used as an adjunct to face and neck lift to extract submental fat through minimal incisions, facilitate smooth and efficient removal of lateral cervical and facial fat, and expedite treatment of prominent nasolabial folds.

HISTORY

As early as 1932 Maliniac[1] emphasized the relationship of fat to facial appearance. He identified "emaciation of the subcutaneous fat" as an "important" sign of aging yet pointed out that excessive fat in the cheeks would limit face-lift results. Padgett and Stephenson[2] and Davis[3] also stressed the importance of fat removal in face and neck lift.

The fatty double chin, in particular, attracted the attention of plastic surgeons, and many advocated direct excision of submental fat and skin through a variety of incisions in the anterior cervical area.[1,4-9] All skin excision, however, resulted in significant scarring.

In two important articles Millard, Pigott, and Hedo[10] and Millard et al.[11] demonstrated that extensive removal of cervical fat could dramatically improve face-lift results. They used a submental incision to excise fat under direct vision. Submandibular and more lateral fat was removed through lateral periauricular incisions. Direct removal of anterior cervical skin was eschewed since the extra skin served to fill in the submental hollow and anterior cervical skin excision left unacceptable scars.

Fat removal in the neck was subsequently reported by many authors as a critical ingredient in achieving superior face-lift results.[12-30] Most surgeons lifted a flap of skin with a thin layer of subcutaneous fat attached and then removed fat from the underlying platysma. Lemmon[21] and Lemmon and Hamra,[22] however, made their initial plane of dissection just superficial to the platysma, lifting a thick flap of cervical skin with all subcutaneous fat attached and then excising fat from the undersurface of the flap. Several authors recommended removal of subplatysmal fat, usually in conjunction with medial platysma plication.[17,26,28,31-33]

Davis,[34] Davis and Cinflone,[35] and Cardoso de Castro[36] emphasized the desirability of creating an oval face by removing fat from the lower cheeks, mandibular area, and jowls. Excision of fat from the cheeks and jowls was also advocated by others.[12,14,15,32,34,35,37-39]

Although fat removal usually involved surgical rejuvenation of the aging face, it soon became apparent that surgical fat reduction could also benefit younger patients.[10,17,26,28,33,38,40-44] Connell and Gaon[17] went so far as to create full face-lift flaps in a young woman to gain exposure to the lateral neck. After defatting the neck, they sutured the flaps back without excising skin, an unorthodox approach demonstrating the unequivocal importance they attached to fat sculpting.

Once the safety and efficacy of liposuction on the body was demonstrated, it was inevitable that this modality would be applied to the face and neck. In his first publication in the English literature Illouz[45] reported that the face and neck were treated in 4% of his liposuction patients. Fournier and Otteni[46] also described liposuction of these areas. In 1983 Teimourian[47] reported a series of 46 patients on whom he used adjunctive liposuction for face and neck lifts. Other surgeons also described favorable results using adjunctive liposuction in rhytidectomy.[48-53] Liposuction of the neck through limited incisions, with or without platysma plication, was also reported.[50,51,54,55]

An increased interest and facility in removing superficial face and neck fat also stimulated a renewed interest in buccal fat pad excision. Most authors used an intraoral approach,[55-60] but removal through a face-lift incision was also advocated.[30,61,62]

AESTHETIC AND ANATOMIC CONSIDERATIONS

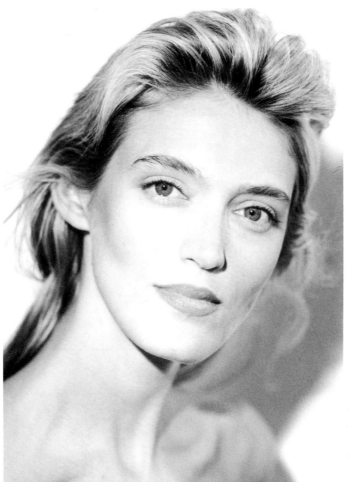

Photo by Richard Imrie

Facial contour in healthy young adults gracefully reflects the underlying musculoskeletal framework. The malar eminences and overlying soft tissue mass give strength and emphasis to the midlateral face, whereas the lower face is defined by the shape and prominence of the mandible, which also delineates the border between the lateral face and neck.

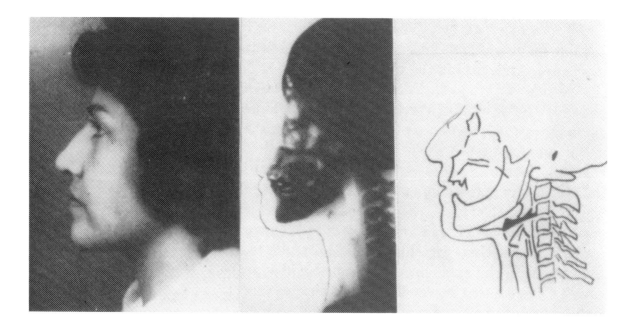

A high, posteriorly placed hyoid provides a sharp, clean neckline. Marino, Galeano, and Gondolfo[63] first described the importance of hyoid positioning in determining submental contour. With the face in neutral position, the hyoid should be no lower than the mentum to produce a 90-degree cervicomental angle. Neck and facial muscles also add fullness, particularly in those who have well-developed masseters or bulky cervical strap muscles.

More than any other soft tissue parameter, the volume and disposition of fat determine cervicofacial contour. Fat is found in both superficial and deep locations.

Superficial Fat

The superficial fat lies between the skin and the subjacent platysma–subcutaneous musculoaponeurotic system (SMAS). The superficial fat may be particularly abundant in the neck, especially in the submental area. In the face the superficial fat is evenly distributed and is usually less than 5 mm thick. The fat is traversed by multiple small neurovascular bundles that provide blood supply and sensibility to the skin. No major blood vessels or motor nerves cross the superficial fat.

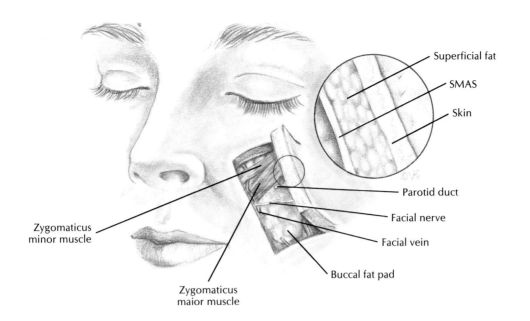

Superficial fat

SMAS

Skin

Zygomaticus
minor muscle

Parotid duct

Facial nerve

Facial vein

Buccal fat pad

Zygomaticus
maior muscle

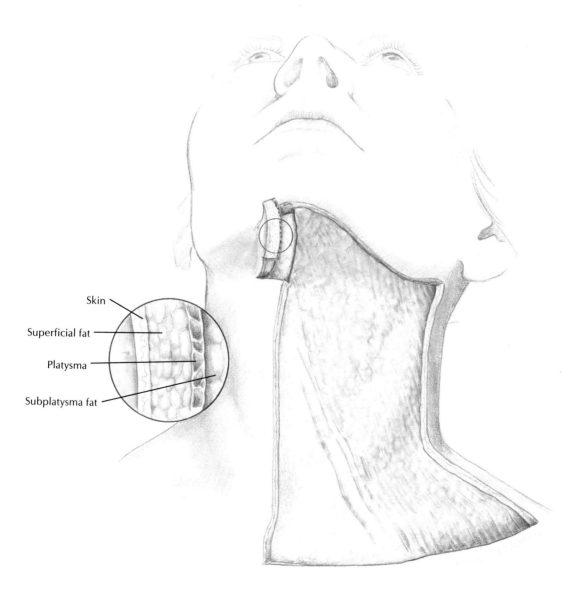

Skin

Superficial fat

Platysma

Subplatysma fat

Deep Fat
Neck

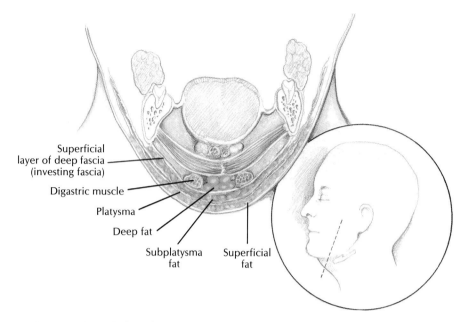

Superficial
layer of deep fascia
(investing fascia)

Digastric muscle

Platysma

Deep fat

Subplatysma
fat

Superficial
fat

A coronal section through the submental region shows subcutaneous fat superficial to the platysma (light yellow) and subplatysmal fat (dark yellow), which is both superficial and deep to the investing fascia.

Considerable amounts of fat may lie between the platysma and the superficial layer of the deep cervical fascia (investing fascia). This fat is usually most prominent in the submental area and is superficial to the anterior bellies of the paired digastric muscles. Fat also lies between the digastric muscles deep to the superficial layer of investing fascia. This deeper fat should not be disturbed since its removal will create an undesirable submental hollow. Additional subplatysmal fat may exist more laterally in the submandibular area, although fat here is usually not as abundant as in the submentum.

The submental vein runs just beneath the medial platysma. No other important structures lie in the medial subplatysmal fat, but the marginal mandibular and cervical branches of the facial nerve are found laterally, as are the submandibular gland and other structures of the suprahyoid triangle. The medial subplatysmal fat can be suctioned or removed under direct vision. More lateral subplatysmal fat can be suctioned, but the cannula should be directed away from the area directly adjacent to the mandible to avoid injury to the marginal mandibular nerve.

Face

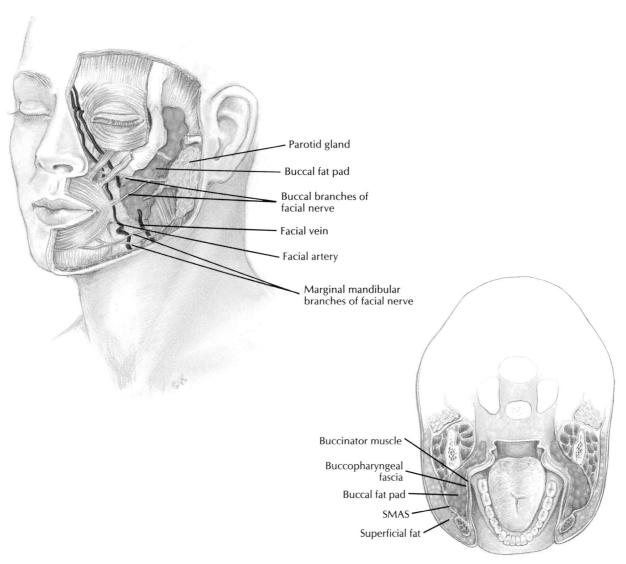

Parotid gland

Buccal fat pad

Buccal branches of facial nerve

Facial vein

Facial artery

Marginal mandibular branches of facial nerve

Buccinator muscle

Buccopharyngeal fascia

Buccal fat pad

SMAS

Superficial fat

The deep facial fat consists largely of the buccal fat pad.[64] This discrete collection of fat extends anteriorly from behind the mandibular ramus into the cheek in the space deep to the SMAS and superficial to the bucco-pharyngeal fascia and the immediately subjacent buccinator muscle and buccal mucosa. The buccal branches of the facial nerve course over its superficial aspect, supplying the muscles of facial expression. The sensory buccal nerve branches of the fifth cranial nerve run deep, supplying the oral mucosa. The facial vein runs through the anterior portion of the fat pad, and the terminal portion of the parotid duct passes through it en route to the oral cavity.

A very full buccal fat pad gives a rounded appearance to the cheek, particularly its lower half. A leaner fat pad leaves a hollow beneath the malar eminence, emphasizing the so-called high cheek bones many women and men desire as a becoming facial attribute.

Nasolabial Fold

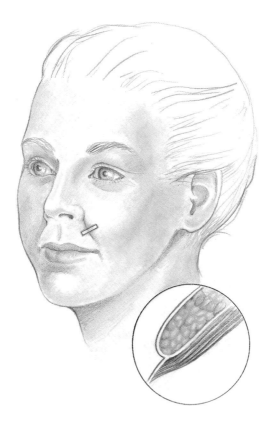

The nasolabial crease is formed by the insertion of muscle fibers into the skin and is a normal landmark even in the youthful face. The nasolabial fold, lateral to the crease, is formed largely of redundant skin and underlying fat.[65-71] Although a slight fullness in this area is normal, a large hanging fold accentuates the crease and is considered an undesirable sign of age. Conversely, complete obliteration of the nasolabial fold and/or crease gives a flat, expressionless look to the face and carries the stigma of "one face lift too many."

PATIENT TYPES AND TREATMENT OPTIONS
Neck

Younger patients with relatively tight skin and minimal to moderate volumes of excess cervical fat are best treated by liposuction of the neck. The ideal patient will meet the following criteria: less than 40 years old; tight, elastic cervical skin; and cervical fat volume of less than 100 cc.

Patients who do not meet these requirements may also benefit from liposuction alone, but results will begin to deteriorate as the criteria are expanded.

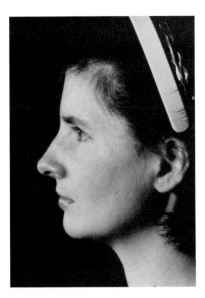 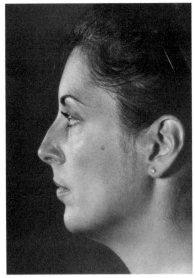 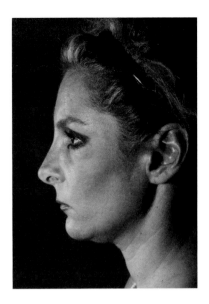

These three young women all have small amounts of excess submental fat and tight skin. Although the patient on the right is over 40 years of age, she meets the other criteria so well that she is still an excellent candidate for liposuction.

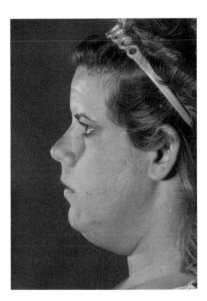 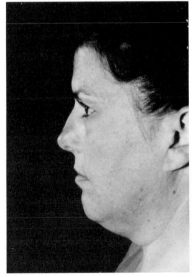

Both of these women have large volumes of fat in the submental area. Despite their relative youth (32 and 38 years old), it is unlikely that their stretched-out cervical skin will shrink enough to conform to the reduced volumes created by liposuction. Some residual laxity must be expected.

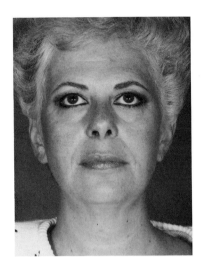 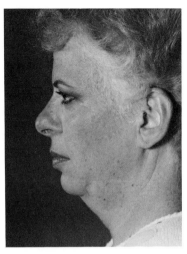

This 47-year-old woman fails to meet any of the criteria for successful liposuction. She is over 40, she has a large volume of excess fat, and her skin is lax.

Patients in early middle life may still benefit from neck liposuction without face lift, but they usually require ancillary procedures in the anterior neck to obtain satisfactory results. These additional procedures may include (1) direct removal of subplatysmal fat, (2) tightening of the anterior platysma, and (3) wide undermining and redraping of the cervical skin.

Men, because of their thicker skin and more prominent musculature, frequently require platysma plication and extensive skin undermining to obtain maximal results without a face lift.[55] In fact, rarely can outstanding results be obtained in men with liposuction alone.

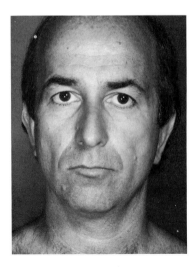 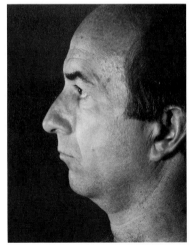

This 48-year-old man requested liposuction to improve the appearance of his neck. Although slight excess fat and relatively good skin elasticity for his age made him a candidate for liposuction, hypogenia and a low hyoid precluded creation of a 90-degree cervicomental angle. As with most men, thick skin and muscular bulk also limit the amount of refinement.

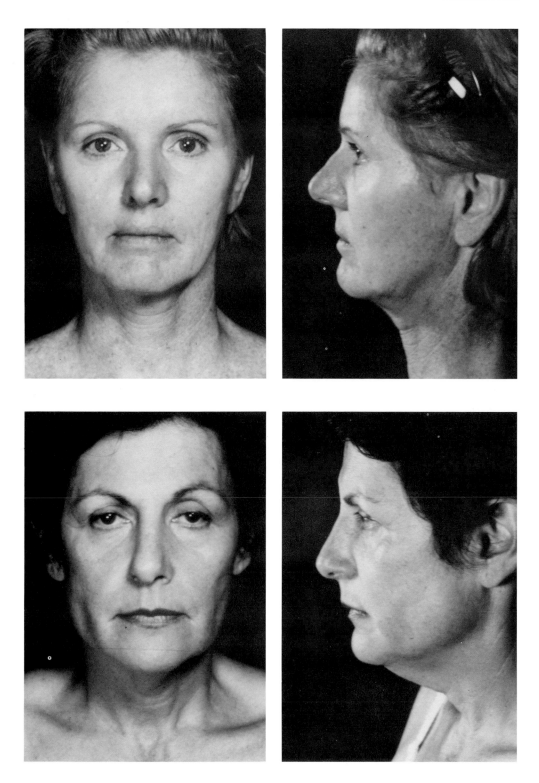

When excess fat in the neck is accompanied by lax wrinkled skin or aging changes extend to the face, face and neck lift are required to effect a satisfying change. Adjunctive liposuction of the neck can facilitate the operation and obviate the need for a direct open approach to the anterior neck for fat removal.

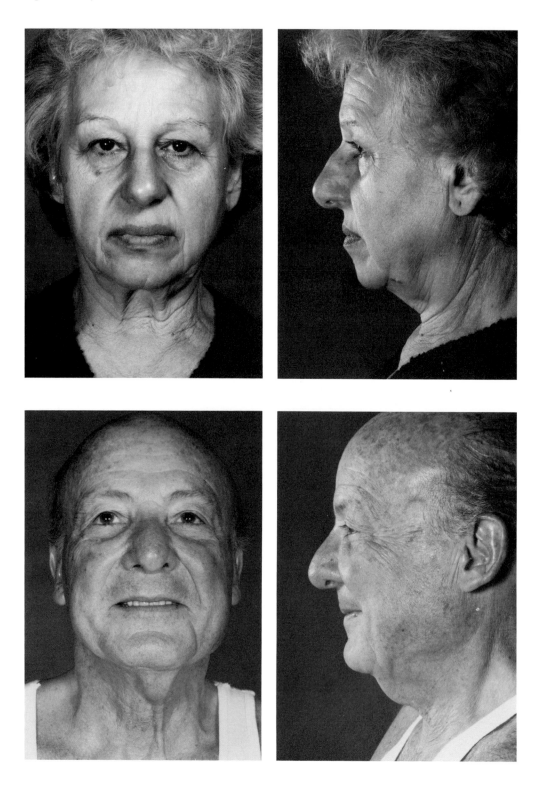

When platysmal bands stretch from the upper neck to below the thyroid cartilage or large amounts of fat are deep to the platysma, creation of a clean, sharp cervicomental angle mandates face and neck lift with an approach to the anterior platysma through a 4 cm incision in the submental crease. Treatment of platysmal bands and/or excision of deep fat is performed under direct vision.

Face

Fat removal in the face should be approached with caution. An oval-shaped face with strong malar eminences is desirable and may be achieved in some patients by liposuction of the lower third of the face. The surgeon should bear in mind, however, that a round, full face is a sign of youth and good health, whereas a thin, drawn face is associated with illness or aging. Liposuction of the face and buccal fat pad excision should be reserved for those patients who clearly have excess and superfluous fat.

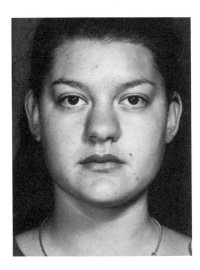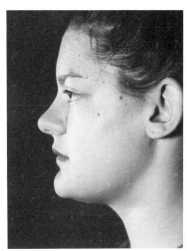

This 17-year-old patient has a full face. Although fat removal would reduce contour, the fullness of her other facial features makes thin cheeks inappropriate.

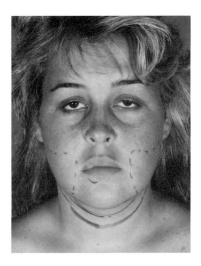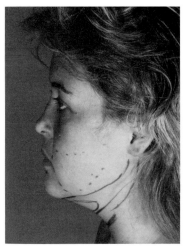

On the other hand, this 28-year-old, moderately overweight woman has full cheeks and relatively fine facial features. She is a more suitable candidate for facial fat contouring and is shown with face and neck markings prior to surgery.

Full cheeks can be treated with liposuction or buccal fat pad excision at the time of face lift. Liposuction is also useful in conjunction with face lift for ameliorating heavy nasolabial folds and jowls.

In evaluating patients for facial fat contouring, the surgeon should also consider skeletal contouring options such as malar augmentation, chin augmentation, and genioplasty.

PATIENT EVALUATION AND COUNSELING
Physical Examination

Overall skin condition is noted with attention directed to laxity and hanging folds of skin, particularly along the mandible (jowls), in the nasolabial fold area, and in the neck.

Although a single cadaver study found submental fat volumes to be 15 to 27 cc[4] and clinical studies of fat removed by liposuction have reported volumes of 10 to 100 cc,[51,68] I have removed as much as 200 cc from patients with very fat necks.

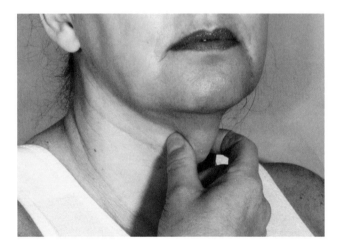

A pinch test should demonstrate a 2 cm thickness of subcutaneous cervical fat prior to neck liposuction. It is sometimes difficult on physical examination to differentiate supraplatysmal and subplatysmal fat. If the surgeon gently pinches the submental soft tissues and then asks the patient to forcefully stick out her tongue, the tongue thrusting will contract the platysma and force deep fat in an upward direction. This maneuver is helpful but not foolproof. A search for anterior platysmal bands should be made, although large fat deposits may obscure a lax platysma. The bulk and thickness of the deep neck musculature should be assessed carefully, particularly in men.

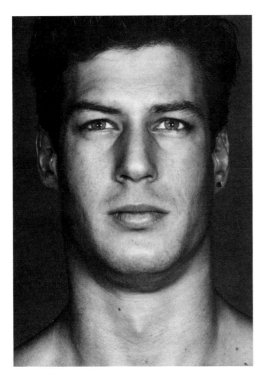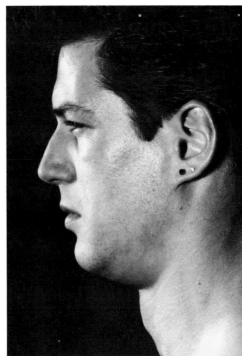

This professional male model sought liposuction to thin his neck and create a more pronounced cervicomandibular definition. The fatty layer was sparse. Neck fullness was caused by muscle bulk, and liposuction did nothing to improve appearance.

The hyoid should also be palpated. If it lies below the level of the mentum or is very anterior, an acute cervicomental angle is impossible to achieve.[73]

Excessive subcutaneous fat volume in the face can be seen as overly full cheeks. Bimanual palpation with one finger in the mouth and another on the skin surface sometimes permits evaluation of the buccal fat pad, but fullness secondary to subcutaneous fat or to the buccal fat pad generally cannot be distinguished. Pinching the nasolabial folds will help differentiate lax skin from significant fat.

Defining Patient Goals

Patients seek the idealized face and neck of youthful movie stars and fashion models. Younger patients are frequently looking for a "type change." They want to transform round, full faces and heavy necks to thinner, more angular visages. They want to "look different." Older patients more frequently want their youthful appearance restored. They don't want to look different; they want to look younger.

The goals of younger and older patients are mirrored in differences in physical attributes as well as differences in the surgeon's approach to evaluation and treatment. Younger patients' needs can frequently be met by fat volume reduction. Older patients may come to the office requesting liposuction as treatment for a sagging, fat neck. They have seen or heard in the media that liposuction is safer, simpler, easier, and less costly than a face lift. Older patients, however, almost always require operations that tighten the skin and musculofascia.

By no means the least consideration is simply what operation the patient is willing to accept. Although a face lift may provide the optimal result, some patients may not be willing to undergo the procedure. In fact, they may be entirely satisfied with the limited result achieved by a simpler procedure. The surgeon, on the other hand, is reluctant to proceed when he knows the result will be suboptimal. It requires considerable time and skill for the surgeon to educate patients to the differences between liposuction and lifting procedures, but it is time well spent. The choice of operation should be a joint decision by surgeon and patient. The surgeon is obligated to offer and explain alternatives but should clearly state his recommendation and not hesitate to refuse to operate if he feels the result will be inferior.

Informed Consent

The patient should be fully informed of the nature of the operation and the location and length of all incisions. The submental incision will be approximately ¼ inch in length unless it is necessary to remove subplatysmal fat or tighten the platysma, in which case it will be 3 to 4 cm. Although I tell the patient that scars are unpredictable and may hypertrophy, I also explain that these scars usually heal well and are in inconspicuous locations.

A tight, stiff, or "woody" feeling in the neck is common after surgery. Diminished sensation is usually temporary, but may last 3 months or longer. Areas of hardness and temporary irregularities, which are usually palpable but only sometimes visible, are common and last about 6 to 8 weeks. Hematomas and infections are rare, but they should be mentioned nonetheless. The patient should also be told of the possibility of injury to a branch of the facial nerve. In my experience, motor nerve injuries associated with liposuction are always temporary and usually resolve in less than a month.

LIPOSUCTION WITHOUT FACE LIFT
CERVICAL LIPOSUCTION
Markings

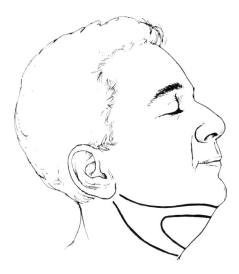

The patient is marked while standing or sitting. A line is drawn just below and parallel to the inferior border of the mandible. Another line is drawn at the lower limit of excess fat accumulation as determined visually and by the pinch test. The central submentum, which usually contains the greatest concentration of fat, is also marked. The accuracy of markings is confirmed by pinch and by a visual check for symmetry. Access incisions are placed in the submental crease and behind each earlobe.

Operative Technique

Local anesthesia with minimal or no sedation is sufficient when suction is used without full face and neck lift since the operation rarely lasts more than 20 minutes. Subcutaneous tissues are generously infiltrated with the following solution:

8.4% sodium bicarbonate	4 ml
1% lidocaine in 1:100,000 epinephrine	40 ml
Physiologic saline solution	120 ml
0.25% lidocaine with 1:400,000 epinephrine	164 ml

Ten minutes after lidocaine infiltration I visually inspect and pinch the tissues to determine the baseline appearance and feel for comparison with untreated adjacent areas.

Volumes to be removed range from 20 to 200 cc. I use a 2.4 or 3.0 mm Mercedes Type cannula. Although much has been written about whether to use a one-hole or multiport cannula and whether to have the port facing the platysma or skin, I find these arguments irrelevant. What *is* relevant is smooth resection in a systematic fashion. Checking the thickness of the skin and subcutaneous layer frequently is a must. I get consistently satisfactory results with the Mercedes Type cannula, but comparable results can be achieved with other instruments.

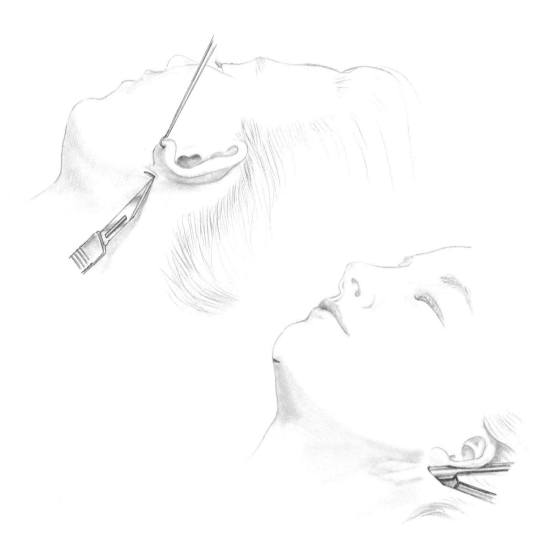

Stab incisions are made in the submental crease and behind each earlobe. Using a Stevens scissors to separate the skin from the tightly adherent sternocleidomastoid fascia helps to establish the plane of tunneling from the lateral incisions. Spreading should extend beyond the anterior border of the muscle, keeping the scissors between the skin and platysma. Establishing the correct plane at this time facilitates suctioning and decreases the probability of injuring the marginal mandibular branch of the facial nerve.

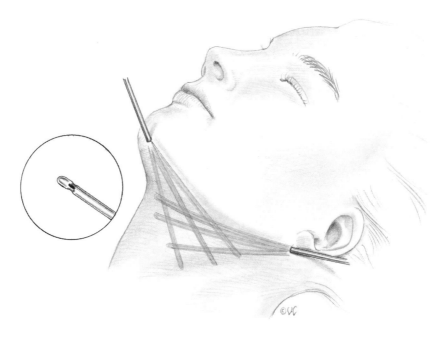

Suctioning begins through the submental incision. The entire anterior neck is treated in a systematic fashion, but more time is concentrated on the submental area since this is the region of greatest fat deposition. The cannula is kept just beneath the skin. After about half the volume to be removed has been suctioned via the submental incision, I turn the patient's head and suction from the right retrolobular crease, removing an additional 25% of fat. The cannula should reach to the midline from the lateral access incision, creating a crisscross or grid dissection. Next, I suction from the left retrolobular area, again removing about 25% of the total expected volume. I check the skin frequently for smoothness of the subcutaneous layer.

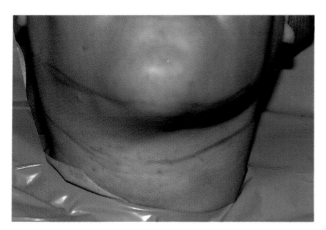 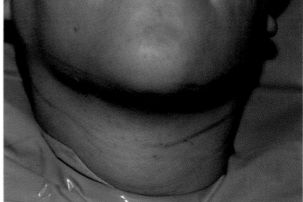

In the photograph on the left the left side of the patient's neck has been suctioned. In the photograph on the right both sides of the neck have been treated.

The end point is reached when there is a noticeable contour reduction with a uniformly smooth surface, the pinch thickness is about 1 cm, and the collection bottle holds the expected volume.

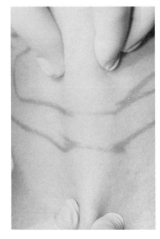

Pinch test before liposuction in submental and adjacent areas.

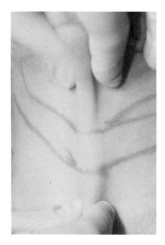

Areas are of approximately equal thickness after liposuction.

Comparison of pinch thickness with a nearby untreated area is the most important parameter, but all of the above maneuvers help in determining the end point. Courtiss[72] recommends that all connections between the platysma and subcutaneous tissues be divided with a scissors after completion of suction. I prefer to leave the fibrous connections intact unless I want to release the skin for redraping or require additional exposure for ancillary procedures. The skin retains more sensibility and heals more quickly if connections to the platysma are left intact.

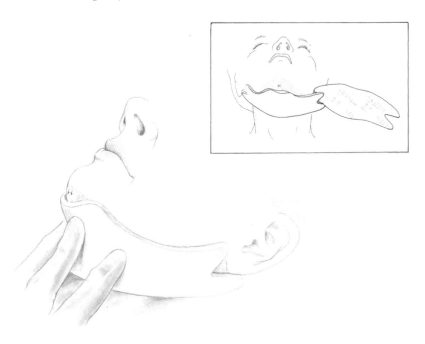

Incisions are closed with one or two absorbable sutures. A ¼-inch thick adhesive-backed foam sponge (Reston) is cut to size and placed over the anterior neck up to the ears to provide firm compression and support.

Results

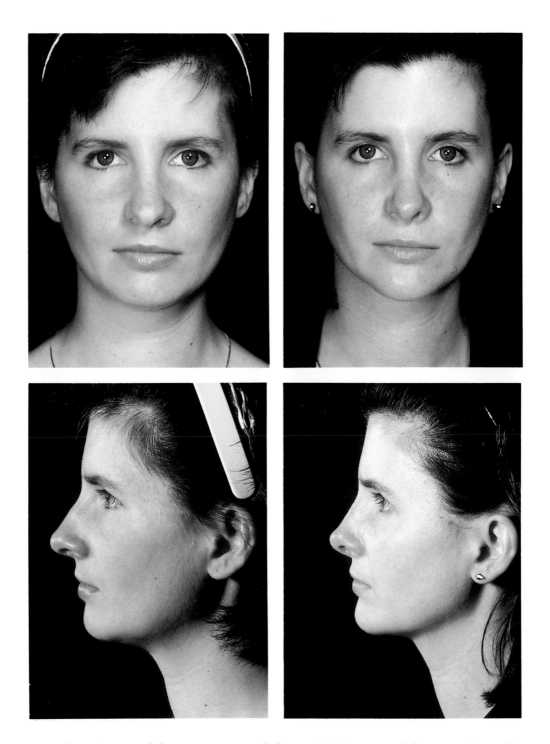

Less than 25 cc of fat was removed from this 27-year-old woman's neck. Changes in neck contour are subtle but noticeable. Rhinoplasty and allo-plastic chin augmentation were performed simultaneously.

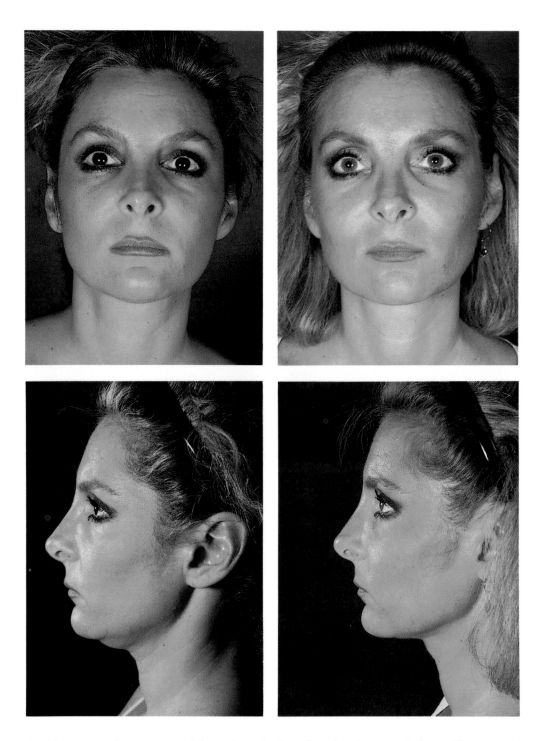

A 43-year-old woman with a sharply localized submental fat collection is shown before and 5 months after removal of 25 cc of fat.

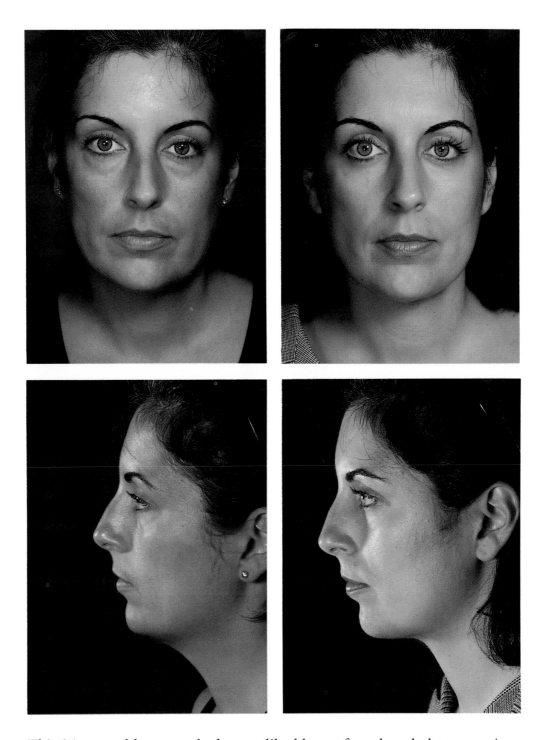

This 36-year-old woman had never liked her soft neck and obtuse cervico-mental angle. She requested an "Audrey Hepburn" look and is shown before and 8 months after liposuction of 30 cc from the neck along with simultaneous bilateral lower lid blepharoplasty. Her neck is thinner and more elegant.

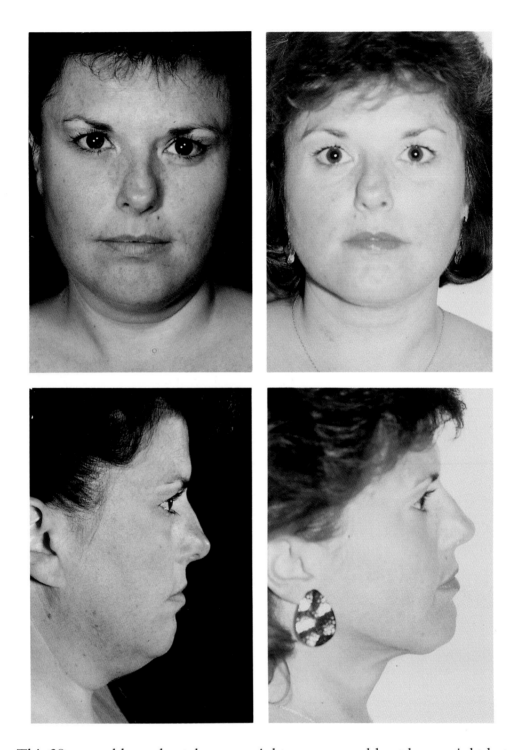

This 38-year-old, moderately overweight woman could not lose weight but wanted a thinner neck. She is shown before and 6 months after liposuction of 200 cc from the neck. Although she shows dramatic improvement, such large-volume removals usually result in some skin redundancy.

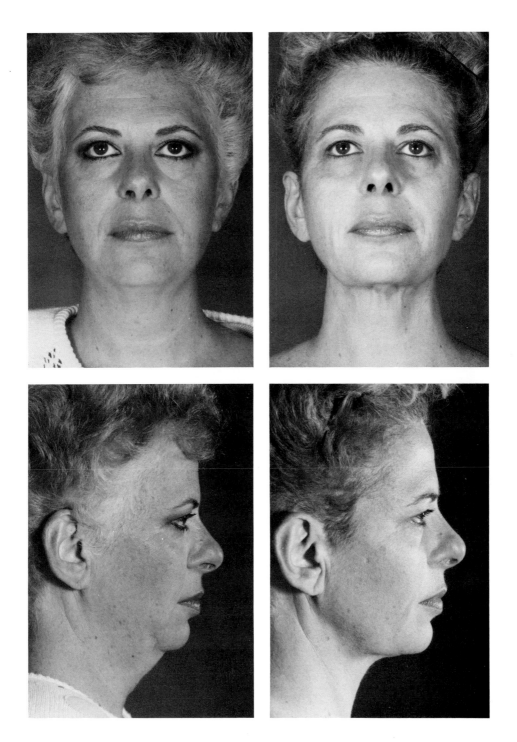

This 47-year-old woman is shown before and 8 months after liposuction of 100 cc of fat from the neck. I had recommended a face lift, but she had refused. Her age, skin laxity, and large fat volume all mitigated against a good result from liposuction alone. She was disappointed with the result.

CERVICAL LIPOSUCTION COMBINED WITH OPEN APPROACH TO ANTERIOR NECK
Operative Technique

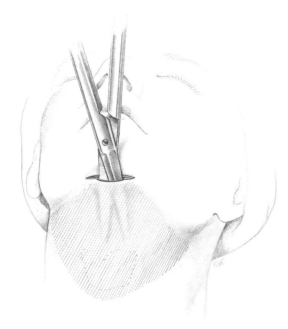

If the surgeon believes there is residual subplatysmal fat after suctioning or if the platysma requires treatment, the submental stab incision is extended to a length of 3 to 4 cm. Rees face-lift scissors are used to divide all fibrous connections between skin and platysma to below the thyroid cartilage and to the mandibular angle. A small fiberoptic lighted retractor helps with hemostasis.

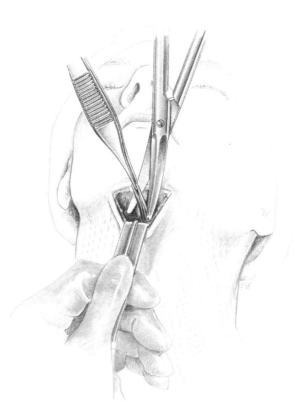

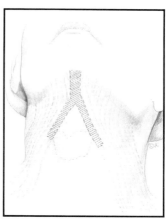

If the platysma decussates in the submental area, a narrow strip of muscle is excised from the midline so that the muscle does not bunch when the left and right platysma are sutured together. Excision of the midline muscle strip exposes the subplatysmal fat.

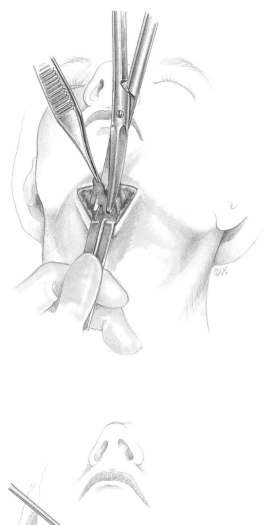

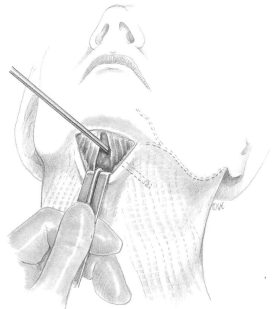

The medial portion of subplatysmal fat is removed under direct vision with the scissors. Lateral subplatysmal fat is suctioned using the 1.8 or 2.4 mm cannula. The cannula should be kept against the undersurface of the platysma and away from the mandibular body and ramus to avoid injury to the marginal mandibular nerve. Overresection of fat from the submentum will leave a depression and should be avoided.

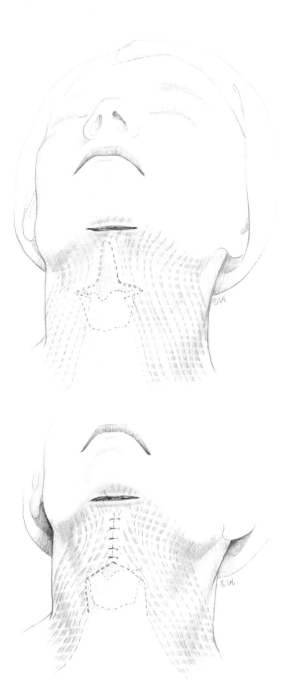

After removal of subplatysmal fat, wedges of muscle may be excised from the anterior borders of the platysma at the level of the thyroid cartilage to interrupt prominent anterior platysmal bands. The platysma may also be divided transversely as far laterally as necessary to increase mobility. This division should leave intact the superficial layer of cervical investing fascia that lies just deep to the platysma. The anterior platysma is then sutured to itself in the midline using 3-0 polydioxanone sutures (PDS; Ethicon Inc., Somerville, N.J.). The platysma is, in effect, cinched around the central upper neck, forming a tightened anterior supporting hammock.

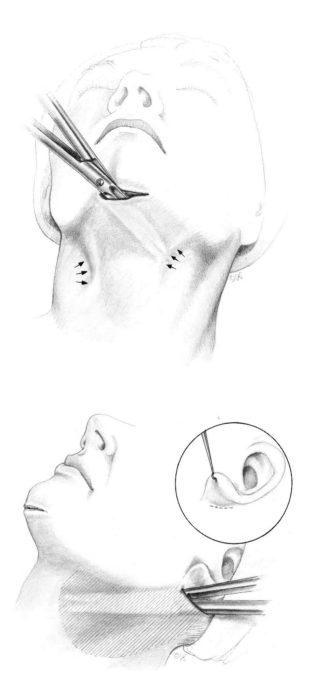

Platysma plication draws lateral skin medially and causes dimpling. Lateral undermining with the scissors is continued until the skin is free and can redrape smoothly. If necessary, undermining may be carried out from the retrolobular incisions to completely free the entire upper neck skin and permit smooth redraping. After a final check for coagulation of bleeders, wounds are closed with interrupted 5-0 nylon. A Reston sponge is placed on the neck (see p. 130).

Results

Although most liposuction patients do not need preoperative fat imaging, a discrete mass in the neck should be investigated prior to surgery to define its precise location and extent.

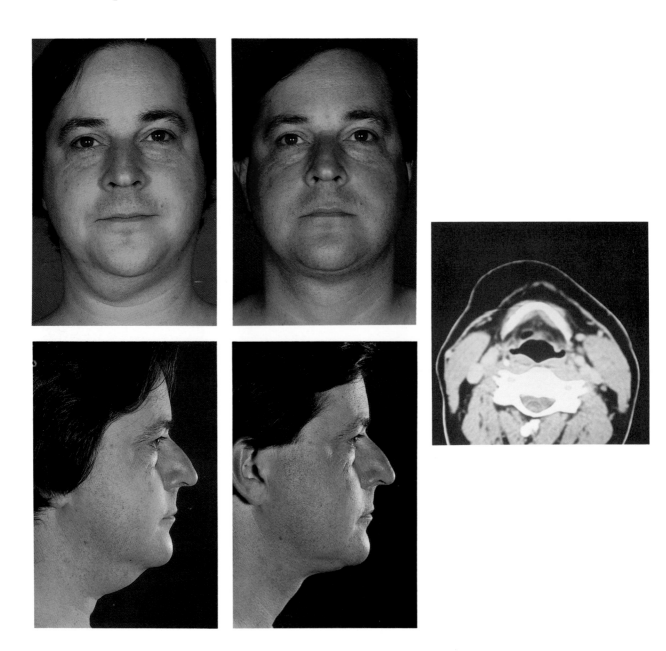

This 41-year-old man had a slowly growing mass in his right anterior cervical area for 15 years. The findings on a CT scan were consistent with a lipoma superficial to the platysma. He is shown before and 6 months after liposuction of 20 cc from the supraplatysmal space. The lipoma was removed under direct vision through a 4 cm submental incision. A small amount of subplatysmal fat was also removed prior to anterior platysma plication.

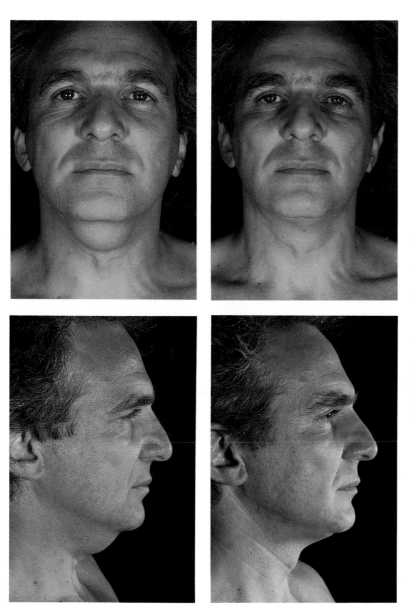

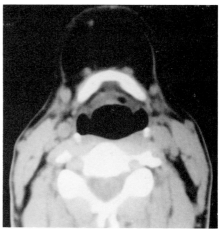

This 46-year-old man had a slowly enlarging fullness of the submentum for 10 years. The findings on a CT scan were consistent with a lipoma deep to the platysma. I removed the lipoma under direct vision through a submental incision. Liposuction was not required. The central platysma decussation was excised and the anterior platysma plicated. Complete scissors undermining from bilateral retroauricular incisions permitted smooth skin redraping. He is shown before and 8 months after surgery.

The surgeon can use adjunctive techniques to achieve a clean, crisp cervicomental angle in patients who would not benefit from liposuction alone. These additional procedures are useful in a wide variety of patients, but I find them particularly helpful in treating men.[55]

BUCCAL FAT PAD EXCISION AND FACIAL LIPOSUCTION

Because suction of the superficial facial fat can cause grooving, dimpling, and other surface irregularities, removal of the deep buccal fat pad is my first choice for facial fat contouring in young people. Buccal fat pad excision leaves the superficial fat undisturbed, providing a smooth layer to disguise any irregularities. Buccal fat pad excision via the intraoral approach has the added advantage of leaving no scars on the skin. Unfortunately, removal of the buccal fat pad changes the external contour very little in some patients, and additional removal of superficial fat is required.

Since there is no way to determine in advance whether the cheek fullness is due to deep or superficial fat, I tell all patients they will undergo buccal fat pad excision and be evaluated on the operating table for further intervention. If the change following excision of the deep fat is sufficient, the operation is terminated. If additional fat removal is required, I proceed with liposuction. Since the buccal fat pad has already been excised, less superficial fat has to be suctioned to achieve the desired contour change.

Markings

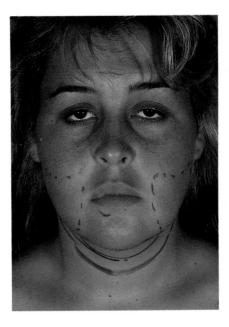 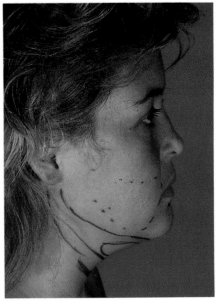

The preparotid area and more medial midcheek area are marked while the patient is standing or sitting. Most excess fat in the face will be found in these contiguous areas. The areas over the malar eminences, mandibular body, and ramus usually require emphasis rather than contour reduction. Fat should be excised from these areas only in rare instances. Fat removal alone will not improve sagging jowls or a full nasolabial fold, and patients requiring treatment of these problems need face lift.

Operative Technique

Local anesthesia is achieved by infiltrating 0.25% lidocaine with 1:400,000 epinephrine into the subcutaneous cheek tissues. One or two milliliters of the same solution is infiltrated into the buccal mucosa just below the maxillary gingivobuccal sulcus in the second molar area.

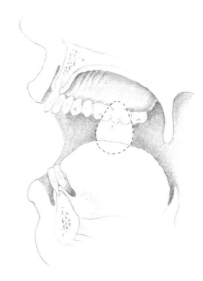

The cheek portion of the buccal fat pad is shown "ghosted in" against the buccal mucosa.

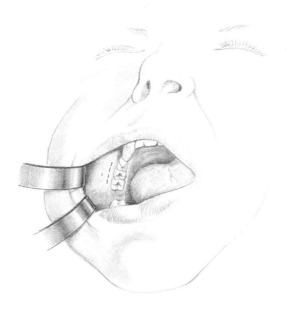

A 1.5 cm incision is made opposite the maxillary second molar halfway between the gingivobuccal sulcus and the parotid duct papilla. This incision is made parallel to the sulcus and extends only through the mucosa.

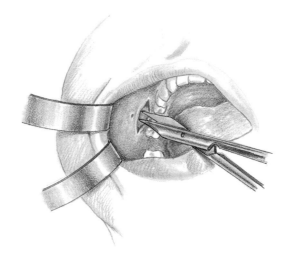

Since the thin layer of buccinator muscle is subjacent to the mucosa, spreading the muscle fibers with a Stevens scissors exposes the underlying buccinator fascia.

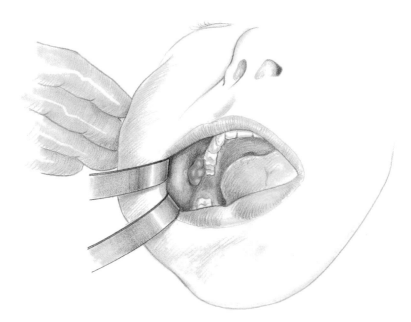

The fascia is penetrated with the point of the scissors; this releases the buccal fat pad, which can then be teased out through the incision. Gentle pressure on the cheek aids in expressing the fat intraorally so that it can be grasped with a hemostat. Small amounts of local anesthesia injected into the base of the fat reduces the pain caused by traction. The excess is excised over a clamp, and the fat stump is cauterized before being released and allowed to retract into the cheek.

All of the fat that can be expressed easily into the mouth is removed. Attempts to reach in and pull out additional fat may damage the facial vein or buccal branches of the facial nerve. Less than 5 gm of tissue is removed in most instances. The external cheek should be checked with the fat drawn into the mouth to determine if the amount of fat removed is appropriate. If the cheek appears too hollow, some of the fat should be replaced. The incision is closed in one layer with 4-0 interrupted chromic sutures.

For most patients, buccal fat pad excision alone does not produce a sufficient diminution in contour, and I also perform facial liposuction. Only minuscule amounts are removed, and the total is always less than 5 cc for both sides together. I use a 1.8 or 2.4 mm Mercedes Type cannula.

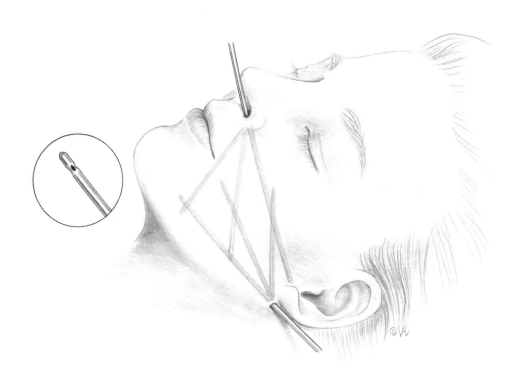

Stab incisions in the retrolobular area and nasal vestibule provide access to most of the face. The cannula is kept close to the skin as crisscrossing tunnels are made. Care is taken not to remove too much fat from any one area; cautious conservatism is the key to obtaining a smooth reduction and avoiding contour irregularities. Incisions behind the ear are closed with one or two absorbable sutures. The nasal incisions do not require closure, and dressings are not necessary.

Results

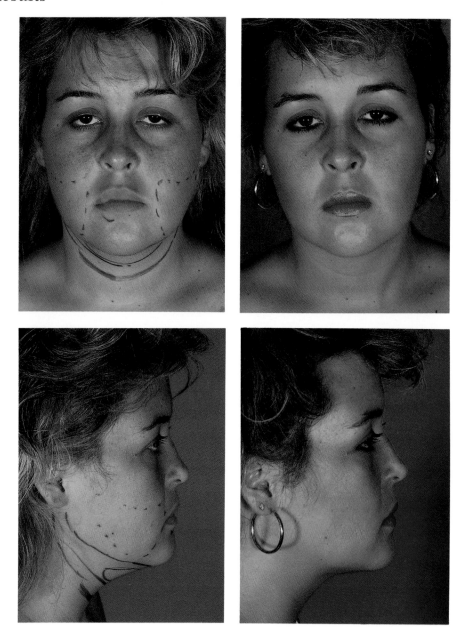

This 28-year-old woman was moderately overweight. She had previously undergone liposuction of the abdomen and thighs and wished to have a more angular, thinner looking face and neck. She is shown marked for face and neck liposuction (no markings are necessary for buccal fat pad excision) and 3 months following buccal fat pad excision and liposuction of the face and neck. Although her weight did not change, her facial features were more chiseled. She was pleased with the change since it made her look thinner.

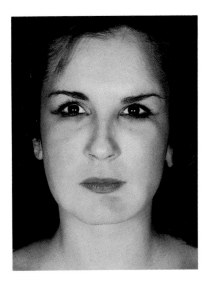 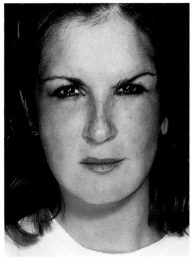

This 26-year-old woman had silicone injections in the right side of her face. She found the resultant cheek swelling disfiguring, and direct removal through a cheek flap had been attempted previously. Buccal fat pad excision combined with liposuction of the superficial fat reduced bulk and made her look more symmetric. She is shown 1 year after surgery.

POSTOPERATIVE CARE AND RECOVERY
Neck

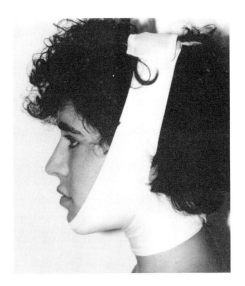

The Reston sponge is removed in 7 days and the patient wears a chin/neck strap at night for an additional 2 weeks. When the Reston sponge is first removed, the results in the neck are usually quite dramatic. Within a few hours, however, the skin, freed from its restraint and support, will swell, and some of the original result will be lost. This change in contour is temporary, and the acute cervicomental angle will be restored gradually. Swelling may not fully resolve for 6 weeks. This point should be made clear to the patient when the dressing is removed.

Postoperative pain is minimal, and patients generally require no medication after the first 24 hours. Tightness, stiffness, and diminution in sensibility are noticeable for several weeks. As swelling recedes, the patients will feel and may be able to see irregular areas of induration. Complete softening and resolution may require 3 months. Despite the rather prolonged course, the patient is presentable in a week. She may resume all nonsports activities when the Reston sponge is removed at 1 week or earlier. Sports may be resumed at 3 weeks if only liposuction was performed and at 6 weeks if the platysma has been sutured.

Face

External compression of the cheeks is difficult without packing the oral cavity. Therefore no dressings are used for the face. The patient is instructed to apply ice compresses for 24 hours to minimize edema. Although she is told to rest for 24 hours after surgery, activities are not restricted thereafter except for sports, which are prohibited for 2 weeks. As in the neck, induration and visible irregularities are common but generally resolve between the third and sixth weeks. Patients with an intraoral incision from buccal fat pad excision are limited to a liquid diet for 24 hours, after which their oral intake is unrestricted. Patients rinse their mouth out gently with saline solution after meals and resume toothbrushing after 5 days. Swelling may be considerable, and results may not be apparent for 6 weeks.

LIPOSUCTION COMBINED WITH FACE AND NECK LIFT
Operative Technique

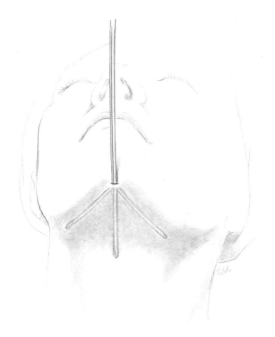

For the face-lift patient with excess submental fat, anterior cervical suctioning is the first step. The technique is similar to that described on pp. 127-130. A single submental stab incision is used. Fat is removed aggressively in the central area but is left undisturbed adjacent to the inferior border of the mandibular body and angle so that subsequent SMAS-platysma elevation does not bring defatted areas over the mandible, reducing projection and flattening an area that should be prominent.

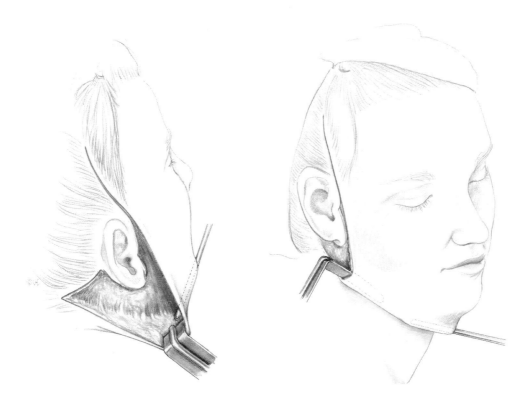

After the subcutaneous central neck fat is suctioned, the lateral face-lift incision is made, and skin flaps are elevated over the temporal area, cheek, and lateral neck. Lateral neck dissection is facilitated by having the assistant place a cannula in the submental incision and direct it toward the surgeon. The assistant presses up gently against the skin flap to improve lateral neck exposure.

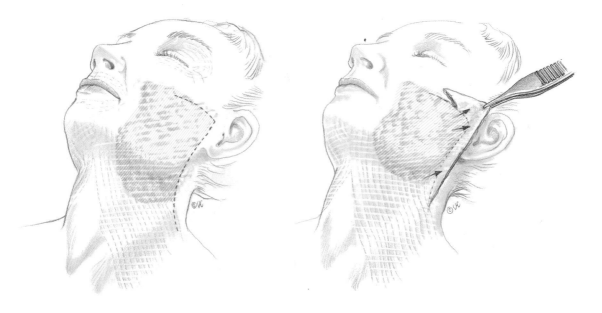

After the skin flaps are elevated, the SMAS–platysma is lifted as a separate layer, pulled back and up, and sutured into a more superolateral position, tightening the neck and lower face.

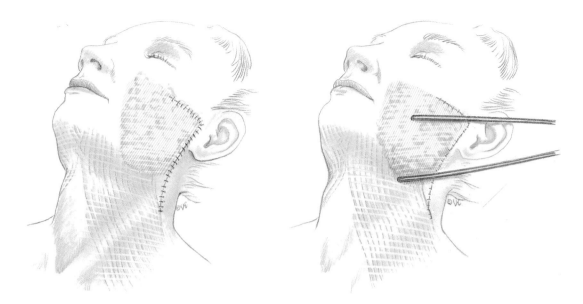

When the SMAS-platysma has been repositioned, the upper lateral cervical area below the inferior border of the mandibular angle can be defatted to emphasize the prominence of the mandible. I use an open suction technique with a 6 mm single-port cannula. The cannula is also used to remove excess cheek fat to accentuate the malar eminence. It is easy to overresect, and fat removal in the cheek should be particularly conservative.

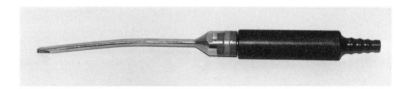

The aperture is at the very end of the cannula, which is slightly bent so that the entire opening is easily pressed against the fat, facilitating vacuuming under the open flap.

This method of contouring a fat neck during face lift is rapid and efficient. It avoids a long submental incision and retains some direct neurovascular supply to skin in the submental area. Since the anterior cervical skin remains attached to the platysma, pulling back on the lateral platysma and SMAS also redrapes the neck skin and deepens the cervicomental angle. This technique is compatible with a variety of techniques for elevation of the SMAS-platysma.

Results

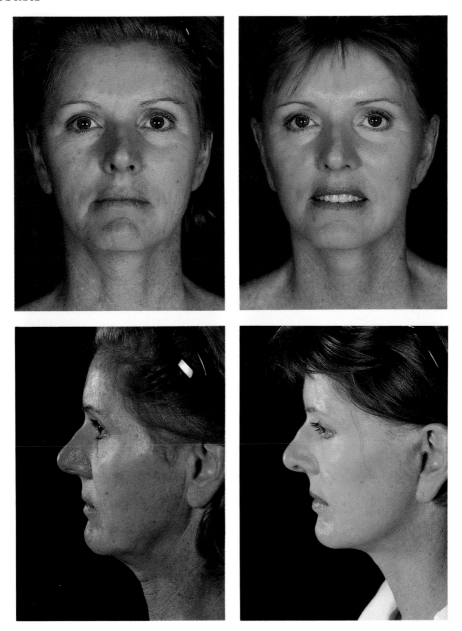

A 47-year-old woman is shown before and 13 months after face and neck lift with submental liposuction. The anterior platysma was not disturbed. A lower lid blepharoplasty and perioral peel were performed simultaneously. The lateral SMAS-platysma was elevated as a unit. The tension from pulling upward and backward on this deep tissue layer was transmitted to the submental and submandibular skin, creating a tightening and upward lift in the anterolateral neck. Up and back rotation of this layer also helped define the mandibular angle.

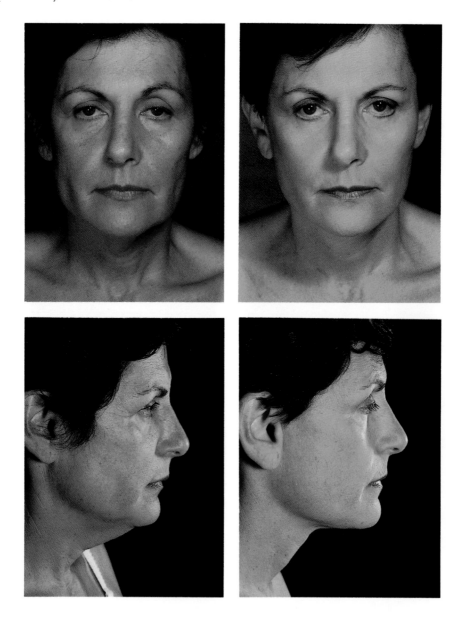

This 47-year-old woman had a neck lift with submental liposuction. The anterior platysma was not disturbed. She also underwent bilateral upper and lower blepharoplasty. Liposuction of the anterior neck permitted extensive fat removal with minimal disturbance of the connections between platysma and skin in the anterior cervical area. Consequently, postero-superior traction on the SMAS-platysma layer was readily transmitted to the anterior neck skin, deepening the cervicomental angle without the necessity of an open approach to the anterior platysma. The patient is shown before and 13 months after surgery.

OPEN APPROACH TO ANTERIOR CERVICAL AREA DURING FACE LIFT

Patients with very prominent and lax anterior platysmal bands or patients with large subplatysmal fat collections require more than just suction in the submental area. The anterior neck is treated as described on pp. 136-139.

Results

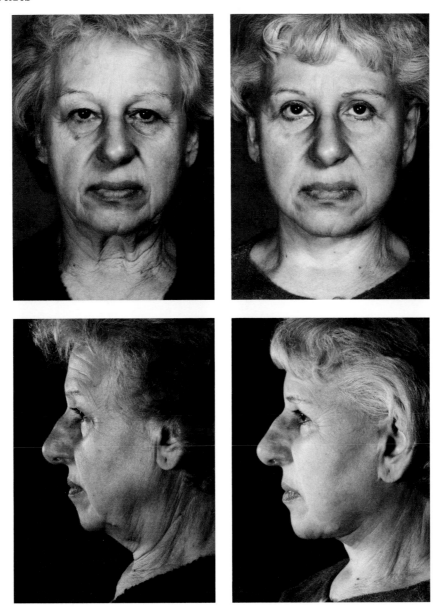

This 65-year-old woman had lax anterior cervical skin, about 40 cc of submental fat, and prominent anterior platysmal bands extending below the thyroid cartilage. After preliminary submental suctioning, I approached the anterior platysmal bands through a 4 cm transverse submental incision. I excised the midline platysmal decussation, divided the anterior bands at the level of the thyroid cartilage, and then sutured the anterior platysma to itself in the midline to create a central cinching effect and deepen the cervicomental angle. There was insufficient subplatysmal fat for removal. I then performed a lateral face and neck lift with elevation of the SMAS-platysma as a separate layer. She also had bilateral upper and lower blepharoplasty. She is shown before and 1 year after surgery.

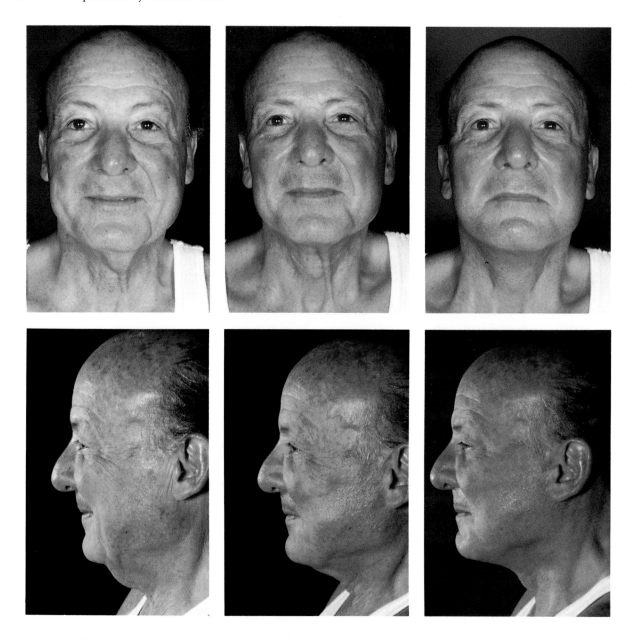

This 71-year-old man had lax cervicofacial skin, excess submental and facial fat, and prominent, stretched anterior platysmal bands, particularly on the left. Treatment included a face and neck lift. The SMAS-platysma was elevated as one layer from the lateral approach. The submental area was treated with closed suction. At 6 months (center) the patient's appearance was improved, but laxity of the anterior platysma, which I had not addressed at surgery, was unacceptable. Dissatisfied with the result, I suggested a secondary operation, which the patient readily accepted. He is seen on the right 1 year after an open submental procedure in which I excised strips of anterior platysma, removed wedges of platysma at the level of the thyroid cartilage, suctioned about 10 cc of subplatysmal fat, and cinched the anterior platysma to itself. I also redraped and tightened the skin from the lateral face-lift incisions.

BUCCAL FAT PAD EXCISION DURING FACE LIFT

Patients with very fat cheeks may benefit from buccal fat pad excision during face lift.

Operative Technique

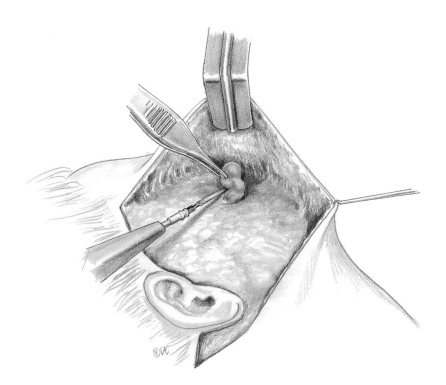

Elevation of the SMAS beyond the anterior border of the parotid gland exposes the area of the buccal fat pad just beyond the masseter muscle and the anterior border of the mandibular ramus. The buccal fat pad is found by piercing the tissues just beyond the mandible with the closed points of the dissecting scissors. The small rent is enlarged by spreading the scissors in a vertical plane to avoid damage to the buccal branches of the facial nerve. If the buccal fat is abundant, it will protrude into the operative field. It is easily distinguished from the surrounding subcutaneous fat by its darker color and smooth, glistening surface. Placing a finger inside the mouth and against the buccal mucosa and applying gentle pressure aids in bringing the fat into the operative field, where it is gently teased out and excised over a clamp. Attempts to extract the buccal fat by reaching into the pad with an instrument risk damage to the facial nerve or branches of the facial artery and vein. As with the intraoral approach, meticulous hemostasis will minimize hematomas.

TREATING NASOLABIAL FOLDS AND JOWLING DURING FACE LIFT

Prominent nasolabial folds are composed of redundant skin and fat. Liposuction removes only fat, not skin, and attempts to obliterate the nasolabial fold or jowls with liposuction alone can only worsen the patient's appearance.

Operative Technique

Liposuction is, however, a useful adjunct to face lift in treating nasolabial folds and jowling. I have modified the approach of Millard, Yuan, and Devine[65,66] to this area by using the suction cannula as a technical aid. Ellenbogen et al.[67] have also described fat excision from the nasolabial fold using curettes.

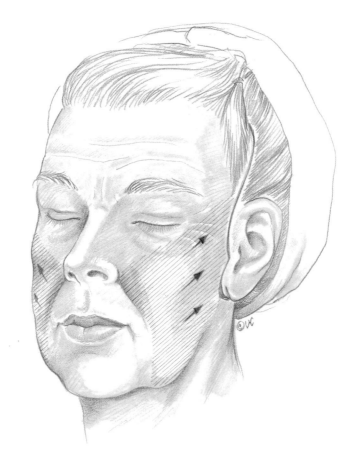

Flattening of the fold and jowl is achieved by extracting the underlying fat and pulling up on the excess skin. The direction of pull should be perpendicular to the nasolabial crease, which dictates face-lift dissection over the malar eminence all the way to the fold so that the skin can be redraped and the fold flattened. The technique is applicable with dissection of the superficial subcutaneous tissues as originally described by Millard, Yuan, and Devine[65] or with a thicker flap as described by Lemmon[21] and Hamra.[20]

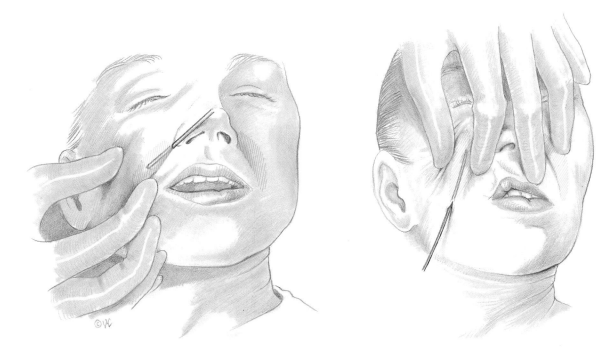

Closed suction of the nasolabial fold is the first step. Two stab wounds are made at the superior and inferior ends of the nasolabial crease. These twin access incisions require no suturing and heal with an inconspicuous scar. I use a 1.5 mm cannula and remove as much fat as necessary, usually 1 or 2 cc.

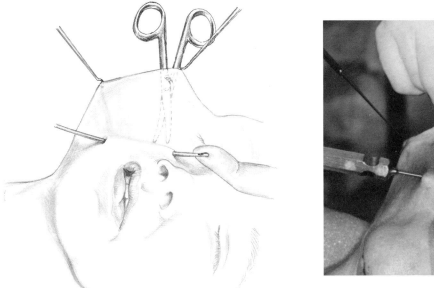

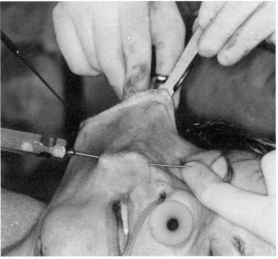

After the nasolabial fold is suctioned, the submental area is treated as necessary. The lateral face-lift incision is made, and the cheek flap is elevated. Dissection over the malar eminence to the fold can be tedious since the curve of the face obscures visualization of the fold and crease. The cheek flap is dissected as far as the surgeon can conveniently view the area.

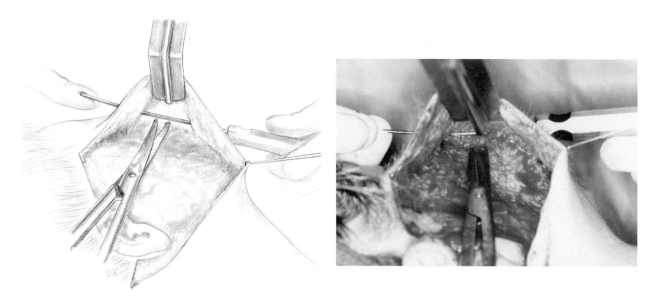

The nasolabial fold is then elevated to the visual plane using the suction cannula placed subcutaneously beneath the fold through the stab incisions in the nasolabial crease. In effect, the fold is skewered and then elevated with the cannula. Once the tissues have been raised, the fibrous bands between the skin of the nasolabial fold and the underlying fascia are easily divided. Bleeders in this area can also be readily seen and controlled.

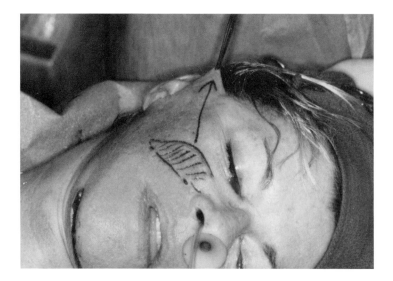

The skin is redraped in a superolateral direction, the excess is excised, and the flap is sutured into position.

Results

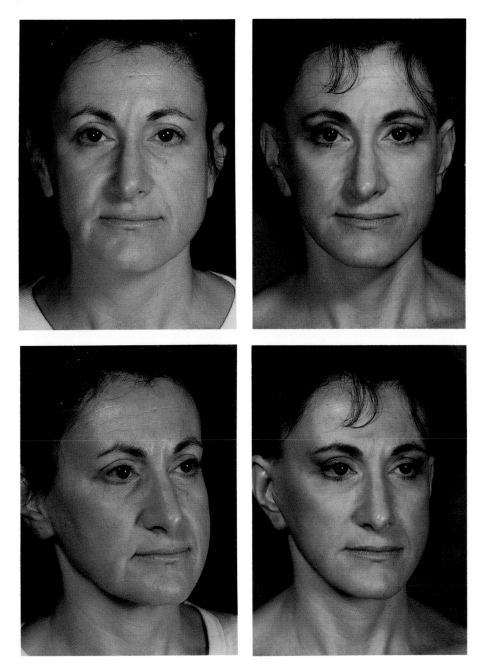

This 49-year-old woman's principal concern was the fullness of her naso-labial folds. I treated her with face and neck lift. Since she had no excess neck fat or severe platysmal bands, neither suction nor an open approach was required for the submental area. The first step in the operation was suction of the nasolabial folds. The lateral cheek flaps were raised as thick composite flaps including the SMAS-platysma and skin as one unit. Most important, the flaps were undermined extensively over the malar eminence to the nasolabial fold. She is shown before and 1 year after surgery.

POSTOPERATIVE CARE AND RECOVERY

Recovery following face lift is more prolonged than after liposuction alone or liposuction with adjunctive procedures through limited incisions. Details of recovery can be found in standard textbooks.[73] In general, patients can expect to remain confined at home for a week. They come to the office on the fourth and seventh postoperative days for suture removal. Sometime in the second week the patient will begin to look presentable enough to venture out for short periods, albeit with makeup and other cover-ups. Almost all patients can return to nonsports activities by postoperative day 14, but lesser bruising may persist for another week and slight edema usually lasts 6 weeks. Sports can be resumed at 6 weeks.

COMPLICATIONS AND UNAESTHETIC RESULTS
Liposuction

When suction is used as an adjunct to a face lift, it is difficult to determine if a particular adverse sequela is caused by suction or by some other aspect of the operation. Nevertheless, treatment remains the same. As with all aesthetic procedures, postoperative problems from suction of the face and neck should be classified as either true surgical complications or unaesthetic results.

Skin Pigmentation

Pigmentation is usually transient and fades gradually, but some residual discoloration may be permanent. This problem can be due to rough cannula manipulation causing microbleeding into the dermis and deposition of iron pigment breakdown products of blood. Unevacuated gross hematomas will, of course, have the same effect.

Skin Penetration

Penetration of the overlying skin with the tip of the cannula can occur, particularly if the area is scarred from previous surgery or cystic acne. Healing with inconspicuous scars is the usual course.

Necrosis

Because the closed suction method causes only minimal disruption of the blood supply to the overlying skin, necrosis is rare if there are no precipitating causes such as hematoma or infection.

Hematoma

Microhematomas and bruising are common and resorb spontaneously. Small hematomas, varying from 2 to 20 cc, may not become apparent until several days after surgery when swelling has subsided. The clot usually liquefies in the second week, after which the surgeon can aspirate the blood through a 14-gauge needle. Alternatively, the blood can be expressed through a small stab incision over the most dependent portion of the hematoma. Narrow-gauge flexible tubing can be inserted through the stab incision and the blood irrigated out with copious amounts of sterile saline solution (the fill tubing for inflatable mammary implants works well for this purpose). A small suction cannula attached to an aspirator can also be used.

It is advisable to remove even small collections thoroughly. If left in situ, they will organize into solid masses forming troublesome swellings that take months to resolve. During this lengthy resolution the overlying skin may retract and pucker prior to resuming its normal state many months later. Prolonged or permanent discoloration can result from hemoglobin breakdown products deposited in the skin.

Large, expanding hematomas should be treated promptly and aggressively since they may result in skin necrosis. If they occur in the neck, they may threaten the airway. Prompt drainage and irrigation through an adequate sized dependent incision is usually sufficient treatment. If the incision is placed in a line of minimum skin tension, it usually heals with an inconspicuous scar. Although the surgeon may be reluctant to create yet another incision in a patient who has only had liposuction, the consequences of undrained or inadequately drained hematomas can be devastating and far worse than the additional small scar from a well-planned drainage. If bleeding persists after drainage, the source must be exposed by enlarging the drainage incision or by a standard face- and neck-lift approach.

Infection

Infections are rare. They should be treated with antibiotics appropriate to the organism. In the presence of frank pus, dependent drainage is mandatory to avoid progression to necrosis of overlying skin or deep cervical abscess. There is no evidence that prophylactic antibiotics reduce the already minuscule infection rate for liposuction.

Nerve Injury

All patients undergoing liposuction experience hypesthesia in treated areas. The subjective sense of numbness is temporary, and patients routinely report full return of sensibility. Nevertheless, careful, objective testing may reveal permanent sensory deficits.[72] Hypesthesia is not, strictly speaking, a complication since it is a universal sequela. Liposuction, not surprisingly, causes fewer sensory symptoms than full face lift.

Motor nerve injuries from liposuction most frequently involve the marginal mandibular branch of the facial nerve and are almost always neuropraxic. Spontaneous return of function in a few days or weeks is the usual course.

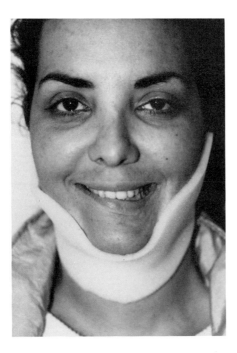 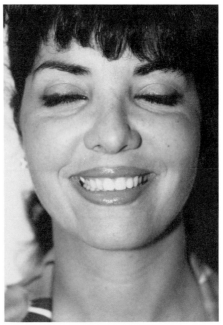

This 35-year-old woman had weakness of her right lower lip the day after cervical liposuction. Recovery was complete by 4 weeks.

More prolonged recovery calls for neurologic consultation and electrodiagnostic studies. If no improvement occurs after 6 months, nerve exploration and microsurgical repair should be considered.

Scars

Hypertrophic scars and keloids are not usually a problem since the incisions for liposuction are only about ⅛-inch long and placed in inconspicuous areas. If a scar is troublesome, intralesional injection of dilute corticosteroid solution offers relief. With time, however, most problems relating to these small scars will resolve spontaneously.

Aesthetic Sequelae

The face is more prone to irregularities, grooving, depressions, underresections, and overresections than the neck, and the surgeon must exercise particular care when suctioning the face.

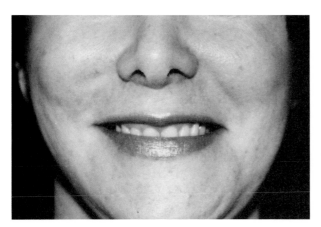 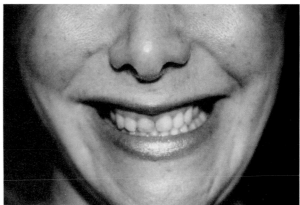

Grooving adjacent to the right nasolabial crease was apparent 2 weeks after liposuction in this patient. The problem resolved along with swelling at 2 months.

Use of fine cannulas and multiple access incisions and removing only small volumes will minimize undesirable sequelae.

Buccal Fat Pad Excision
Hematoma

Expanding hematomas can occur from branches of the external facial vessels.[60] They are heralded by swelling and pain and should be promptly evacuated through the incision. Meticulous hemostasis with the electrocautery minimizes the incidence of hematomas.

Infection

Infections are rare and abscesses rarer still. Cellulitides are treated with appropriate antibiotics. Abscesses should be drained and cultured prior to antibiotic therapy.

Nerve Injury

Injuries to the facial nerve during buccal fat pad excision involve the buccal branches. Trauma to the nerve branches is more likely if fat is excised via the face-lift approach, which traverses the plane of the nerves. Delicate dissection with spreading in the direction of the nerve fibers avoids injury. Cauterization should be well away from the plane of the nerve branches. Upper lip weakness should be treated expectantly as it will almost certainly resolve.

———————————————— REFERENCES ————————————————

1. Maliniac JW. Is the surgical restoration of the aged face justified? Med J Rec 135:321-324, 1932.
2. Padgett EC, Stephenson KL. Plastic and Reconstructive Surgery. Springfield, Ill.: Charles C Thomas, 1948, p 632.
3. Davis AD. Obligations in the considerations of meloplasties. J Int Surg 24:568-571, 1955.
4. Adamson JE, Horton CE, Crawford HH. The surgical correction of the "turkey gobbler" deformity. Plast Reconstr Surg 34:598-605, 1964.
5. Cannon B, Pantazelos H. W-plasty approach to the submandibular lipectomy. In Transactions of the Fifth International Congress of Plastic Surgeons. London: Butterworth, 1971, p 1113.
6. Cronin TD, Biggs TM. The T-Z plasty for the male "turkey gobbler" neck. Plast Reconstr Surg 47:534-538, 1971.
7. Gurdin MM, Carlin GA. Aging defects in the male: A regional approach to treatment. In Masters FW, Lewis JR, eds. Symposium on Aesthetic Surgery of the Face, Eyelids, and Breast. St. Louis: CV Mosby, 1972, pp 52-57.
8. Johnson JB, Hadley RC. The aging face. In Converse JM, ed. Reconstructive Plastic Surgery, 1st ed. Philadelphia: WB Saunders, 1962, pp 1328-1330.
9. Morel-Fatio D. Cosmetic surgery of the face. In Gibson T, ed. Modern Trends in Plastic Surgery. London: Butterworth, 1964, pp 221-222.
10. Millard DR Jr, Pigott RW, Hedo A. Submandibular lipectomy. Plast Reconstr Surg 41:513-522, 1968.
11. Millard DR Jr, Garst WP, Beck RL, Thompson ID. Submental and submandibular lipectomy in conjunction with a face lift in the male or female. Plast Reconstr Surg 49:385-391, 1972.
12. Aston SJ. Platysma muscle and rhytidoplasty. Ann Plast Surg 3:529-539, 1979.
13. Aston SJ. Platysma-SMAS cervicofacial rhytidoplasty. Clin Plast Surg 10:507-520, 1983.
14. Cardoso de Castro C, Aboudib JH Jr. Extensive cervical and lower face lipectomy: Its importance and anatomical basis. Ann Plast Surg 4:370-375, 1980.
15. Cardoso de Castro C. Extensive mandibular and cervical lipectomy. Aesthetic Plast Surg 5:239-248, 1981.

16. Connell BF. Contouring the neck in rhytidectomy by lipectomy and a muscle sling. Plast Reconstr Surg 61:376-383, 1978.

17. Connell BF, Gaon A. Surgical correction of aesthetic contour problems of the neck. Clin Plast Surg 10:491-505, 1983.

18. Guerrerosantos J. The role of the platysma muscle in rhytidoplasty. Clin Plast Surg 5:29-49, 1978.

19. Guerrerosantos J, Espatllat L, Morales F. Muscular lift in cervical rhytidoplasty. Plast Reconstr Surg 54:127-131, 1974.

20. Hamra ST. The deep-plane rhytidectomy. Plast Reconstr Surg 86:53-61, 1990.

21. Lemmon ML. Superficial fascia rhytidectomy. Clin Plast Surg 10:449-478, 1987.

22. Lemmon ML, Hamra ST. Skoog rhytidoplasty: A five-year experience with 577 patients. Plast Reconstr Surg 65:283-297, 1980.

23. Pangman WJ, Wallace RM. Cosmetic surgery of the face and neck. Plast Reconstr Surg 27:544-550, 1961.

24. Owsley JQ. SMAS-platysma face lift. Clin Plast Surg 10:429-440, 1983.

25. Pennisi VR, Capozzi A. The transposition of fat in cervicofacial rhytidectomy. Plast Reconstr Surg 49:423-427, 1972.

26. Souther SG, Vistnes LM. Medial approximation of the platysma muscle in the treatment of neck deformities. Plast Reconstr Surg 67:607-613, 1981.

27. Souza Pinzo EB. Importance of cervicomental complex treatment in rhytidoplasty. Aesthetic Plast Surg 5:69-75, 1981.

28. Weisman PA. Simplified technique in submental lipectomy. Plast Reconstr Surg 48:443-446, 1971.

29. Wolfe SA, Fusi S. Treatment of the particularly fatty neck and the short-interval secondary facelift. Aesthetic Plast Surg 15:195-201, 1991.

30. Peterson RA. The role of the platysma muscle in cervical lifts. In Goulian D, Courtiss EH, eds. Symposium on Surgery of the Aging Face. St. Louis: CV Mosby, 1978, pp 115-126.

31. Cardoso de Castro C. The value of anatomical study of the platysma muscle in cervical lifting. Aesthetic Plast Surg 8:7-11, 1984.

32. Connell BF. Surgical technique of cervical lift and facial lipectomy. Aesthetic Plast Surg 5:43-50, 1981.

33. Singer R. Improvement of the "young" fatty neck. Plast Reconstr Surg 73:582-589, 1984.

34. Davis J. The other facet of face lifting: Facial sculpture. In Marchac D, Hueston J, eds. Transactions of the Sixth International Congress of Plastic and Reconstructive Surgeons. Paris: Masson, 1976, p 452.

35. Davis J, Cinflone J. Facial lipectomy. Aesthetic Plast Surg 5:107-113, 1981.

36. Cardoso de Castro C. The anatomy of the platysma muscle. Plast Reconstr Surg 66:680-683, 1980.

37. Feldman JJ. Corset platysmaplasty. Plast Reconstr Surg 85:333-343, 1990.

38. Guerrerosantos J. Surgical correction of the fatty fallen neck. Ann Plast Surg 2:389-396, 1979.

39. Hugo NE. Rhytidectomy with radical lipectomy and platysmal flaps. Plast Reconstr Surg 65:199-205, 1980.

40. Bloch S, Dibbell DG. Submental lipectomy in the young adult. Aesthetic Plast Surg 4:101-105, 1980.

41. Ellenbogen R, Karlin JV. Visual criteria for success in restoring the youthful neck. Plast Reconstr Surg 66:826-837, 1980.

42. Johnson JB. The problem of the aging face. Plast Reconstr Surg 15:117-121, 1955.

43. Weisman PA. One surgeon's experience with surgical contouring of the neck. Clin Plast Surg 10:521-541, 1983.

44. Wilkinson TS. The submental tuck. In Goulian D, Courtiss EH, eds. Symposium on Surgery of the Aging Face. St. Louis: CV Mosby, 1978, pp 111-114.

45. Illouz Y-G. Body contouring by lipolysis: A 5-year experience with over 3000 cases. Plast Reconstr Surg 72:591-597, 1983.

46. Fournier PF, Otteni FM. Lipodissection in body sculpturing: The dry procedure. Plast Reconstr Surg 72:598-609, 1983.

47. Teimourian B. Face and neck suction-assisted lipectomy associated with rhytidectomy. Plast Reconstr Surg 72:627-633, 1983.

48. Baker TJ, Gordon HL. Surgical Rejuvenation of the Face. St. Louis: CV Mosby, 1986, pp 137-145.

49. Connell BF. Neck contour deformities. Clin Plast Surg 14:683-692, 1987.

50. Avelar J. Fat suction of the submental and submandibular regions. Aesthetic Plast Surg 9:257-263, 1985.

51. Lewis CM. Lipoplasty of the neck. Plast Reconstr Surg 76:248-257, 1985.

52. Owsley JQ. The SMAS-platysma face lift. Perspect Plast Surg 4(1):1-23, 1990.

53. Topia A, Ferreira B, Eng R. Liposuction in cervical rejuvenation. Aesthetic Plast Surg 11:95-100, 1987.

54. Pitman GH. Suction lipectomy of the face and body: Precision and refinement. In Riley WB, ed. Plastic Surgery Educational Foundation Instructional Courses. St. Louis: CV Mosby, 1988, pp 71-106.

55. Pitman GH. Face and neck contouring by fat removal. In Courtiss EH, ed. Male Aesthetic Surgery. St. Louis: Mosby–Year Book, 1991, pp 304-315.

56. Carbonell A, Salavert A, Planas J. Resection of the buccal fat pad in the treatment of hypertrophy of the masseter muscle. Aesthetic Plast Surg 15:219-222, 1991.

57. Epstein LI. Buccal lipectomy. Ann Plast Surg 5:123-130, 1980.

58. Krupp S. Buccal lipectomy reappraisal and case report. Eur J Plast Surg 9:40-42, 1986.

59. Stuzin JM, Wagstrom L, Kawamoto HK, Baker TJ, Wolfe SA. The anatomy and clinical applications of the buccal fat pad. Plast Reconstr Surg 85:29-37, 1990.

60. Ortiz-Monasterio F, Olmedo A. Excision of the buccal fat pad to refine the obese midface. In Kaye BL, Gradinger GP, eds. Symposium on Problems and Complications in Aesthetic Plastic Surgery of the Face. St. Louis: CV Mosby, 1984, pp 91-98.

61. Adamson JE, Tosko AE. Progress in rhytidectomy by platysma-SMAS rotation and elevation. Plast Reconstr Surg 68:23-33, 1981.

62. Aston SJ. Refinements in rhytidectomy. Plastic Surgery Educational Foundation. Videotape No. 822, 1988.

63. Marino H, Galeano EJ, Gondolfo EA. Plastic correction of the double chin: Importance of the position of the hyoid bone. Plast Reconstr Surg 31:45-50, 1963.

64. Gaughran GRL. Fasciae of masticator space. Anat Rec 129:383-400, 1957.

65. Millard DR, Yuan RTW, Devine JW Jr. A challenge to the undefeated nasolabial folds. Plast Reconstr Surg 80:37-46, 1987.

66. Millard DR, Mullin WR, Hunsaker RH. Evaluation of a technique designed to correct nasolabial folds. Plast Reconstr Surg 89:356-365, 1992.

67. Ellenbogen R, Wethe J, Jankauskas S, Collini F. Curette fat sculpture in rhytidectomy: Improving the nasolabial and labomandibular folds. Plast Reconstr Surg 88:433-442, 1991.

68. Barton FE Jr. The SMAS and the nasolabial fold. Plast Reconstr Surg 89:1054-1057, 1992.

69. Barton FE Jr. Rhytidectomy and the nasolabial fold. Plast Reconstr Surg (in press).

70. Rubin LR, Mishriki Y, Lee G. Anatomy of the nasolabial fold. The keystone of the smiling mechanism. Plast Reconstr Surg 83:1-8, 1989.

71. Zufferey J. Anatomic variation of the nasolabial fold. Plast Reconstr Surg 89:225-231, 1992.

72. Courtiss EH. Suction lipectomy of the neck. Plast Reconstr Surg 76:882-889, 1985.

73. Rees TD. Aesthetic Plastic Surgery, vol 2. Philadelphia: WB Saunders, 1980, p 703.

—————————— SUGGESTED READINGS ——————————

Bichat F. Anatomie générale, appliquée a la physiologie et a la médecine. Paris: Grosson, Gebon, & Cie, 1982.

Bosse JP, Papillon J. Surgical anatomy of the SMAS at the malar region. In Transactions of the Ninth International Congress of Plastic and Reconstructive Surgeons. New York: McGraw-Hill, 1987, pp 348–349.

Bourquet J. La disparition chirurgicale des rides et plis du visage. Acad Med Paris, October 14, 1919.

Connell BF. Cervical lift: Surgical correction of fat contour problems combined with full width platysma muscle flaps. Aesthetic Plast Surg 1:355–362, 1975.

Dingman RO, Grabb WC. Surgical anatomy of the mandibular ramus of the facial nerve based on the dissection of 100 facial halves. Plast Reconstr Surg 29:266–272, 1962.

Dubin B, Jackson IT, Halim A, Triplett WW, Ferreira M. Anatomy of the buccal fat pad and its clinical significance. Plast Reconstr Surg 83:257–262, 1989.

Furnas DW. The restraining ligaments of the check. Plast Reconstr Surg 83:11–16, 1989.

Guerrerosantos J. Neck lift: Simplified surgical technique, refinements, and clinical classification. Clin Plast Surg 10:379–404, 1983.

Hetter GP. Lipoplasty of the face and neck. In Hetter GP, ed. Lipoplasty: The Theory and Practice of Blunt Suction Lipectomy, 2nd ed. Boston: Little, Brown, 1990, pp 249–269.

Hoffman S, Simon BE. Complications of submental lipectomy. Plast Reconstr Surg 60:889–894, 1977.

Illouz Y-G, de Villers YT. Body Sculpturing by Lipoplasty. New York: Churchill Livingstone, 1989, pp 297–320.

Jost G, Levet Y. Parotid fascia and face lifting: A critical evaluation of the SMAS concept. Plast Reconstr Surg 74:42–51, 1984.

Kaye BC. The extended face lift with ancillary procedures. Ann Plast Surg 6:335–346, 1981.

Mitz V, Peronie M. The superficial musculoaponeurotic system (SMAS) in the parotid and cheek area. Plast Reconstr Surg 58:80–88, 1976.

Mladick RA. Lipoplasty combined with facial rhytidectomy. In Hetter GP, ed. Lipoplasty: The Theory and Practice of Blunt Suction Lipectomy, 2nd ed. Boston: Little, Brown, 1990, pp 270–283.

Newman J, Dolsky RL, Mai ST. Submental liposuction with chin augmentation. Arch Otolaryngol 110:454–457, 1984.

Owsley JQ. Platysma-facial rhytidectomy. Plast Reconstr Surg 60:843–850, 1977.

Rees TD, Aston SJ. A clinical evaluation of the results of submusculoaponeurotic dissection and fixation in face lifts. Plast Reconstr Surg 60:851–859, 1977.

Ruess W, Owsley JQ. The anatomy of the skin and fascial layers of the face in aesthetic surgery. Clin Plast Surg 14:677–682, 1987.

Skoog T. Plastic Surgery. Philadelphia: WB Saunders, 1974, pp 300–330.

Snyder GB. Submental rhytidectomy. Plast Reconstr Surg 62:693–697, 1979.

Tideman H, Bosanquet A, Scott J. Use of the buccal fat pad as a pedicled graft. J Oral Maxillofac Surg 44:435–440, 1986.

Vistnes LM, Souther SG. The anatomical basis for common cosmetic anterior neck deformities. Ann Plast Surg 2:381–388, 1979.

Wilkinson TS. The repair of a submental depression occurring after rhytidectomy. Plast Reconstr Surg 57:33–35, 1976.

Chapter 7

ARMS

Less than 5% of all liposuction involves the upper extremities,[1,2] and brachioplasty constitutes less than 0.2% of all cosmetic surgery procedures.[3] The infrequency of upper extremity cosmetic surgery reflects a relatively low level of patient concern about this area as well as the limited surgical options.

From the patient's perspective, the arms do not have the same intense psychosexual connotations as hips, thighs, and buttocks. Recent fashion trends, moreover, emphasize broader shoulders and a fuller upper body to minimize the apparent size of the hips and thighs. Preoccupation with health and fitness has also made more muscular arms on women acceptable if not desirable.

From the surgeon's point of view, the skin of the arms is thinner and more mobile than skin on the lower extremities. Therefore arm contour adjusts poorly to major fat volume depletions. When brachioplasty is performed, even the most favorable scar is noticeable unless the patient keeps her arms at her side.

Despite these limitations, selected patients will benefit from skillfully performed surgical reduction of the brachial silhouette. For these women, liposuction has increased the ability of the surgeon to slim the arms with minimal scarring.

HISTORY

Early descriptions of brachioplasty were reported by Correa Iturraspe and Fernández,[4] Gillies and Millard,[5] and Clarkson.[6]

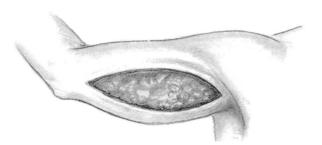
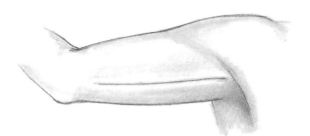

Lewis (1973), Baroudi (1975)

Lewis[7] and Baroudi[8] reduced bulk and ptosis by elliptical excisions of skin and fat along the longitudinal axis of the inner aspect of the arm. Guerrerosantos[9,10] and Grazer and Klingbeil[11] added a large Z-plasty to break up the scar in the axilla. The Z-plasty, of course, further narrowed the transverse dimension of the upper arm.

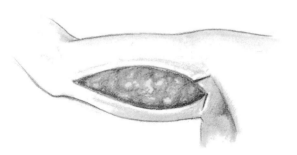
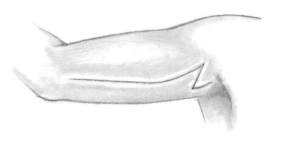

Guerrerosantos (1978, 1979), Grazer and Klingbeil (1980)

Guerrerosantos[9,10] urged a superficial dissection to protect the brachial vein and its accompanying lymphatics and cutaneous nerves. He also emphasized locating the final scar so that it lay against the thorax when the arms were hanging in a rest position.

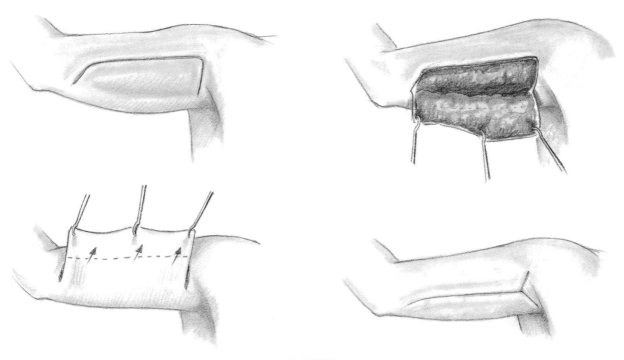

Juri (1979)

McCraw[12] and Teimourian[13] addressed the issue of increased tissue in the proximal aspect of the arm by advocating a T closure with the transverse portion of the T in the axilla and the longitudinal portion running down the inner aspect of the arm. Juri's quadrangular flap also resulted in a T closure.[14]

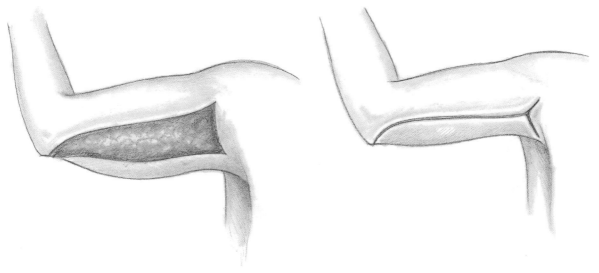

Regnault (1983)

Regnault[15] and Regnault and Daniel[16] used a "fish tail" type excision with a Y closure to excise tissue near the axilla and still keep the scar confined to the axilla and arm.

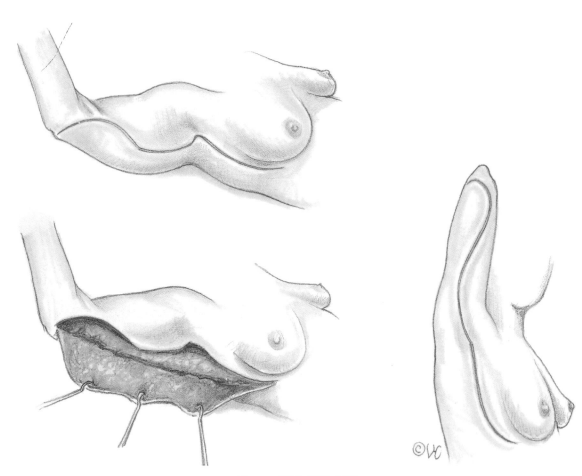

Pitanguy (1975, 1980, 1981)

For massive excess tissue extending onto the chest wall, Zook,[17] Pitanguy,[18-20] and Hallock and Altobelli[21] used excisions extending from the elbow through the axilla and onto the lateral thoracic wall beneath the breast.

All authors acknowledged the very significant scarring that could only be hidden by long-sleeved garments. Attempts to reduce the scarring included Franco's curved closure with the concavity facing posterior[22] and Lewis' and Borges' W-plasty closures.[7,23] Transverse excisions limited to the axilla[13,15] or outer aspect of the elbow[7,24] avoided longitudinal scars down the arm but accomplished little.

With the advent of liposuction, several authors reported its use to reduce fullness.[13,25-27] Although contour diminution by liposuction is limited, the minimal scarring and low morbidity recommend the procedure for properly selected patients.

AESTHETIC AND ANATOMIC CONSIDERATIONS

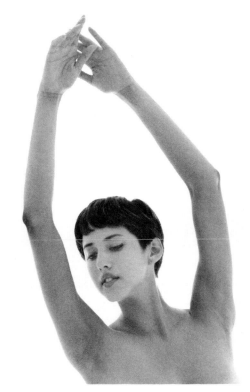

Photo by Richard Imrie

The ideal, youthful feminine arm is lean and tapers smoothly from axilla to elbow. In obese patients the arm is full and bulky, particularly in the proximal area; with age, the brachial skin becomes lax and gradually loses tautness.

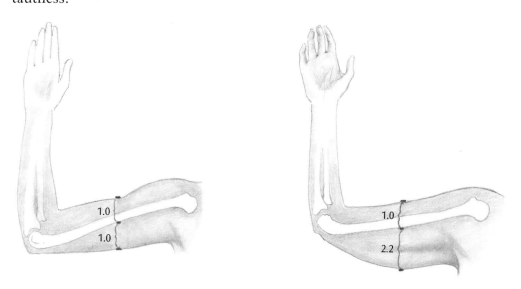

Glanz and González-Ulloa[28] described the coefficient of Hoyer as the ratio of the superior and inferior parts of the arm when the arm is held out from the body at a 90-degree angle. The inferior border of the humerus is used as a reference base. In a 10-year-old girl the coefficient is 1:1.0. By age 70 it increases to 1:2.2.

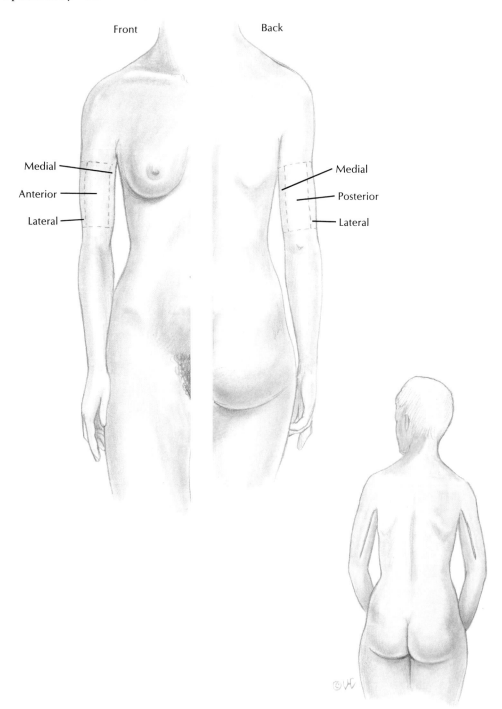

Incorrect placement of scar

Nomenclature relating to the surface of the arm should be precise in order to describe accurately the location of incisions. Guerrerosantos' classification is practical and useful.[9,10] He divides the arm into four surfaces. With the subject upright and the arm hanging in the rest position, the medial surface lies against the thorax; the external or lateral surface is opposite the medial surface, the anterior surface is forward, and the posterior surface is to the rear. A common error in planning can leave scars on the more visible posterior surface.

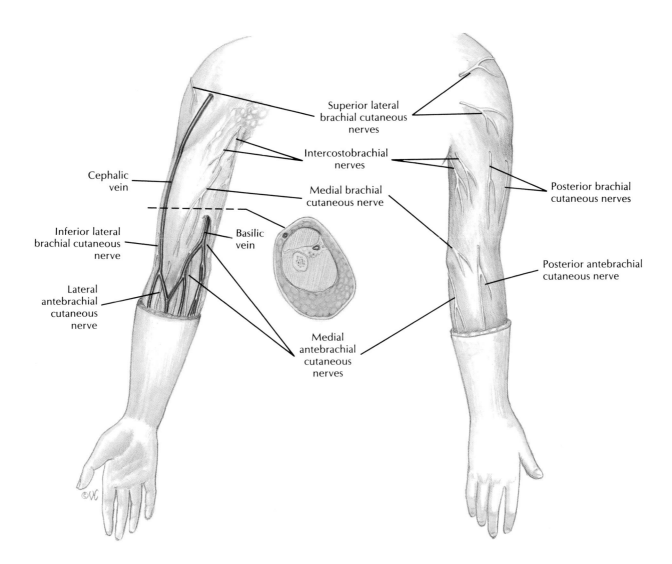

The subcutaneous fat, which is most abundant on the posterior aspect of the arm, lies between the skin and the muscle investing fascia.

Sensory nerves at risk during brachioplasty include the intercostobrachial, medial brachial cutaneous, and medial antebrachial cutaneous. The latter accompanies the basilic vein as it emerges from the deep fascia in the lower half of the arm. The cephalic vein, which is superficial to the deep fascia throughout the arm, is generally out of the field of surgical resection, as are the superior lateral brachial cutaneous nerve (branch of the axillary nerve), the inferior lateral brachial cutaneous nerve, the posterior brachial cutaneous nerve, and the posterior antebrachial cutaneous nerve. The brachial artery and major nerve trunks are deep to the investing fascia. Lymphatics are distributed throughout the arm, but a large group of superficial lymphatics are concentrated along the course of the basilic vein.

CLASSIFICATION AND TREATMENT OPTIONS

I divide surgical patients into three groups.

Group	Condition of Skin and Fat	Treatment Options
I	Minimal to moderate fat excess; taut skin	Liposuction only
II	Minimal to moderate fat excess; loose skin	Liposuction plus skin excision
III	Loose skin secondary to weight loss or senile laxity	Skin excision only

The massively obese are not candidates for surgery.

PATIENT EVALUATION AND COUNSELING
Physical Examination

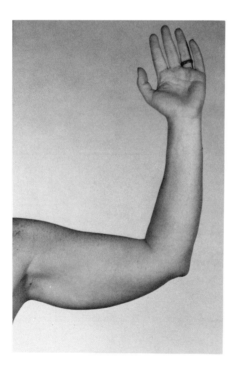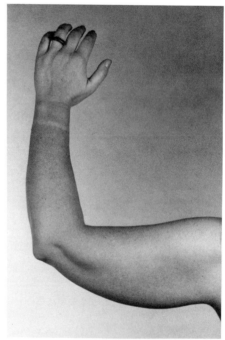

The bulk of subcutaneous fat is on the posterior aspect of the arm and is most noticeable when the arm is held out at a 90-degree angle. A few patients will have significant subcutaneous fat deposits in other brachial areas, most often the lateral and anterior and less often the medial. The deltoid area can also be the site of a large subcutaneous fat collection.

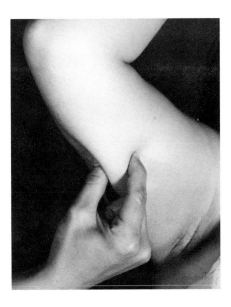

Patients are examined upright with arms held out at 90 degrees to evaluate volume of fat and degree of skin laxity. The skin is gently pinched between the fingers to assess thickness of the fat. At least 2 cm of pinch should be demonstrable if the patient is to benefit from liposuction.

Defining Patient Goals

Patients seek help for one or more of the following reasons: their arms are bulky, the soft tissues are loose, or the skin is wrinkled. Generally the appearance of their arms is less troubling when their hands are held at their sides. Raising the arms to point or engage in athletic activities is embarrassing because it emphasizes bulk and/or flaccidity. Patients will often avoid wearing short-sleeved or sleeveless garments.

The normal or slightly overweight patient with excessive bulk due to fat (group I) can be successfully treated with liposuction and should be encouraged to proceed so long as she is aware of the limitations inherent in the procedure and the relatively subtle nature of the expected improvement.

The patient with excessive bulk and loose skin (group II) can also be successfully treated with liposuction. Although there is more fat to remove than in group I patients, the loose skin shrinks poorly, and volume reduction must be conservative. These patients should be educated to expect a limited result. Skin excision can effectively reduce contour in group II patients, but since their skin is relatively smooth due to excess fat, they will only rarely accept a brachioplasty scar as the necessary trade-off for greater contour reduction.

The patient most likely to accept and benefit from a brachioplasty scar is the patient with little subcutaneous fat whose skin is already markedly wrinkled and furrowed from age or weight loss (group III).

Informed Consent

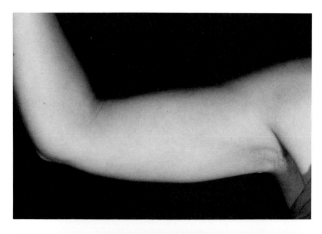

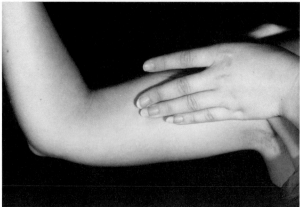

Under the best of circumstances, liposuction of the arms will produce only a modest degree of improvement. To demonstrate this to the patient I stand her in front of a wall mirror and pull up on the skin of the arm to show the expected degree of improvement. Most patients accept an honest explanation of what can and cannot reasonably be expected and are grateful for a realistic assessment of expected results. A large number will opt for a subtle change in contour.

As for liposuction of any area, the patient should be informed in advance of the potential for increased wrinkling, skin irregularities, and contour defects following surgery.

When brachioplasty is indicated, the surgeon should explain clearly the permanent nature of the scarring. Although the scar fades with time, it is a permanent, visible reminder of surgery.

LIPOSUCTION
Markings

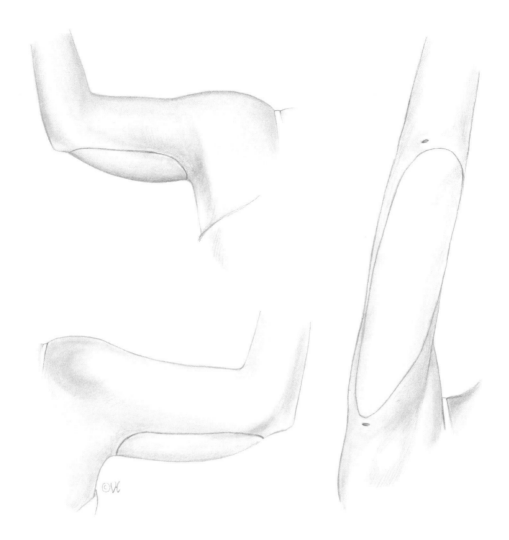

The posterior brachial area is treated most frequently. The patient is marked in the standing position with arms held out 90 degrees from the shoulders. Areas of excess fat are outlined as well as two access incisions: one near the medial epicondyle and one in the axilla. If necessary, additional access incisions can be added at convenient and inconspicuous locations.

Operative Technique

If only the arms are treated, local anesthesia is satisfactory. I infiltrate generous volumes of 0.05% lidocaine with 1:1,000,000 epinephrine.

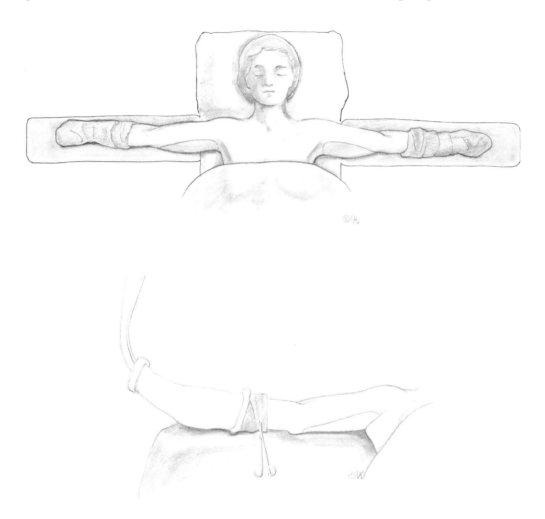

The patient is placed supine on the operating table with arms extended to 90 degrees. An intravenous catheter is inserted in a foot vein, and monitoring devices are placed on the lower extremity. The entire upper extremity, shoulder area, and adjacent anterolateral thorax are prepped. If lower extremity venous access is contraindicated, a hand or wrist vein may be used and a sterile stockinette placed over the intravenous line.

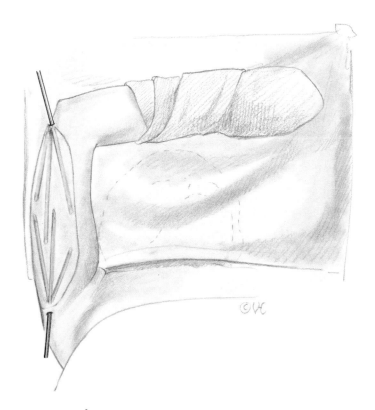

A 2.4 or 3.7 mm Mercedes Type cannula, approximately 20 cm in length, is used for suctioning. Volume of aspirate ranges from 100 to 200 cc. A 20 cm cannula permits creation of crossing tunnels from proximal and distal access incisions.

An assistant holds the patient's arm to maintain its position. If a general anesthetic has been used, the shoulder should not be abducted beyond 90 degrees from the sagittal plane to avoid brachial plexus traction injury.

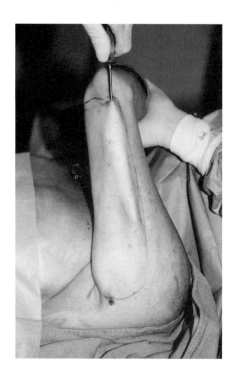

I begin suctioning from the distal access incision. Half of the estimated total volume is removed, concentrating on those areas that seem to have the most fat but proceeding in a systematic fashion to treat the entire distal two thirds of the arm. Although the ulnar nerve is in close proximity to the medial epicondyle, it is deep to the investing fascia and should not be at risk.

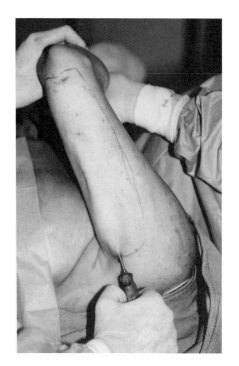

The patient's upper body is rolled slightly for access to the incision near the axilla. I then treat the proximal two thirds of the arm, stopping periodically to check for thickness of the subcutaneous layer and smoothness of excision. The area of maximum overlap of the cannulas will be the central third of the arm, which is usually the area of maximal fat deposition. Care must be exercised not to overresect in this area.

The identical procedure is performed on the other arm. As with all bilateral areas, attainment of symmetry is aided by comparison of volumes from right and left sides. With the patient supine a visual comparison of both sides can be made.

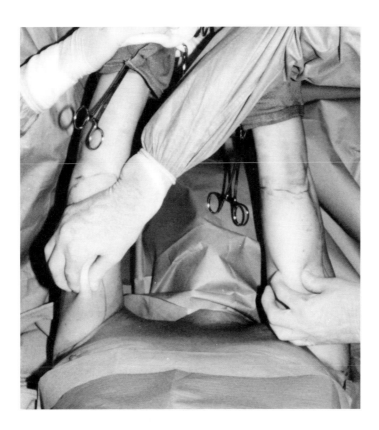

The exact thickness of skin at the end point varies depending on the patient's age, weight, body habitus, and other clinical factors. Generally, however, it is prudent to maintain a pinched skin thickness of no less than 1 cm. Note the bilateral pinch test after treatment of the right arm but before liposuction of the left arm.

Postoperative Care and Recovery

After wound closure a 4-inch thick elastic bandage is wrapped around the arm to provide gentle compression. Alternatively, a ¼-inch thick foam compression sponge (Reston) can be placed over the treated area.

The patient is instructed to rest in bed and keep her arms elevated on pillows for 24 hours. Forty-eight hours after surgery she is examined in the office, and skin staples and the dressing are removed. Sedentary activities are generally unrestricted after the first 48 hours. Sports activities may be resumed in 2 weeks.

Results

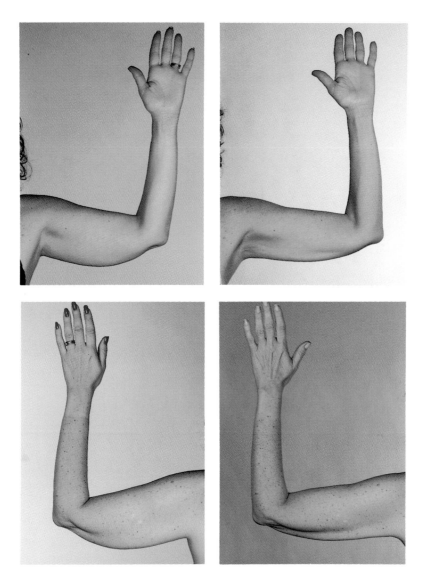

This 48-year-old, 5-foot 5-inch, 140-pound woman had undergone success-ful liposuction of her torso and lower extremities. She returned seeking contour reduction of her arms. There was a notable thickness of the bra-chial silhouette with the arms at 90 degrees. The skin was loose but not wrinkled, and pinch thickness of the posterior arm was 3 cm. I told the patient that liposuction would reduce arm fullness, but the results would be more subtle than those obtained in the torso and lower extremities. I mentioned that brachioplasty was an alternative but that the resultant scar-ring would be unacceptable given the overall good quality of her skin.

She is shown before and 16 months after liposuction of 150 cc from the posterior aspect of each arm. Her improvement is manifest as a straighten-ing of the inferior brachial border. The apparent overall size reduction is due to slight differences in photographic technique used for pre- and post-operative views.

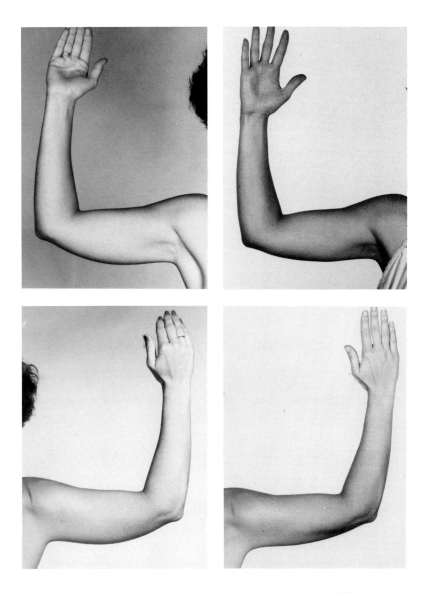

This 34-year-old, 5-foot 5-inch, 125-pound woman had liposuction of her torso and lower extremities. She returned asking for reduction of her arm silhouette because her slight upper arm fullness was an embarrassment when wearing short sleeves. The pinch thickness was 2.5 cm over the posterior arm. The skin was moderately loose. She is shown before and 9 months after liposuction of 150 cc from the posterior aspect of each arm. The rather subtle straightening of the inferior border of her arm pleased the patient, who felt more confident when wearing short-sleeve and sleeveless styles.

BRACHIOPLASTY
Markings

Excision is planned so that the final scars are on the medial aspect of the arm and are not visible from behind when the arms are at the side. The patient is marked standing with arms held up at right angles from the body.

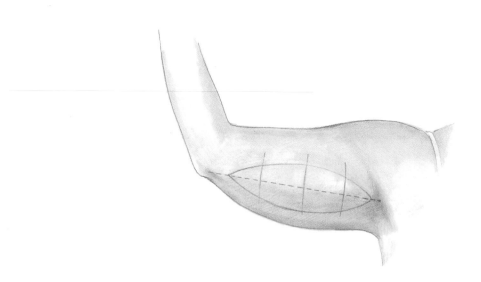

A reference line indicating the position of final closure is drawn along the brachial groove running from the medial epicondyle to the apex of the axilla. The planned excision is drawn as an eccentric ellipse with the brachial groove as its central axis. The length and width of the ellipse depend on the planned excision and are determined by pinching the skin to ascertain the degree of laxity. Most often the proximal end of the ellipse begins at the axilla and extends as far down the arm as necessary, usually ending proximal to the medial epicondyle. Transverse lines drawn along the ellipse assist in alignment of skin during closure.

Operative Technique

Anesthesia, positioning, and draping are identical to that for brachial liposuction.

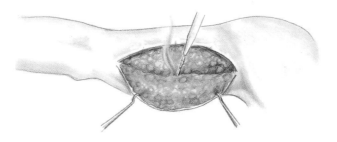

The skin is divided along the superior line of the ellipse, and an electrocautery is used to raise an inferiorly based flap. The plane of dissection is through the superficial fat. The deep fat is left undisturbed to protect the basilic vein and accompanying lymphatics and to preserve maximal skin sensibility.

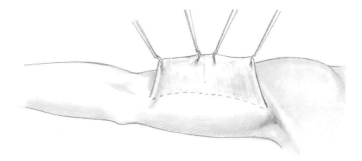

The flap is undermined as far as the preoperative estimate of the extent of resection. Additional dissection is neither necessary nor desirable. The flap is then pulled in an upward direction, and the contour of the lower border of the arm is observed to estimate the correct level of excision. The effect should be one of smooth diminution of size with no central constriction.

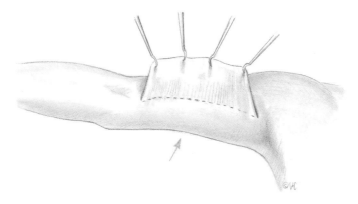

Excessive tension on the flap will constrict the central third of the arm. If an area of constriction is present, flap tension is decreased.

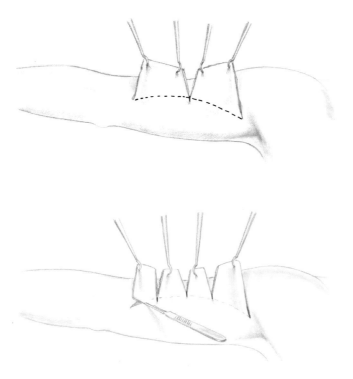

The excess is cut away in a segmental fashion.

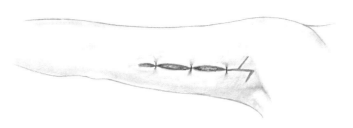

Deep tissues are closed with 0 chromic sutures.

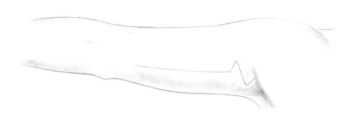

The skin is closed with running subcuticular 3-0 polydioxanone sutures (PDS). If necessary, a Z-plasty in or near the axilla can be used to prevent contracture and further reduce the transverse dimension of the upper arm.

Postoperative Care and Recovery

Light dressings are secured with loosely wrapped compressive bandages. The patient is instructed to rest with arms elevated on pillows for 48 hours before she resumes limited activities. Vigorous sports using the arms are prohibited for 6 weeks.

Results

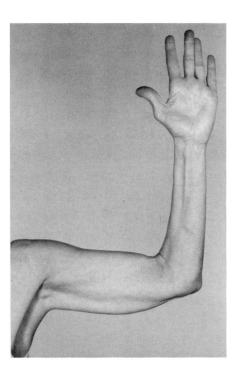

This 66-year-old, 5-foot 3-inch, 105-pound woman complained of looseness and wrinkling of upper arm skin, particularly redundant skin proximal to the elbow. The pinch thickness was less than 2 cm over her posterior arm, and the skin was flaccid with wrinkling near the elbow. Although she was classified a group III patient, I judged her concern to be inordinate relative to objective findings and asked her to defer surgery. Over the course of 2 years it became apparent that excess skin was such an emotional burden that a brachioplasty scar would be relatively unimportant in comparison.

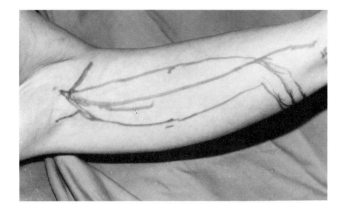

I planned a medial brachial skin excision to extend behind the elbow to remove as much skin as possible in that region.

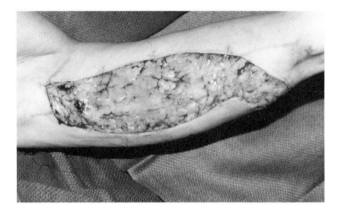

Very little fat was present and the surgical specimen was predominantly skin.

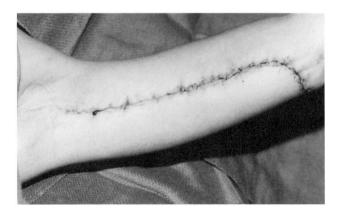

Closure did not require a Z-plasty.

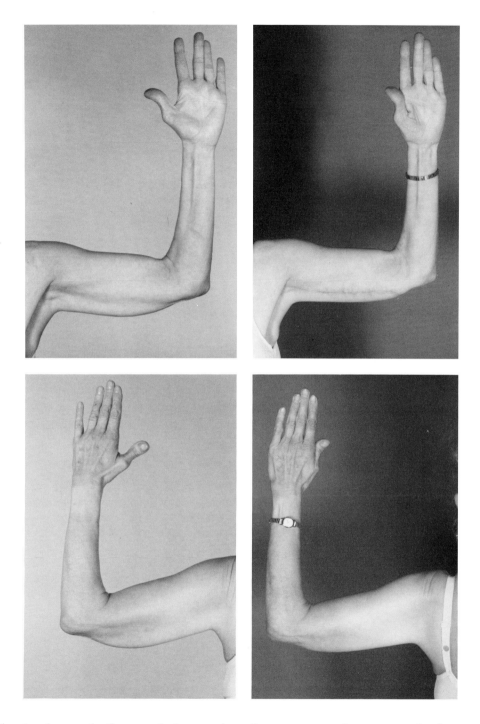

She is shown before and 6 months after surgery. As expected, the scar concerned her not at all. Although scarring was not a problem for this patient, should she have a secondary procedure, I would design the excision to relocate the scar more anteriorly so that it would be less visible when she had her hands at her sides.

SUCTION COMBINED WITH BRACHIOPLASTY

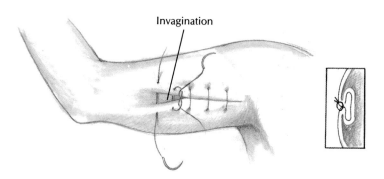

Grazer[26] treats patients for combined skin and fat excess without raising a flap. He removes the fat by closed suction and then uses the tailor-tack principle[29] to estimate the amount of excess skin.

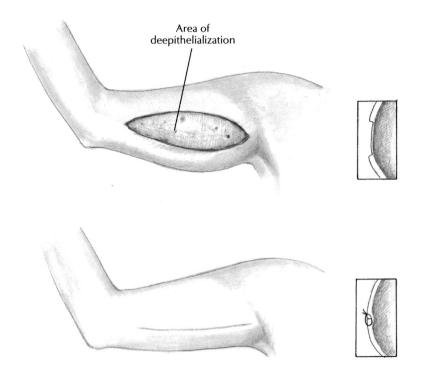

He deepithelializes the excess skin and then buries the deepithelialized segment with plication sutures to reduce the skin envelope. If there is excess tension at closure, he performs additional suctioning to reduce volume. The simplicity of this technique is appealing, and preservation of neurovascular connections between the fascia and skin is theoretically advantageous.

COMPLICATIONS AND UNAESTHETIC RESULTS
Liposuction

The posterior arm is subject to waviness, irregularities, and contour depressions.[25] The skin is relatively thin with a paucity of attachments from the deep fascia to the dermis. Consequently, reduction in fat volume produces only a limited amount of skin shrinkage, predisposing to wrinkling and puckering.

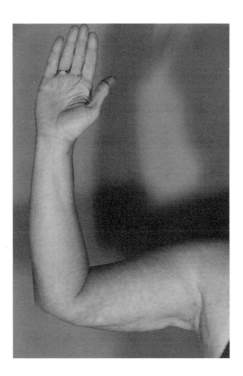

One year earlier this 50-year-old woman had undergone liposuction of the posterior arm. Overresection and failure to taper the excision with adjacent medial and lateral areas resulted in a noticeable depression near the axilla and wrinkling of the posterior arm skin. Use of fine cannulas and conservatism in volume can help prevent such problems. I performed circumferential arm liposuction to reduce overall bulk, but the increased skin laxity and irregularities could only be corrected by brachioplasty, an option she refused.

Brachioplasty

Hematomas and seromas are uncommon. Excessive skin resection with tight closure can result in suture-line dehiscence, marginal wound slough, and prolonged edema of the distal extremity. Edema will be aggravated if the basilic vein or its accompanying lymphatics are divided.

Unaesthetic results include poor scar placement with the scar visible from behind, hypertrophic scarring, transverse skin furrowing caused by excessive skin resection, and central constriction with bulging at the ends of the wounds when a disproportionately large amount of tissue has been excised centrally.

──────────── REFERENCES ────────────

1. Illouz Y-G. Body contouring by lipolysis: A 5-year experience with over 3,000 cases. Plast Reconstr Surg 72:591-597, 1983.
2. Pitman GH, Teimourian B. Suction lipectomy: Complications and results by survey. Plast Reconstr Surg 76:65-69, 1985.
3. American Society of Plastic and Reconstructive Surgeons. Membership survey, July 8, 1991.
4. Correa Iturraspe M, Fernández JC. Dermolipectomía braquial. La Prensa Med 41: 24-32, 1954.
5. Gillies H, Millard DR. The Principles and Art of Plastic Surgery. Boston: Little, Brown, 1957, p 404.
6. Clarkson P. Lipodystrophies. Plast Reconstr Surg 37:499-503, 1966.
7. Lewis JR. Atlas of Aesthetic Plastic Surgery. Boston: Little, Brown, 1973, pp 271-278.
8. Baroudi R. Dermatolipectomy of the upper arm. Clin Plast Surg 2:485-494, 1975.
9. Guerrerosantos J. Arm-lift. In Courtiss EH, ed. Aesthetic Surgery: Trouble, How to Avoid It and How to Treat It. St. Louis: CV Mosby, 1978, pp 232-246.
10. Guerrerosantos J. Brachioplasty. Aesthetic Plast Surg 3:1-14, 1979.
11. Grazer FM, Klingbeil JR. Body Image: A Surgical Perspective. St. Louis: CV Mosby, 1980, pp 357-378.
12. McCraw LH. Surgical rehabilitation after massive weight reduction. Plast Reconstr Surg 53:349-352, 1974.
13. Teimourian B. Suction Lipectomy and Body Sculpturing. St. Louis: CV Mosby, 1987, pp 163-192.
14. Juri J, Juri C, Elias JC. Arm dermolipectomy with a quadrangular flap "T" closure. Plast Reconstr Surg 64:521-525, 1979.
15. Regnault P. Brachioplasty, axilloplasty, and preaxilloplasty. Aesthetic Plast Surg 7: 31-36, 1983.
16. Regnault P, Daniel RK. Upper extremity. In Regnault P, Daniel RK, eds. Aesthetic Plastic Surgery. Boston: Little, Brown, 1984, pp 693-704.
17. Zook EG. The massive weight loss patient. Clin Plast Surg 2:457-466, 1975.
18. Pitanguy I. Correction of lipodystrophy of the lateral thoracic aspect and inner side of the arm and elbow dermosenescence. Clin Plast Surg 2:477-483, 1975.
19. Pitanguy I. Aesthetic plastic surgery of the upper and lower limbs. Aesthetic Plast Surg 4:363-372, 1980.
20. Pitanguy I. Aesthetic Plastic Surgery of the Head and Body. New York: Springer-Verlag, 1981, pp 153-159.

21. Hallock GG, Altobelli JA. Simultaneous brachioplasty, thoracoplasty, and mammoplasty. Aesthetic Plast Surg 9:223-235, 1985.
22. Franco T. Aesthetic surgery of the upper and lower limbs. Aesthetic Plast Surg 4:245-256, 1980.
23. Borges AF. W-plasty dermolipectomy to correct "bat-wing" deformity. Ann Plast Surg 9:494-501, 1982.
24. Kostianovsky AS. Aesthetic surgery of the elbow. Aesthetic Plast Surg 5:163-167, 1981.
25. Burkhardt BR. Lipolysis of the arms. In Hetter GP, ed. Lipoplasty: The Theory and Practice of Blunt Suction Lipectomy. Boston: Little, Brown, 1984, pp 211-217.
26. Grazer FM. Body contouring. In McCarthy JG, ed. Plastic Surgery. Philadelphia: WB Saunders, 1990, pp 3981-3988.
27. Illouz Y-G, de Villers YT. Body Sculpturing by Lipoplasty. New York: Churchill Livingstone, 1989, pp 281-282, 353-356.
28. Glanz S, González-Ulloa M. Aesthetic surgery of the arm. Aesthetic Plast Surg 5:1-17, 1981.
29. Widden PG. Tailor-tack mastopexy. Plast Reconstr Surg 62:347-354, 1978.

Chapter 8

BREAST AND CHEST WALL

Liposuction has significantly improved our ability to treat gynecomastia. It permits more rapid, efficient, and controlled tissue removal, facilitating consistently good results without some of the drawbacks of open surgical excision. In particular, it has largely eliminated contour irregularities as a complication. It has also decreased the incidence of hematoma and has reduced the number of patients who require skin excision beyond the confines of the areola.

The uses of liposuction for female breast reduction are much more circumscribed, and although the technique can facilitate procedures in extremely fatty breasts, its use for women has not had the same impact as for men.

Finally, liposuction has been used to treat excess fatty deposits of the extramammary chest wall. Results are limited since the excess fat is frequently accompanied by obesity and/or skin laxity.

TREATMENT OF GYNECOMASTIA

Gynecomastia is the unilateral or bilateral development of female-like breasts in a man. The word is derived from the Greek *gyne,* meaning "woman," and *mastos,* meaning "breast." The incidence of gynecomastia in adults has been reported to be 32% by Carlson[1] and 36% by Nuttall.[2] It is seen frequently as a transient phenomenon during puberty and is a normal part of male adolescence. After performing approximately 2000 examinations at a Boy Scout summer camp over a 3-year-period, Nydick et al.[3] found an incidence of 38.7% in 13- to 17-year-olds. The peak incidence (14.6%) was found at 14 to 14½ years. In only 27.1% of the boys did enlargement persist through two summers and in 7.7% through three summers.

197

History

Paulus Aegeneta[4] (625-690 B.C.) is credited with first describing surgical intervention for gynecomastia. In the first half of the twentieth century almost all surgical solutions for gynecomastia involved scars extending beyond the areola, and at least one surgeon[5] recommended excision of the nipple and areola altogether, stating that "the nipple is of little consequence to the male patient."

In 1928 Dufourmentel[6] reported treating gynecomastia through an incision limited to the areola-skin junction. Perhaps because Dufourmentel's article was largely concerned with the female breast, his technique was not widely adopted until Webster's publication on the use of a "semicircular intraareolar incision" for gynecomastia.[7] Webster's detailed report on treatment of 32 breasts in 17 patients had such impact that the periareolar incision became the standard of care. Webster recommended leaving a thick layer of tissue just beneath the areola to prevent a central depression, careful tapering at the periphery of the excision to prevent abrupt contour irregularities, and suture approximation of residual breast tissue beneath the areola also to prevent central depression. Of note, 4 of his 17 patients required drainage or aspiration of seromas or hematomas.

To improve operative exposure Barsky, Kahn, and Simon[8] recommended an "inverted omega" scar with short horizontal arms running out from either side of an inferior semicircular periareolar scar. Other surgeons subsequently proposed straight-line incisions contained within the areola. Pitanguy[9] described an incision through the transverse diameter of the nipple-areola complex, and Eade[10] advocated an incision limited to the radius of the areola. The short length of Eade's incision mandated a largely blind sharp dissection to excise breast tissue and resulted in a high incidence of postoperative hematoma. Balch[11] avoided a scar on the chest altogether by using a transaxillary approach.

Several surgeons addressed the problem of removing excess skin while still confining the ultimate scar to the border of the areola. Letterman and Schurter's superior crescent excision permitted removal of a limited amount of skin and upward movement of the nipple-areola complex with a scar restricted to the superior half of the periareola.[12] Huang, Hidalgo, and Lewis's "apple core" technique[13] and Davidson's excision of a "donut" of skin around the areola[14] were also attempts to reduce skin and still keep the scar confined to the periareola.

For larger skin excisions and ptotic breasts approaching female size, surgeons were willing to accept scars beyond the confines of the areola. Several authors recommended pedicled transpositions of the nipple-areola combined with extensive skin resections[15-18] modeled after the oblique reduction technique of Dufourmentel and Mouly.[19] Others preferred transverse skin excisions and elevation of the nipple as a free graft.[20,21]

With the advent of liposuction, it became apparent that the fatty component of the breasts could be reduced through minuscule incisions. Teimourian and Perlman[22] were the first to publish their experience, and others followed.[23-25] All recommended liposuction of the fatty component and, if necessary, removal of residual glandular tissue by direct excision. Rosenberg[26] reported removal of glandular material by liposuction, but his technique was criticized as inadequate.[25,27]

Surgeons using liposuction relied on skin redraping and retraction by intact connective tissue bands to reduce the skin envelope.[22-25] Cohen[27] and Cohen, Pozez, and McKeown[28] recommended liposuction, open glandular removal, and extensive skin undermining beneath the inframammary crease to permit optimal redraping and obviate the need for skin resection, even for large skin redundancies.

Anatomic Considerations and Pathophysiology

In the normal adult male breast, glandular tissue is limited to the area directly beneath the nipple and areola and is usually not palpable as a discrete mass.[29] The nipple-areola complex usually varies from 2 to 4 cm in diameter. It is most commonly located over the fourth interspace but may be as high as the fourth rib or as low as the fifth interspace. Although some fullness in the chest is acceptable, particularly in muscular men, the desired male chest is generally flat and featureless save for the nipple-areola complexes.

Swelling associated with gynecomastia may occur as a circumscribed, firm, glandular mass of varying size just beneath the areola or may be a diffuse, fatty fullness of the chest with ill-defined margins. Aiache[30] has described extensive glandular enlargement extending well beyond the areola in body builders who use anabolic steroids.

In glandular hyperplasia the microscopic appearance depends on the duration of the condition.[31] Gynecomastia of recent onset will show a highly cellular or proliferative stroma containing many ducts. Proliferation does not progress to tubular or acinar formation. Patients with long-standing gynecomastia have little ductal proliferation and extensive stromal fibrosis. Once the fibrotic state has been reached, gynecomastia is unlikely to spontaneously regress even after removal of the inciting cause. If the mass is associated with obesity, the characteristic histologic finding is fat.

The cause of gynecomastia is uncertain, but most authorities attribute it to stimulation of breast tissue by excess circulating estrogens or estrogen-like substances. Detailed reviews of this subject can be found in several publications.[1,28,32-34]

Common associated physiologic conditions include puberty and senescence. Obesity may contribute to gynecomastia at any age. Associated pathologic conditions include Klinefelter's syndrome and other causes of hypogonadism. Hyperthyroidism is the most common associated endocrine disorder. The condition is also seen in patients with alcoholic cirrhosis and in patients who are refed after starvation. Tumors are a rare cause of gynecomastia, but some patients with testicular tumors will develop gynecomastia, as will those with malignant adrenal cortical tumors or pulmonary carcinoma secreting human chorionic gonadotropin. A multitude of drugs, legal and illegal, have also been associated with gynecomastia. Digitalis compounds, clomiphene, spironolactone, phenytoin, and diazepam are some of the agents known to cause breast enlargement. Marijuana is the best documented of the illicit causes. Anabolic steroid abuse among body builders has also been associated with glandular hyperplasia.[30]

Successful medical management is directed at finding the underlying cause and treating the condition, if possible. Treatment with various drugs has been tried, but serious side effects have limited the utility of drug therapy.

In most patients the cause is never discovered. If the duration of the disease has been long and the condition is asymptomatic, extensive laboratory investigation is generally unproductive, and the cause may be ignored in otherwise healthy patients.[1]

Classification and Treatment Options

The classification of Simon, Hoffman, and Kahn[20] was once the most useful. They categorized male breast enlargements as small, moderate, and marked, with the last category requiring extra-areolar skin excisions. Cohen's more recent four-category classification distinguished gynecomastia of largely fat origin from gynecomastia that is predominantly glandular.[27] Cohen's categorization also identified those patients with ptosis.

I find classifications based on the presence of fat vs. glandular material unnecessary. It is usually impossible to make this assessment preoperatively, and since the patient is prepared for liposuction and possible glandular excision prior to surgery, the distinction is unnecessary.

Of more importance is the preoperative identification of patients who will require extra-areolar skin excision. Even before liposuction was used, the vast majority of patients required no skin excision. In 117 patients treated by Von Kessel et al.[35] and 70 patients treated by Simon, Hoffman, and Kahn,[20] extra-areolar incisions were needed in only 7.5% and 14.3% of patients, respectively.

Although Cohen, Pozez, and McKeown[28] believe that liposuction and glandular excision combined with extensive sharp dissection beneath the submammary fold can eliminate the need for skin excision in all patients, my own experience and that of others[23,25] is that occasional patients with severe ptosis will still require skin removal to achieve a flat chest. These patients should be identified at the time of initial examination to avoid unsatisfactory results and the need for secondary procedures.

Initially I use liposuction alone to remove the fatty component of gynecomastia. If a residual glandular mass persists after suction, I make an inferior semicircular periareolar incision for glandular resection. If the breasts are ptotic, circumferential excision around the areola with a purse-string type closure[36] permits skin reduction with scars still confined to the periareola.

Preoperative Evaluation and Counseling
Indications

The indication for surgery is the presence of a persistent mass that becomes embarrassing to the patient. Some men refuse to go to the beach and will not wear tight-fitting shirts. Although adolescent gynecomastia is usually self-limited, if the mass persists after 2 years and is emotionally disabling to the patient, surgery is indicated.

History and Physical Examination

The age of onset and duration of the condition are important. Prepubertal gynecomastia is rare and deserves investigation. Adolescent gynecomastia is common but usually transitory and generally is neither investigated nor treated. Gynecomastia during and after middle age is usually related to testicular involution and/or obesity. A careful drug history is mandatory for all patients.

The presence of a unilateral or bilateral mass is the hallmark of gynecomastia. If the tumor is mostly glandular, the mass will be firm, discrete, and centered under but not always limited to the subareola. It is usually nontender. A hard and/or fixed mass is suggestive of carcinoma and should be biopsied prior to definitive treatment. If there is a significant component of fat, the mass will be softer and more diffuse. It is sometimes difficult to differentiate between fat and glandular tissue at the initial examination, but the preoperative distinction is largely academic since all patients should be prepared for liposuction followed by open excision for glandular material when necessary.

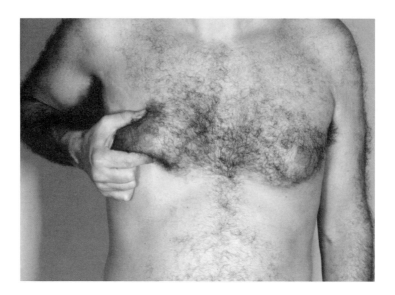

The pinch test is an important diagnostic aid since it will help distinguish between excess subcutaneous tissue fullness and fullness from a well-developed pectoralis major.

The testes should be examined since either testicular enlargement or atrophy can be associated with gynecomastia.

Informed Consent

Preoperative asymmetry should be pointed out to the patient since perfect postoperative asymmetry may not be obtainable. All patients are also told that the initial surgical treatment is liposuction, but if glandular tissue remains after liposuction, it will be removed with open dissection. The access incision sites for suction and the potential periareolar incision for glandular removal are outlined on the chest wall. When extra-areolar scars are planned, their length and location are detailed. The possibility of secondary surgery is also explained in advance.

Some diminution in nipple-areola sensibility is inevitable and patients should be told of this in advance.

Liposuction
Markings

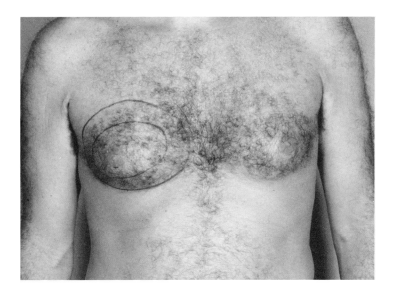

The patient is marked in the standing position. Concentric circles are used to create a topographic demarcation of the areas to be treated. Access incisions are also marked.

Operative Technique

I routinely use general anesthesia. After anesthesia is induced, the entire area is infiltrated with large volumes of 0.05% lidocaine with 1:1,000,000 epinephrine. Enough solution is used to distend the tissues. The patient is positioned supine with arms at his side.

Suction volumes vary with the size of the area to be aspirated but commonly range from 75 to 250 cc. I use 3.7 mm diameter Mercedes Type cannulas for the more peripheral areas and 2.4 mm diameter cannulas to remove tissue in the subareolar region. The smaller cannulas more easily penetrate the fibrous glandular tissue beneath the areola. I do not believe that significant amounts of glandular material can be aspirated, but the associated fat is more easily removed with the smaller cannulas.

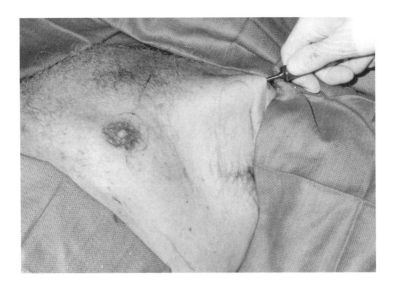

Ten minutes after infiltration stab incisions are made at the 6 o'clock position of the skin-areola junction and in an axillary crease. Suction is carried out first from the axilla. Pretunneling or establishment of the plane by sharp dissection is not necessary, and the tip is directed and redirected in a radial fashion to reach 3 to 5 cm beyond all involved areas. Although the majority of suctioning is in the central, fullest areas, the entire anterior chest should be reached as well as the upper abdomen in some patients. The cannula is kept close to the fascia.

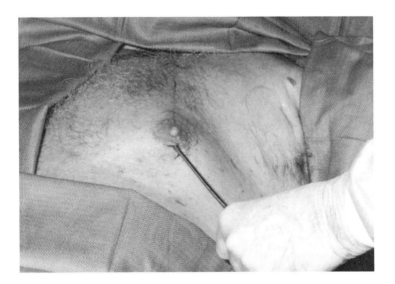

After half the expected volume has been removed, I place the cannula in the areolar incision and suction the entire area again. An incision in an existing inframammary crease can also be used.

The chest skin is assessed by the diminution in contour and by the pinch test. When larger volumes are aspirated, particularly in patients with potential skin excess, contour is assessed with the patient in a sitting position.

Glandular Resection

After suctioning is completed, the area is palpated; if a firm glandular mass is still present, the periareolar stab wound is extended around the areola to the 3 and 9 o'clock positions at a depth of 10 to 15 mm.

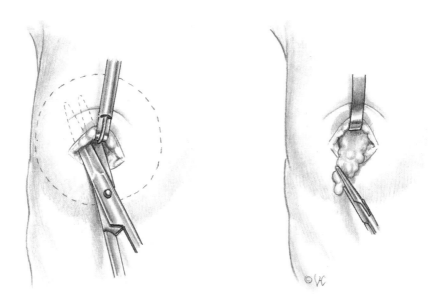

The nipple–areola complex and surrounding skin are undermined sharply 3 to 5 cm beyond the areola, the extent depending on the size of the glandular mass. A 10 to 15 mm thickness of tissue is left on the undersurface of the flap. It is particularly important to leave a thick flap directly beneath the nipple–areola.

With the use of a lighted fiberoptic retractor and a headlight, the glandular mass is excised, taking care to taper the edges of the excision. The fascia over the pectoralis major is left intact. If the residual mass is large, it may be divided into two segments before it is delivered from the wound. A two-layer skin closure followed by application of a light dressing and a Jobst support garment completes the procedure. Unless the glandular resection is very large, I do not drain the wound.

Postoperative Care

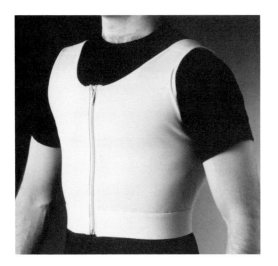

Skin sutures are removed 4 to 5 days after surgery. Patients will experience considerable swelling, which may persist for as long as 12 weeks. Wearing of the support garment is a critical component of postoperative care. Patients are instructed to wear the garment continuously for 6 weeks, at which time they are examined. If still swollen, they continue to wear the garment until the swelling subsides. Bruising follows a course similar to that of liposuction in other areas. Patients generally return to sedentary activities 72 hours following surgery.

Results

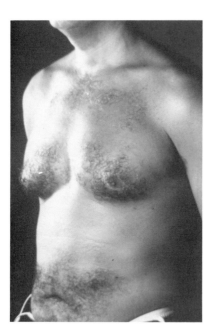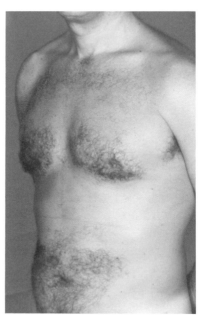

This 42-year-old physician had had enlargement of the chest since puberty. At 5 feet 10 inches and 186 pounds he was 15 pounds above what he considered his ideal weight. Examination revealed soft and full breast tissue without a discrete, palpable glandular mass. He is shown 6 months after liposuction of 200 cc from each breast.

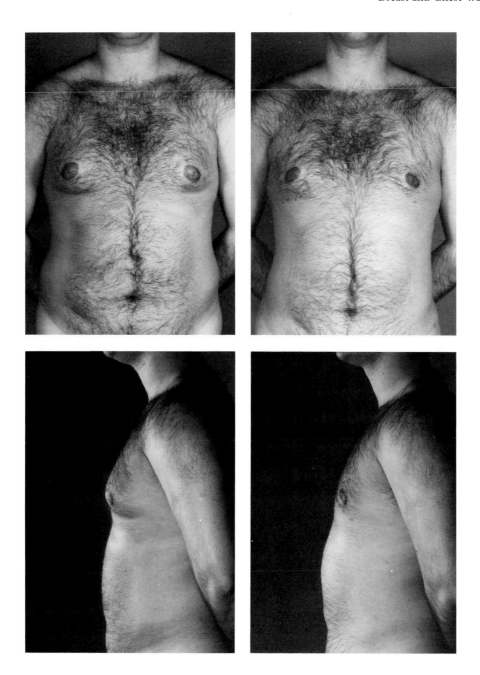

Since adolescence this 29-year-old man had had excessive fullness of the chest. Recent weight gain accentuated the problem. On preoperative examination an apparent glandular mass in addition to diffuse fullness was noted. A volume of 250 cc was suctioned from each breast; the right breast was explored through an inferior periareolar incision, but no residual glandular material was found. The results 5 months after surgery show improvement. The right side was slightly larger than the left before and after surgery.

Complications and Unaesthetic Results

Hematomas and seromas were once frequent complications of surgery for gynecomastia.[7,10,13] Liposuction has largely eliminated this problem. If open excision is used, careful hemostasis with the aid of a lighted fiberoptic retractor is mandatory. Although drains will not prevent hematomas, they may reduce the incidence of seromas, and suction drains should be placed after extensive dissections. Infection and necrosis are rare.

Hypertrophic Scarring

The scars from the liposuction procedure are generally inconsequential, and it is rare for a periareolar scar to be problematic. It is common, however, for scars outside of the areola to be hypertrophic and conspicuous.

Contour Deformity

A postoperative concavity beneath the nipple-areola and surrounding area is generally seen only with open dissection and failure to leave adequate soft tissue on the nipple-areola flap and surrounding skin. Depressions in more peripheral areas with abrupt contour changes in surrounding untreated areas were commonly seen in the past but are rare after liposuction treatment. Secondary suctioning to taper the periphery can improve this deformity.

Residual Skin

Folding of the skin and nipple-areola can occur following large reductions if the skin envelope does not shrink adequately. Ptotic skin may continue to improve for up to a year after surgery, and early attempts to correct it are ill-advised. This problem is best avoided by extra-areolar skin excision on the few patients who have voluminous skin envelopes. These men are frequently but not always older and have some degree of obesity.

Asymmetry

Almost all patients have some preoperative asymmetry, and minor degrees of postoperative asymmetry are common. Right-to-left differences are most frequently due to musculoskeletal conformation and will not benefit from attempts at correction. An obvious postoperative subcutaneous tissue asymmetry should, of course, be treated with secondary suction and/or glandular excision.

Inadequate Resection

The end point of liposuction is readily determined by pinch and palpation. Underresections are uncommon. Careful intraoperative assessment for residual glandular tissue and its appropriate excision are important technical points in avoiding inadequate resection.

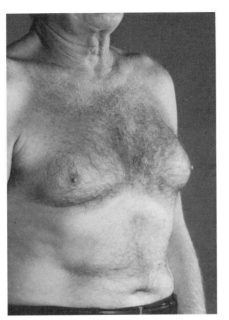 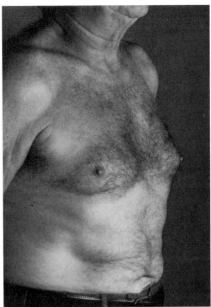

Although this 68-year-old man had a long-standing problem with chest fullness, it became worse in the 10 years prior to consultation. Liposuction of 175 cc reduced breast volume. Glandular material was not excised at the time of surgery, leaving subareolar fullness. He refused an offer of secondary surgery.

TREATMENT OF THE FEMALE BREAST

Liposuction has been applied to volume reduction of the female breast usually as an adjunct to breast reduction or mastopexy.[37-41] According to Teimourian, Massas, and Weigering,[40] the advantages are said to be:

1. Ease of defatting the lateral chest wall and lower chest, particularly in obese patients
2. Ability to remove additional adipose tissue by suction after trial closure without having to take down the closure
3. Maintenance of nipple-areola sensation by combining skin excision with liposuction for volume removal in patients whose breasts are composed largely of adipose tissue
4. Creation of an inframammary fold in breast reconstruction

Liposuction has also been used as a sole modality for breast reduction,[38] but indications are limited to patients whose breasts are mostly fat and who have minimal or no ptosis, an infrequent combination.

I personally do not use liposuction to remove breast tissue in women. The technique is ineffective for removal of glandular tissue, and patients who require mostly fat excision also need skin excision, obviating the advantages of the small scar for liposuction. The remote possibility of missing a malignant tumor or spreading it by the action of the cannula also speaks against use of liposuction in the female breast.

Liposuction can be used adjunctively during breast reduction to remove extramammary fat in areas adjacent to the breast. Fat extending laterally from the breast can be suctioned without lengthening the lateral scar. Of course, if the patient has excessive skin laterally, a direct excision with scars extending past the midaxillary line will be required. The anterior axillary fold may also be suctioned during breast reduction.

OTHER AREAS OF THE CHEST WALL

Additional areas on the thoracic wall that are treated with some frequency include regions adjacent to the anterior and posterior axillary folds and the midback.

Anterior Axillary Fold

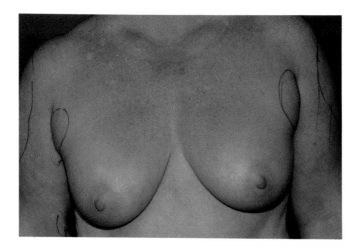

Treatable fullness of the anterior axillary fold is seen most frequently in overweight women and is sometimes a complaint of patients seeking reduction mammaplasty. It is noticeable in bathing attire or when the patient wears off-the-shoulder evening dresses. This patient has also been marked for liposuction of the deltoid area and arms.

The pinch test will distinguish if the fold contains significant fat or is mostly excess skin. A minimal pinch thickness of 1.5 cm is desirable in order to treat this area successfully. If there is lax skin, suction is contraindicated since it will only aggravate the problem.

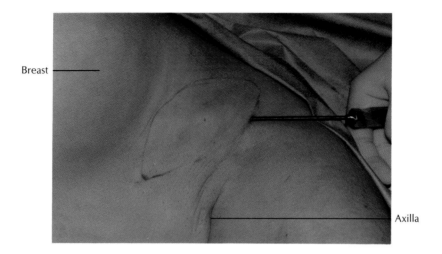

Relatively fine cannulas (2.4 to 3.0 mm in diameter) are used, and volumes are generally less than 10 cc. A single stab incision in a skin crease behind the anterior axillary fold provides sufficient access. The area can be treated using local anesthetics, but since it is usually treated in conjunction with other areas, general anesthesia is more common.

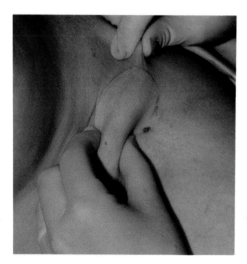 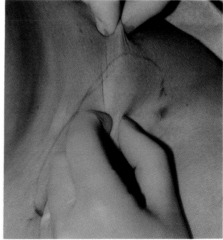

Observation of surface contour and the results of an intraoperative pinch test determine the end point of suctioning.

Following wound closure, a Reston sponge is laid over the treated area for a minimum of 2 days and a maximum of 7 days (not critical after the first 48 hours, so time of removal depends on when the patient returns to the office). Results are generally satisfying. The most common postoperative problems are wrinkling and depressions. These can be avoided by not overresecting and limiting the operation to patients who have sufficient excess fat.

Back and Posterior Axillary Fold Contouring

The area adjacent to the posterior axillary fold and other areas on the posterior thoracic cage can also be treated with liposuction. Patients complain of excess fat hanging over strapless evening attire or above and below brassieres and halter tops. In some patients a roll of fat may extend around to the lateral aspect of the thorax.

The surgeon should use the pinch test to confirm that the problem is related to excess subcutaneous fat, not simply lax skin. The preoperative pinch thickness should be a minimum of 2 cm.

Since the back is usually being treated along with other areas of the trunk and lower extremities, use of the lateral decubitus position is most convenient. More posterior areas are reached by rolling the patient slightly prone. After the first side is completed, the patient is rolled to the opposite lateral decubitus position so the other side can be treated. If only the back is treated, the prone position may be used.

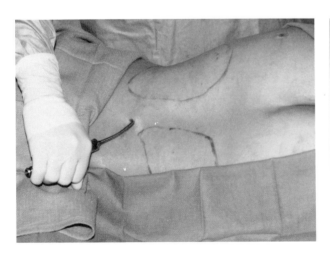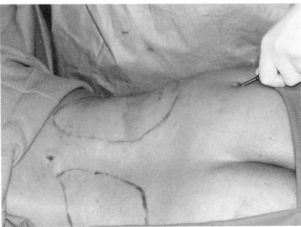

A single midline incision gives access to left and right sides. A second incision may be made in a skin crease or other convenient location. Cannula sizes range from 3.0 to 5.2 mm in diameter, depending on volume removal (usually 50 to 250 cc on each side).

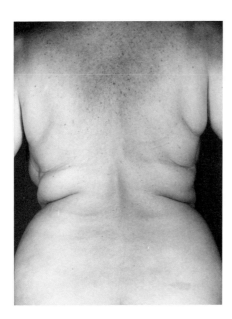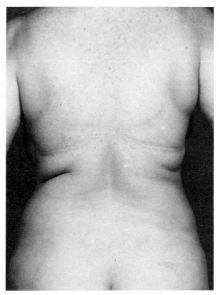

This 47-year-old woman was 20 pounds overweight. She requested liposuction for diminution in the size of her back rolls. Patients whose back rolls are secondary to pure skin laxity due to senile changes or weight loss are generally not helped by liposuction. Moderately overweight patients, however, can expect a significant change. The patient is shown before and 10 months after liposuction of 200 cc from each posterolateral back area. Her hips and thighs were also treated.

REFERENCES

1. Carlson HE. Gynecomastia. N Engl J Med 303:795-799, 1980.
2. Nuttall FQ. Gynecomastia as a physical finding in normal men. J Clin Endocrinol Metab 48:338-340, 1979.
3. Nydick M, Bustos J, Dale JH Jr, Rowson RW. Gynecomastia in adolescent boys. JAMA 178:449-454, 1961.
4. Aegeneta P. The Seven Books of Paulus Aegeneta, vol 2, Book 6, sec. 46. (Translated from the Greek by Francis Adams.) London: London Sydenham Society, 1846, pp 334-335.
5. Menville JG. Gynecomastia. Arch Surg 26:1054-1083, 1933.
6. Dufourmentel C. L'incision areolaire dans la chirurgie du sein. Bull Mem Soc Chir 20:9-14, 1928.
7. Webster JP. Mastectomy for gynecomastia through a semicircular intraareolar incision. Ann Surg 124:567-575, 1946.
8. Barsky AJ, Kahn S, Simon BE. Principles and Practice of Plastic Surgery, 2nd ed. New York: McGraw-Hill, 1964, p 564.
9. Pitanguy I. Transareolar incision for gynecomastia. Plast Reconstr Surg 38:414-419, 1966.
10. Eade GG. The radial incision for gynecomastia excisions. Plast Reconstr Surg 54:495-497, 1974.
11. Balch CR. A transaxillary approach for gynecomastia. Plast Reconstr Surg 61:13-16, 1978.
12. Letterman G, Schurter M. The surgical correction of gynecomastia. Am Surg 35:322-325, 1969.

13. Huang TT, Hidalgo JE, Lewis SR. A circumareolar approach in surgical management of gynecomastia. Plast Reconstr Surg 67:35-40, 1982.

14. Davidson BA. Concentric circle operation for massive gynecomastia to excise the redundant skin. Plast Reconstr Surg 63:350-354, 1979.

15. Pers M, Bretteville-Jensen G. Reduction mammaplasty based on the vertical vascular bipedicle and "tennis ball" assembly. Scand J Plast Reconstr Surg 6:61-68, 1972.

16. Letterman G, Schurter M. Surgical correction of massive gynecomastia. Plast Reconstr Surg 49:259-262, 1972.

17. Bretteville-Jensen MB. Surgical treatment of gynecomastia. Br J Plast Surg 28:177-180, 1975.

18. Welsh F. Handlebar moustache breast reduction. Plast Reconstr Surg 69:544-545, 1982.

19. Dufourmentel C, Mouly R. Plastic mammaire par la méthode oblique. Ann Clin Plast Surg 6:45-58, 1961.

20. Simon BE, Hoffman S, Kahn S. Classification and surgical correction of gynecomastia. Plast Reconstr Surg 51:48-52, 1973.

21. Wray RC, Hoopes JE, Davis GM. Correction of extreme gynecomastia. Br J Plast Surg 27:39-41, 1974.

22. Teimourian B, Perlman R. Surgery for gynecomastia. Aesthetic Plast Surg 7:155-157, 1983.

23. Lewis CM. Lipoplasty: Treatment for gynecomastia. Aesthetic Plast Surg 9:287-292, 1985.

24. Courtiss EH. Gynecomastia: Analysis of 159 patients and current recommendations for treatment. Plast Reconstr Surg 79:740-750, 1987.

25. Mladick RA. Gynecomastia: Liposuction and excision. Clin Plast Surg 18:815-822, 1991.

26. Rosenberg GJ. Gynecomastia: Suction lipectomy as a contemporary solution. Plast Reconstr Surg 80:379-385, 1987.

27. Cohen IK. Discussion of Rosenberg GJ. Gynecomastia: Suction lipectomy as a contemporary solution. Plast Reconstr Surg 80:386, 1987.

28. Cohen IK, Pozez AL, McKeown JE. Gynecomastia. In Courtiss EH, ed. Male Aesthetic Surgery, 2nd ed. St. Louis: Mosby–Year Book, 1991, pp 373-394.

29. Edwards EA. Surgical anatomy of the breast. In Goldwyn RM, ed. Plastic and Reconstructive Surgery of the Breast. Boston: Little, Brown, 1976, pp 37-57.

30. Aiache AE. Surgical treatment of gynecomastia in the body builder. Plast Reconstr Surg 83:61-66, 1989.

31. Nicolis GL, Modlinger RS, Gabrilove JL. A study of the histopathology of human gynecomastia. J Clin Endocrinol Metab 32:173-178, 1971.

32. Crichlow RW, Galt SW. Gynecomastia. In Noone RB, ed. Plastic and Reconstructive Surgery of the Breast. St. Louis: Mosby–Year Book, 1991, pp 98-108.

33. McGrath MH. Gynecomastia. In Jurkiewicz J, Krizek TJ, Mathes SJ, Ariyan S, eds. Plastic Surgery: Principles and Practice. St. Louis: CV Mosby, 1990, pp 1119-1136.

34. Simon BE, Hoffman S. Correction of gynecomastia. In Goldwyn RM, ed. Plastic and Reconstructive Surgery of the Breast. Boston: Little, Brown, 1976, pp 305-325.

35. Von Kessel F, Pickrell KL, Huger WE, Matton G. Surgical treatment for gynecomastia. Ann Surg 157:142-156, 1963.

36. Benelli L. A new periareolar mammaplasty: The "round block" technique. Aesthetic Plast Surg 14:93-100, 1990.

37. Grazer F. Atlas of Suction-Assisted Lipectomy in Body Contouring. New York: Churchill Livingstone, 1991, pp 145-146, 182-185.

38. Mattarasso A, Courtiss EH. Suction mammoplasty: The use of suction lipectomy to reduce large breasts. Plast Reconstr Surg 87:709-717, 1991.

39. Teimourian B. Suction Lipectomy and Body Sculpturing. St. Louis: CV Mosby, 1987, pp 219-251.

40. Teimourian B, Massas E Jr, Weigering CE. Reduction suction lipectomy and suction lipectomy as an adjunct to breast surgery. Aesthetic Plast Surg 9:97-100, 1985.
41. Toledo LS, Matsudo PK. Mammoplasty using liposuction and the periareolar incision. Aesthetic Plast Surg 13:9-13, 1989.

—————————————— SUGGESTED READING ——————————————

Artz JS, Lehman JA Jr. Surgical correction of massive gynecomastia. Arch Surg 113:199-201, 1978.

Gerut ZE. Effective treatment of intraoperative breast prosthesis rupture: New use of the suction assisted lipectomy machine [letter]. Plast Reconstr Surg 80:645, 1987.

Mladick RA, Morris RL. Sixteen months' experience with the Illouz technique of lipolysis. Ann Plast Surg 16:220-232, 1986.

Pinella JW. Creating an inframammary crease with a liposuction cannula [letter]. Plast Reconstr Surg 83:925, 1989.

Sbar S. Unilateral gynecomastia. N Engl J Med 286:1367-1368, 1972.

Chapter 9

ABDOMEN

Liposuction has revolutionized abdominal contouring. In the past, patients who sought contour reduction had only one choice—abdominoplasty. Now superior aesthetic results can be achieved in many patients with liposuction. In addition, small fat deposits, which cannot be treated with abdominoplasty, are ideal for liposuction, which is associated with insignificant scarring, minimal inconvenience, and negligible morbidity. In recent series the majority of patients undergoing abdominal contouring were treated with suction alone.[1-3]

In patients who have abdominoplasty, plastic surgeons have increasingly recognized that variations in abdominal contour require modifications in surgical procedures. Newer techniques use shorter incisions and eliminate umbilical circumscription. Liposuction combined with abdominoplasty has also enhanced our ability to achieve refined results.

Although plastic surgeons now have a much wider range of choices for operative correction of abdominal deformities, the majority of patients are successfully treated by liposuction alone. Of the remainder, most are treated by complete abdominoplasty with umbilical circumscription. In my own practice, liposuction accounts for 70% of abdominal contouring operations. Another 20% of procedures are complete abdominoplasty with umbilical circumscription, and the remaining 10% are divided among the lesser abdominoplasties and procedures for patients after weight loss. In short, our surgical options have increased, but indications for the lesser abdominoplasties remain limited.

217

HISTORY

Demars and Marx[4] are credited with performing the first abdominoplasty in 1890. In the United States Kelly[5,6] described an operation for abdominal fat removal in 1899 and 1910. Other reports followed in quick succession.[7-24] These operations were most frequently performed on obese patients and consisted of removal of large amounts of skin and fat with little or no undermining. Repair of the musculoaponeurosis might or might not be performed, and all manner and combinations of incisions were used (horizontal, vertical, circumferential, combined, fleur-de-lis, etc.). Not infrequently the umbilicus was excised with the specimen. More recent practitioners of these techniques have usually confined their operations to massive weight–loss patients.[25-28]

Although Schepelmann[29] transposed and saved the umbilicus as early as 1924, Vernon's report[30] of "umbilical transplantation upward" focused attention on this important technical point and made it an integral part of subsequent abdominoplasties.

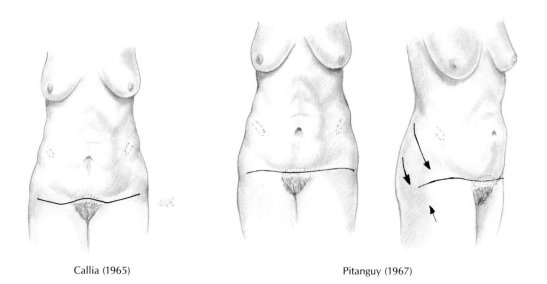

Callia (1965)   Pitanguy (1967)

In 1965 Callia[31] described a low transverse incision with undermining of the upper flap. Pitanguy[32] in 1967 reviewed his first 300 operations using a low transverse incision and umbilical translocation. Pitanguy's incision went straight across the upper portion of the pubic hair onto the upper thighs and then curved downward at the lateral ends to accommodate extra skin from the lateral portion of the upper flap. Pitanguy also emphasized the importance of complete midline musculoaponeurotic plication from xiphoid to pubis. His landmark presentation was enormously influential in popularizing cosmetic abdominoplasty for a whole generation of plastic surgeons.

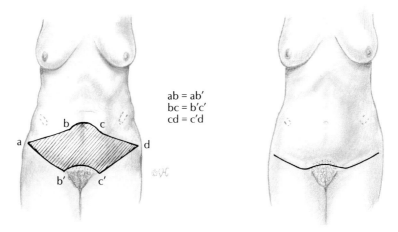

ab = ab'
bc = b'c'
cd = c'd

Serson (1971); Baker, Gordon, and Mosienko (1977)

Serson[33] and Baker, Gordon, and Mosienko[34] proposed excising a geometric pattern of the entire skin segment between the umbilicus and pubis as the first step in abdominoplasty to shorten the operation, facilitate dissection of the superior flap, and ensure a symmetric closure line without dog ears or folds along the edge of the superior flap. This method is possible only when the surgeon is certain that there is sufficient excess skin to permit removal of all the skin between the umbilicus and pubic hairline.

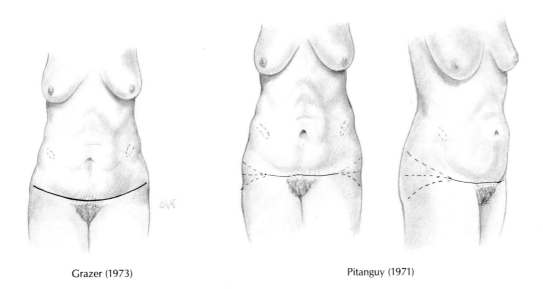

Grazer (1973)   Pitanguy (1971)

Grazer[35] espoused a low transverse "skin-line" incision starting within the pubic hairline and running parallel to the lower abdominal skin fold, curving upward at the end. Pitanguy[36] modified his original incision to include a straight horizontal incision as far as an imaginary line dropped from the anterior superior iliac spines. The lateral extension of this incision could be made in whatever direction best suited the anatomic needs of the particular patient: straight lateral, superolateral, or inferolateral.

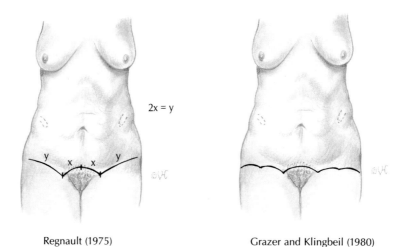

$2x = y$

Regnault (1975)   Grazer and Klingbeil (1980)

Regnault[37] proposed a W-shaped incision to better accommodate the excess skin of the upper flap during closure. On each side the lateral segment of the W ran along the inguinal fold and was about twice the length of the medial segment in the pubic hairline. Grazer and Klingbeil[38] described a modification of the W-shaped incision, the gull-wing incision. It differed from the W incision in that its lateral segments were below the inguinal crease and had a slight upward convexity. They favored the skin-line incision for the more corpulent patient and the gull-wing incision for the thinner patient.

All techniques shared a common feature: the umbilicus was circumscribed and left on its stalk to be brought out through a new, surgically created umbilical opening in the flap. Ideally, the surgeon removed all of the skin between the umbilicus and the transverse suprapubic incision, eliminating the former umbilical site.

If insufficient skin laxity prohibited removal of all of the lower abdominal skin, the umbilical opening was sutured, resulting in a short vertical midline scar in the lower abdomen or a T closure at the bottom of the flap.

Planas[39] proposed a "vest-over-pants" technique to avoid a vertical scar. He first made a transverse incision just above the umbilicus. He then elevated the entire upper abdominal flap as far as the xiphoid and costal margins and pulled the flap down over the lower abdominal skin to see how much of the skin below the umbilicus could be excised without tension. The final closure line lay at the pubic hairline if there was sufficient excess skin. If the flap did not easily reach to the pubic hairline, less lower abdominal skin was excised, and the final closure line was higher. In all cases, however, a midline scar at the former umbilical site was eliminated.

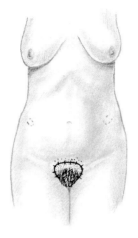
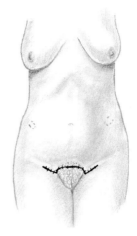

Elbaz (1974)   Glicenstein (1975)

Elbaz's lower abdominal "horseshoe" excision left a scar confined within the pubic hair.[40] The method was ingenious but had limited utility. Glicenstein's procedure was similar, but the scar did not extend as far down the crural crease.[41] Instead, he used short lateral extensions along the inguinal fold.

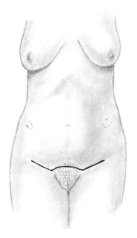
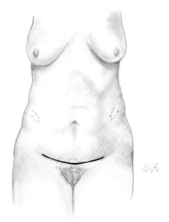

Greminger (1983)   Wilkinson and Schwartz (1986)

Operations to treat the abdomen below the umbilicus included Greminger's "miniabdominoplasty"[42] and Wilkinson and Schwartz's limited abdominoplasty.[43] These incisions did not extend beyond imaginary vertical lines dropped down from the anterosuperior iliac spines. Cardoso de Castro, Cupello, and Cintra[44] also used a short incision to remove fat and skin from the lower abdomen. By careful undermining and the use of long fiberoptic lighted retractors they were also able to tighten the musculature above the umbilicus.

AESTHETIC AND ANATOMIC CONSIDERATIONS

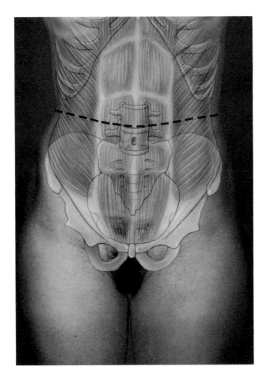 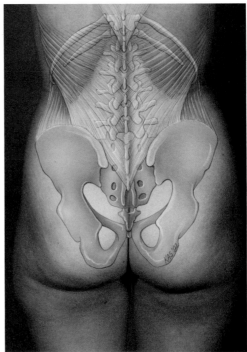

The abdominal wall is bounded superiorly by the costal margin in front and the twelfth rib behind; the pelvic girdle marks the inferior limit. These upper and lower skeletal elements are joined by the lumbar vertebrae, with the abdominal wall forming an enveloping curtain stretched between the rib cage above and pelvic bones below.

In healthy, nonobese men and women the muscular envelope tapers in from the costal margin to define the waist, the narrowest circumference of the torso, before flaring out again to join the pelvic girdle.

The umbilicus, lying at the junction of the midline and a line drawn between the upper iliac crests, punctuates the midanterior abdomen with a gentle depression extending to the fascia. The relative absence of subcutaneous fat in the immediately adjacent area contributes to the concavity.

The flare of the costal margin above and the iliac crest below is separated by the muscular suppression of the waist, which is approximately 1 inch cephalad to the umbilicus. With age, waist definition begins to soften due to skeletal compaction, loss of muscle tone, and increase in fat.

Sex-Specific Factors
Women

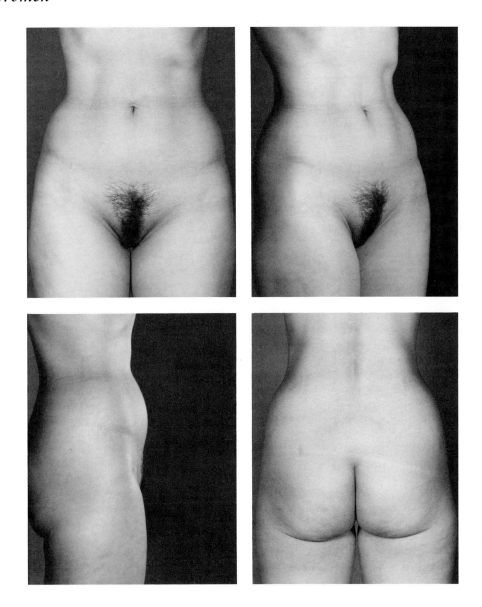

In women the flare of the iliac crests and the pelvic girdle volume are proportionately larger than in men. The resultant fullness of the lower torso in females is accentuated by a more or less voluminous sex-specific subcutaneous fat deposition in the area of the iliac crest (hips).

A subtle rounding of the anterior abdomen is also a secondary sexual characteristic in women. The fullness extends from the xiphoid to just above the pubic hairline, with a depression at the level of the umbilicus. It is more pronounced below the umbilicus and sometimes absent above. Laterally, it extends in a gentle curve as far as a line dropped from the midanterior costal margin. It is formed largely of sex-specific fat and is present even in thin individuals. In overweight women the abdominal fullness becomes excessive and contributes to loss of a youthful figure.

Men

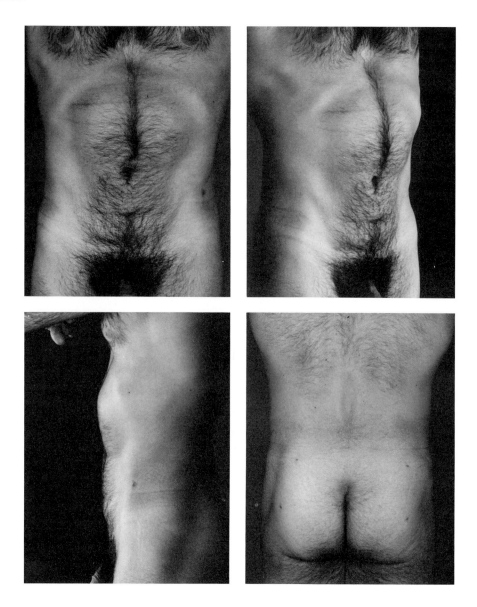

In normal-weight men the anterior abdomen has a flatter appearance because of the relative sparseness of sex-specific fat in this area. The underlying musculature is usually better defined and more easily seen through the thin subcutaneous cover. There is less skeletal flare at the iliac crest, but the circumference of the costal margin and volume of the rib cage are larger than in women. There is no sex-specific excess fat over the hips and less pronounced waist suppression.

Women tend to deposit a large proportion of excess abdominal fat external to the musculature, whereas men tend to deposit more fat within the muscular envelope, making it inaccessible to suction.[45,46] Excess fat in the flank and hip area, including the proverbial "spare tire" in men, is largely subcutaneous and can be suctioned.

Fascia[47]

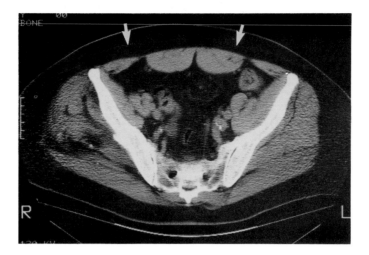

The subcutaneous fat of the abdominal wall is compartmentalized by the superficial fascia, which is usually described as two layers: the superficial Camper layer and the deeper Scarpa layer. A distinct plane separates Camper's and Scarpa's layers in some but not all patients. This plane is most easily identifiable in the lower abdomen, particularly in the obese; see the thin white line (arrows).

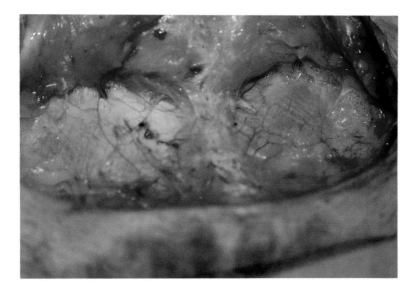

The deep fascia (innominate fascia, fascia of Gallaudet) adheres closely to the underlying musculoaponeurosis and is continuous with the fascia lata of the thigh. It covers a plexus of small arteries and veins on the surface of the anterior rectus sheath.

Musculoaponeurosis[47-52]

The external oblique muscle, the internal oblique muscle, and the transversus abdominis constitute portions of three concentric cylinders enveloping the anterolateral abdominal wall. The aponeuroses or tendinous insertions of these muscles make up the anterior and posterior leaves of the rectus sheath that contain the rectus abdominis muscle. The aponeuroses then continue to the midline, where they meet their opposite counterparts in the linea alba.

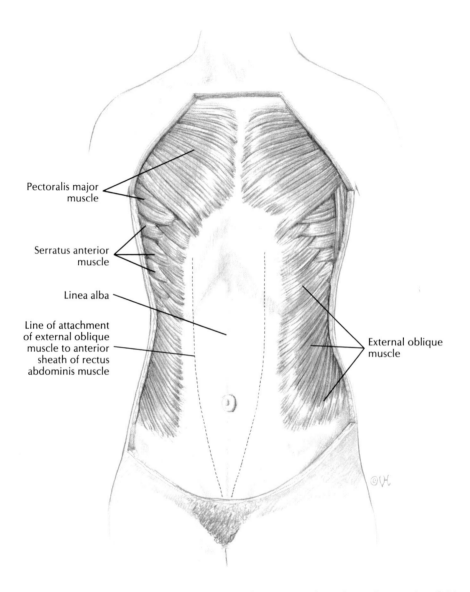

The external oblique muscle originates by muscular slips from the fifth or sixth through the twelfth ribs. Its fibers travel downward and medially, becoming aponeurotic at the lateral edge of the rectus abdominis high in the abdomen. The aponeurosis begins more laterally lower in the abdomen.

The lowermost fibers insert on the iliac crest and help form the inguinal structures, but most of the muscle inserts into the anterior rectus sheath, fusing with the internal oblique and transversus abdominis fibers before continuing to its final insertion at the linea alba.

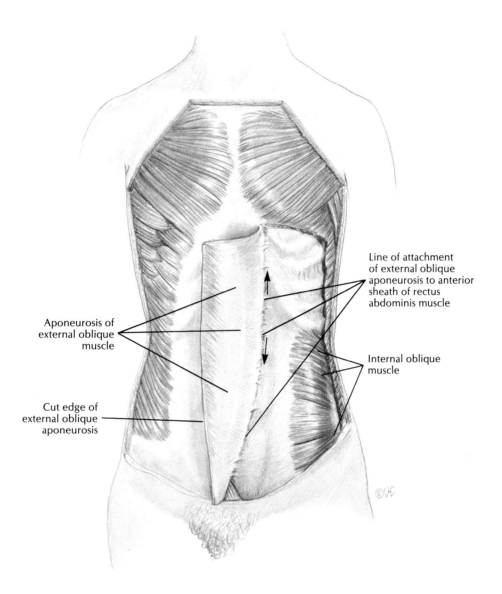

Line of attachment of external oblique aponeurosis to anterior sheath of rectus abdominis muscle

Aponeurosis of external oblique muscle

Internal oblique muscle

Cut edge of external oblique aponeurosis

The internal oblique originates from the posterior spines and transverse processes of the lumbar spine via the lumbodorsal fascia, from the anterior two thirds of the iliac crest, and from the lateral half of the inguinal ligament. It extends superiorly and medially, becoming aponeurotic as it approaches its insertions. The uppermost fibers attach to the three lowest ribs, the middle fibers form the anterior and posterior sheaths before inserting into the linea alba, and the lowest fibers insert on the pubic ramus, contributing to the formation of the inguinal structures.

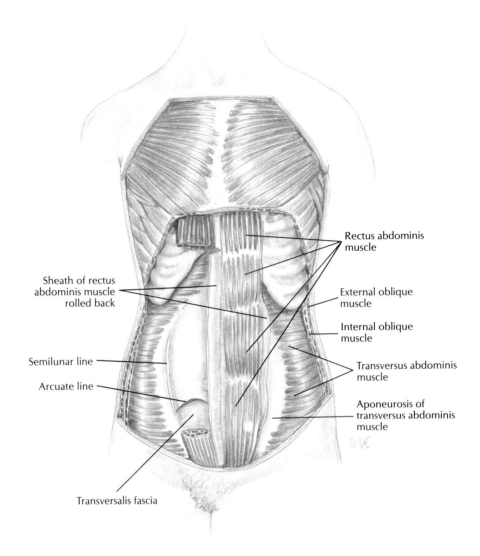

Rectus abdominis
muscle

Sheath of rectus
abdominis muscle
rolled back

External oblique
muscle

Internal oblique
muscle

Semilunar line

Arcuate line

Transversus abdominis
muscle

Aponeurosis of
transversus abdominis
muscle

Transversalis fascia

The transversus abdominis originates from the cartilages of the lower six ribs, from the lumbodorsal fascia, and from the internal line of the iliac crest and the lateralmost inguinal ligament. Its fibers run transversely and fuse with the internal and external oblique aponeuroses, contributing to the anterior and posterior rectus sheaths before inserting in the linea alba. The lowest fibers help form the inguinal structures.

The rectus abdominis muscle extends from its origin on the fifth, sixth, and seventh costal cartilages to its insertion on the symphysis pubis and ramus.[51] It is a long muscle, thin in the anteroposterior dimension and as wide as 3 inches at the rib cage but becoming narrower and thicker as it approaches the pubis. It has three, sometimes four, tendinous inscriptions to which the anterior sheath is adherent.

The rectus sheath is formed by the fusion of the aponeuroses of the external oblique, internal oblique, and transversus abdominis muscles.[49-52] The aponeuroses split at the lateral border of the rectus abdominis (semilunar line) to form anterior and posterior sheaths.

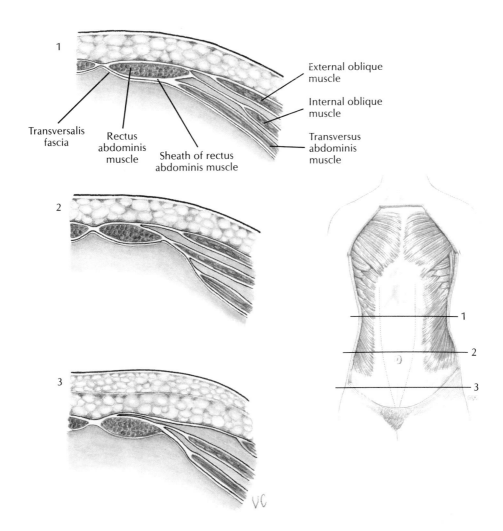

The anterior sheath is formed by the external oblique, the internal oblique, and the transversus abdominis aponeurosis. The internal oblique and transversus abdominis split off some of their fibers to form the posterior sheath. At some point below the umbilicus all fibers pass superficial to the rectus abdominis, and the posterior sheath is absent.

The position of this line of transition, called the *linea semicircularis* or arcuate line, is variable but is most commonly found at the junction of the upper one third and lower two thirds of the distance between the umbilicus and symphysis pubis. Below the linea semicircularis the deep aspect of the rectus muscle rests on transversalis fascia and loose preperitoneal areolar tissue.

The external oblique aponeurosis fuses with the anterior sheath just medial to the semilunar line in the upper portion of the abdomen, but the line of fusion gradually shifts medially until the external oblique aponeurosis almost reaches the midline before fusing with the anterior sheath in the lowest part of the abdomen. Identifying the precise location of the line of fusion is helpful in developing external oblique flaps.

The three large flat abdominal muscles compress the abdomen, depress the thorax, and laterally flex and rotate the vertebral column. The rectus abdominis depresses the thorax and flexes the vertebral column.

Blood Supply

The skin and subcutaneous tissues of the anterolateral abdominal wall are supplied by a rich network of vessels in both the deep and superficial planes with multiple inter- and intraplane anastomoses. Elbaz and Dardour[53] performed anatomic studies on cadavers after radiopaque dye injection to systematize the complex vascular relationships, particularly as they apply to abdominoplasties. The interested reader can find detailed information in other references as well.[51,54-65]

The deep vascular supply to the abdominal wall comes from three main sources:

1. From below, the median axis extends from the deep inferior epigastric artery and, from above, the deep superior epigastric artery, an extension of the internal mammary artery. These vessels anastomose on the deep surface of the rectus abdominis muscle between the umbilicus and the xiphoid. The median axis sends lateral branches to anastomose with branches from the deep intercostal arteries.
2. The superolateral to inferomedial axis includes the deep intercostal arteries T6-12 that travel in the plane between the transversus abdominis and internal oblique until they reach the semilunar line where they anastomose with branches of the median axis. The lower branches also anastomose with branches of the deep circumflex iliac artery.
3. The inferomedial to superolateral axis includes the deep circumflex iliac artery, which has deep anastomoses with the lower intercostal and lumbar arteries.

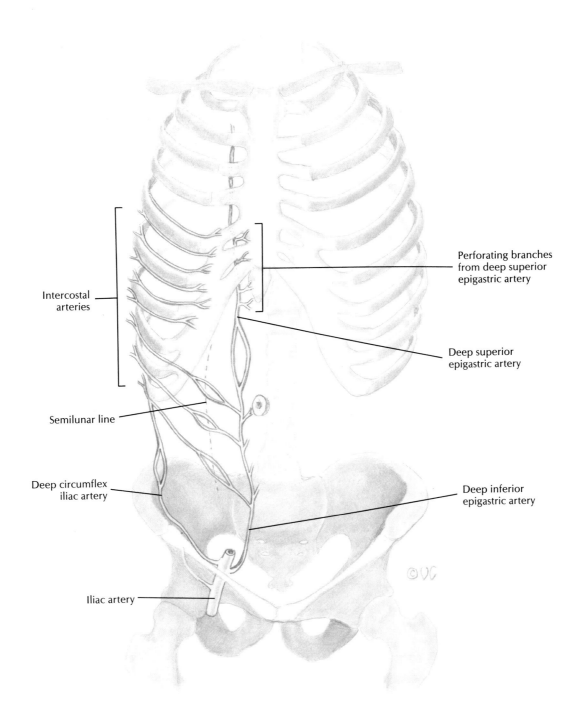

Intercostal
arteries

Semilunar line

Deep circumflex
iliac artery

Iliac artery

Perforating branches
from deep superior
epigastric artery

Deep superior
epigastric artery

Deep inferior
epigastric artery

The superficial blood supply comes from direct cutaneous arteries and perforators from the deep system:

1. The superficial circumflex iliac artery, a direct cutaneous vessel, supplies the inferolateral abdominal skin and anastomoses with superficial branches from the intercostal vessels and perforators from the deep iliac circumflex system.

2. The superficial inferior epigastric artery, also a direct cutaneous vessel, supplies the inferomedial abdominal skin and anastomoses with the superficial circumflex iliac artery and perforators from the deep inferior epigastric artery before proceeding laterally to anastomose with the lateral thoracic artery and superficial branches of the intercostals.

3. Musculocutaneous perforators from the deep inferior epigastric artery supply the inferomedial abdominal skin and anastomose with superficial branches of the intercostal vessels lateral to the semilunar line.

4. Musculocutaneous perforators from the deep superior epigastric artery, a continuation of the internal mammary artery, enter the upper medial abdomen before the deep superior epigastric artery anastomoses with the deep inferior epigastric artery midway between the xiphoid and umbilicus. The deep superior epigastric artery also gives off a superficial superior epigastric artery that runs in the subcutaneous tissues along the lower border of the eighth costal cartilage, anastomosing with the lateral cutaneous branch of the eighth intercostal artery.[56,66] A more medially directed superficial superior epigastric artery is described by Manchot[61]; it branches off the deep vessel and enters the subcutaneous tissues through the upper rectus muscle at the level of the sixth interspace.

5. The intercostal arteries send off musculocutaneous perforators at the level of the slips of origin of the external oblique muscle. These arteries travel in the subcutaneous tissues for a variable distance before anastomosing with superficial perforators from the inferior epigastric and deep circumflex iliac systems.

6. The deep circumflex iliac artery gives several superficial branches to the skin of the lower anterolateral abdominal wall. These branches anastomose with superficial branches from the lower intercostals.

During abdominoplasty the superficial circumflex iliac and superficial inferior epigastric vessels are interrupted. Musculocutaneous perforators from the deep inferior epigastric system are also divided.

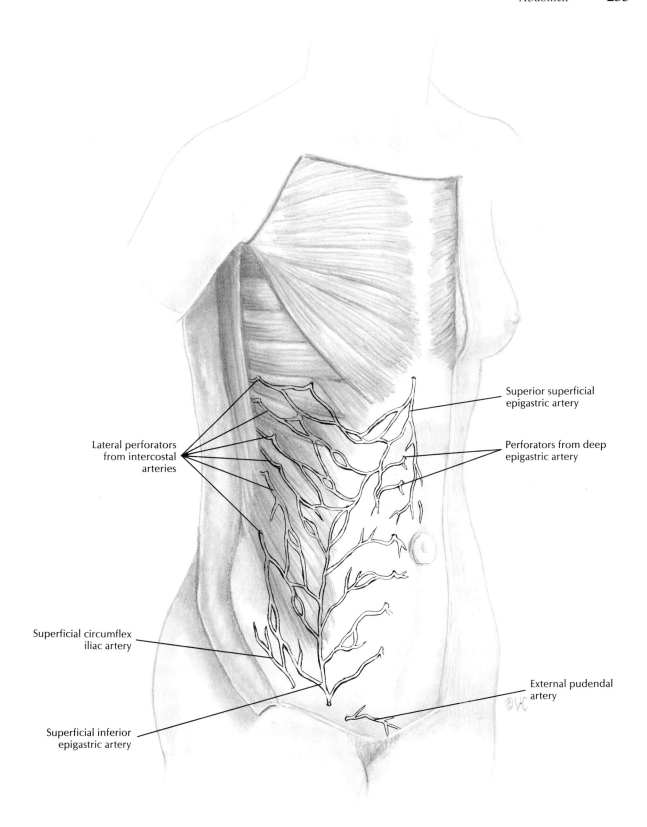

Superior superficial
epigastric artery

Perforators from deep
epigastric artery

Lateral perforators
from intercostal
arteries

Superficial circumflex
iliac artery

External pudendal
artery

Superficial inferior
epigastric artery

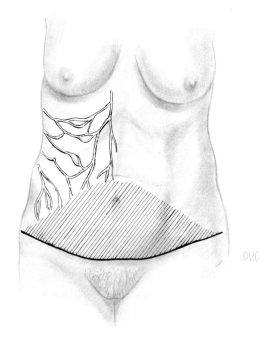

The flap survives on centripetal flow from the superficial branches of the intercostal vessels and from inferior directed flow from the superficial branch of the superior epigastric artery. Anastomoses between the deep circumflex iliac artery and the lower superficial intercostal vessels augment flap blood supply.

Dye studies of intercostal vessels in cadavers demonstrate consistent staining to the semilunar line when T-10 and T-11 are injected.[54] Staining sometimes extends over the rectus muscle and less frequently over the midline. The random pattern of vascularity in the distal central segment of the abdominoplasty flap makes it intolerant of maneuvers that further compromise blood supply. Huger[60] warns against an increased incidence of sloughs if a central wedge is taken from the distal flap with a T closure. This maneuver disrupts flow across the midline and increases the incidence of wound healing problems.[59,67]

PATHOPHYSIOLOGY

Aesthetic deformities of the abdominal wall may involve skin, subcutaneous fat, or musculofascia. Excess subcutaneous fat due to overeating is common in our society. As we pass beyond our twenties and become less physically active, we tend to gain weight. The extra fat accumulates most frequently in the lower abdomen below the umbilicus and is seen, particularly in women, as an exaggeration of the normal sex-specific fullness in this area. Even a small 5- or 10-pound weight gain may be reflected in an unsightly lower abdominal bulge. Fullness in the upper abdomen may be due to fat but is frequently secondary to lower thoracic rib cage bulging combined with skin laxity. In men the extra fat is more diffusely distributed and is more likely to be deep to the musculofascia.

With age, the skin is subject to thinning, stretching, wrinkling, and striae. Some women may retain the youthful appearance of their skin through several pregnancies; but for others the stretched skin never returns to its original state. Major weight gain and subsequent loss, particularly if it is repeated, will also hasten normal aging changes in men and women. Minor signs of aging are confined to the lower abdomen, but more severe changes can involve the entire area from the xiphoid to the pubis. The musculo-aponeurosis also loses its tensile strength. The midline diastasis recti may widen from a few millimeters to several centimeters. No amount of exercise will narrow a widened diastasis or strengthen a weak aponeurosis.

Small, long-standing umbilical hernias may become larger and symptomatic as the abdominal wall weakens. Ventral hernias are uncommon in those who have never had abdominal surgery.

Unsightly scars may occur anywhere on the lower or upper abdomen and may be part of the presenting complaint. Midline scars are often retracted and widened. Low transverse scars may be associated with overhang of the more cephalic skin and subcutaneous tissues.

CLASSIFICATION AND TREATMENT OPTIONS

Several classifications of abdominal deformities have been proposed and operations specifically designed for each deformity.[2,37,68,69] Although these classifications help organize our thinking, patients generally do not fit into neat categories. Each person has a unique combination of problems that requires individual assessment and modifications of operative technique.

Recognizing that patient deformities and surgical options can be of infinite variety, I classify patients into five treatment categories:
- Liposuction
- Complete abdominoplasty with umbilical translocation
- Complete abdominoplasty without umbilical translocation
- Lower abdominoplasty
- Abdominal surgery after major weight loss

The actual surgery may involve one option, a variation on an option, or a combination of options.

TREATMENT CATEGORIES
Liposuction

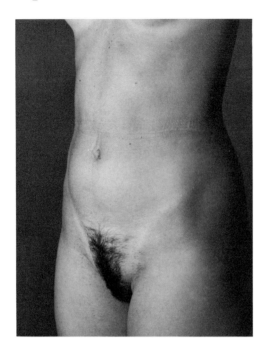 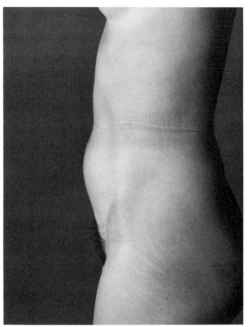

Liposuction is the procedure of choice in patients with excess abdominal subcutaneous fat with little or no skin and muscle laxity. The amount of excess fat may be small or large. The common denominator is that fat removal through minimal incisions will reduce contour.

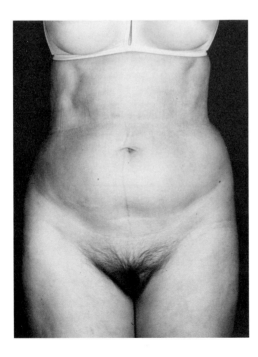 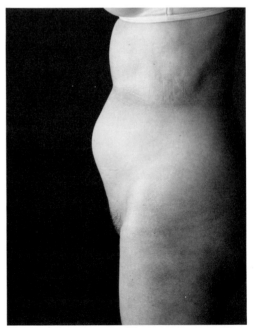

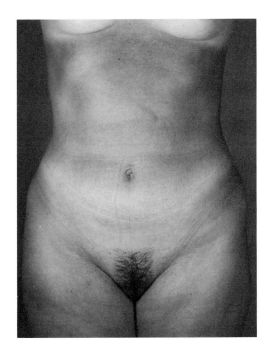
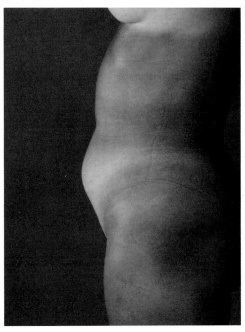

A variety of patients of different ages ranging from those with small to large fat volumes, differing musculoskeletal types, and differing degrees of skin and muscle tone may be treated with liposuction.

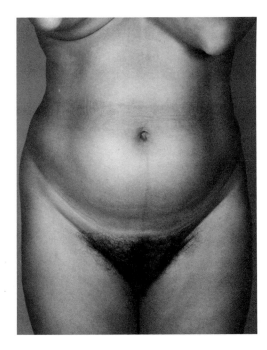
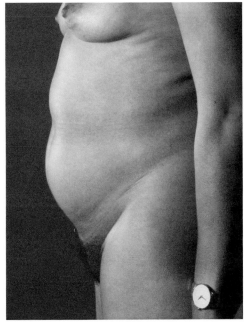

Complete Abdominoplasty With Umbilical Translocation

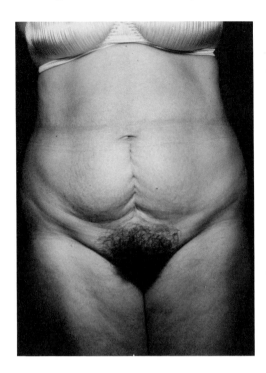
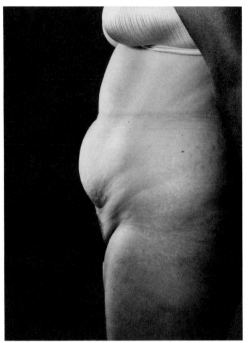

Patients with anterior abdominal muscle laxity, unsightly lower abdominal scars, and large amounts of excess skin involving the upper and lower abdomen are candidates for complete abdominoplasty with umbilical translocation (complete abdominoplasty).

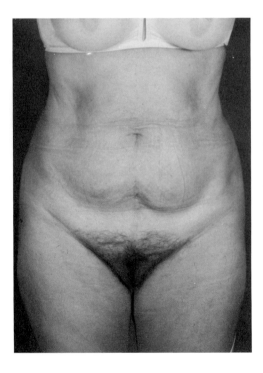
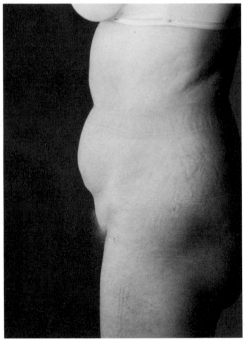

Complete Abdominoplasty Without Umbilical Translocation

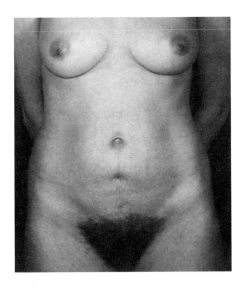 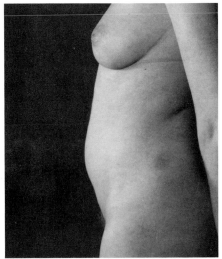

Patients who require upper and lower abdominal fascial tightening and have moderate skin laxity confined largely to the lower abdomen are candidates for complete abdominoplasty without umbilical translocation (modified abdominoplasty).

Lower Abdominoplasty

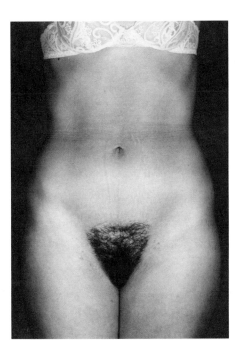 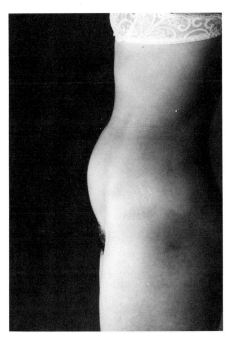

Patients with skin and muscle laxities confined below the umbilicus may benefit from lower abdominoplasty (miniabdominoplasty).

Abdominal Surgery After Weight Loss

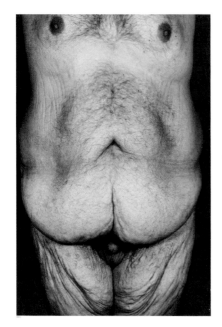 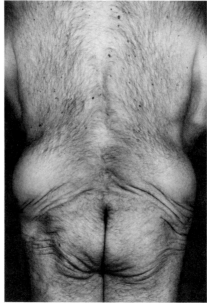 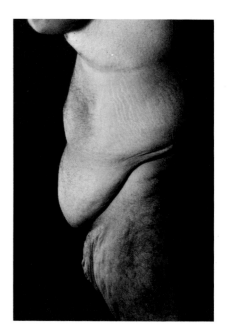

The major problem in patients who have lost large amounts of weight is excess skin that may extend circumferentially around the torso. There may be associated muscle laxity and excess fat despite weight loss.

PATIENT EVALUATION AND COUNSELING
Physical Examination

Although the patient's health status is a concern for any elective cosmetic procedure, it is especially significant if the patient is scheduled for abdominoplasty. Liposuction, particularly of small volumes, is a low-morbidity procedure, but complete abdominoplasty can be associated with significant morbidity and mortality.[70,71] Obesity, in particular, has been identified as a predisposing cause of complications.[72] Abdominoplasty candidates should be at normal or near-normal weight.

The general body habitus is assessed, including abnormal spinal curvatures. Significant scoliosis may produce abdominal asymmetries that should be noted in the chart and pointed out to the patient. Lumbar lordosis can cause lower abdominal protuberance not correctable by abdominal surgery.

All abdominal scars are sketched on the chart for permanent reference. The presence of a scar in an area to be suctioned can cause the cannula to be misdirected and penetrate the abdominal aponeurosis. Midline scars generally have no effect on blood supply to the flap, but subcostal and transverse scars should give pause since they may be associated with diminished distal blood flow.

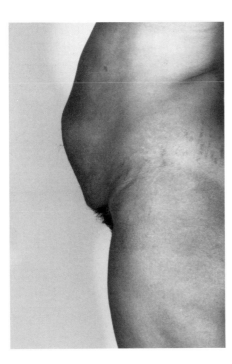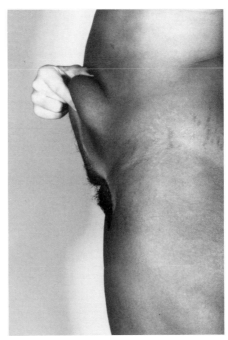

The patient is assessed first in the standing position. If fat and skin hang below the pubic hairline as a panniculus, the skin is too lax for pure suction, and abdominoplasty is indicated. On the left the patient is standing relaxed. On the right the nurse's hand elevates the hanging abdominal panniculus.

The pinch test of the subcutaneous tissues will confirm the presence of excess fat. A 3 cm thickness of tissue indicates the patient is a suitable candidate for abdominal suction. In most men with protuberant abdomens the fat is localized deep to the musculoaponeurosis, making them unsuitable for liposuction (see p. 12). The presence of umbilical or other hernias should be noted.

The abdomen is gently palpated for masses with the patient supine. Palpation while the patient attempts a partial sit-up helps in evaluating the tone and condition of the abdominal musculature and assessing the width of the diastasis recti. The patient is put in a waist-flexed, knees-flexed position with the back supported while the skin between the umbilicus and pubic hairline is gently pinched to estimate if all of the skin below the umbilicus can be excised.

Defining Patient Goals

Younger women seeking abdominal contour surgery frequently request a diminution or flattening of the anterior abdomen, particularly the area below the umbilicus. Older women request, in addition, a restoration or cinching of their waistline. Women at all ages want reduction of overly full hips and tightening of lax skin and/or musculature.

The single most frequent complaint is excess bulging of the lower abdomen. In some women the bulge may be very slight. Society's relentless glorification of youth and fitness induces some women to seek ablation of the normal lower abdominal rounding in favor of a perfectly flat "boyish" abdomen. It is up to the surgeon to educate patients to the aesthetic necessity for gently rounded surfaces in the human form. For most patients, however, the fullness is secondary to varying degrees of obesity and/or muscle laxity and should be corrected.

Elimination of unsightly scars, surface irregularities, wrinkling, and striae is a universal desire. A widened, depressed lower midline scar surrounded by bulging excess fat is a common reason to seek surgery.

Patients may complain that the appearance of their abdomen is satisfactory when they are standing but that sitting causes excessive folds and bulging. Tight clothes become an embarrassment and revealing beach wear an impossibility.

Massive obesity is a contraindication for either procedure. Many patients are looking for a "quick fix." The truly obese should be referred to a reputable weight-loss program. For those who do lose weight there is a high degree of recidivism. Nevertheless, some patients obtain a successful and long-lasting cure for obesity, and efforts are worthwhile for these few.

The surgeon's suggestion of optimal treatment may be unacceptable to the patient because of potential scarring or morbidity. It may be possible to educate some patients to the aesthetic benefits of a more complex procedure, but for others, it is best to offer limited improvement using a simpler procedure the patient can accept.

Informed Consent

I explain the surgical procedure and postoperative course to the patient in clear, simple terms and in considerable detail. I mention alternatives (no surgery, weight loss, liposuction vs. abdominoplasty) but do not overwhelm the patient with multiple procedural possibilities. Although the patient must be aware of alternatives if she is to give a truly informed consent, it is the surgeon's obligation to present a single straightforward and unequivocal recommendation to the patient. I discuss limitations and principal risks as well as expected benefits.

Informed consent for liposuction is described in detail in Chapter 1. In addition, specific points are relevant to treatment of the abdomen. Women with minimal fat accumulations who want perfectly flat abdomens are informed that the risk of surface irregularities increases as less fat is left in the subcutaneous tissues. It should be stressed that anterior abdominal liposuction may increase skin folding when the patient sits. If a large proportion of intra-abdominal fat is beneath the fascia (more common in men but present in some women), the patient should understand that liposuction will not completely reduce bulging. The patient is also shown the position and length of scars, but since these are quite small and usually in the pubic hair or umbilicus, they are rarely a problem.

If the patient is to have abdominoplasty, the location and length of the planned scars, including the umbilical scar, are drawn on the skin. The detailed course of recovery as well as the inconveniences and pain of the postoperative period are explained, particularly as they differ from liposuction. Finally, I mention the serious and special risks peculiar to abdominoplasty. I give patients a detailed information letter on abdominoplasty (see pp. 244-245) that supplements but does not substitute for a full face-to-face discussion.

LIPOSUCTION
Markings

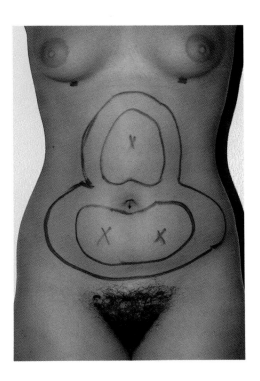

The patient is marked in the standing position, and areas of excess fat are outlined as on a topographic map. Access incisions are marked in the pubic hair, umbilicus, and inframammary creases (occasionally). These well-hidden incisions permit suction of the entire anterior abdomen from multiple sites. The pubic access incisions should be placed so that the cannulas can easily sculpt the fat to emphasize the semilunar line and the "lyre" shape of the normal female lower abdomen.

Abdominoplasty

Abdominoplasty is a surgical procedure on the abdomen for removing excess skin and fat, tightening the muscles, and eliminating or improving the appearance of scars of the lower abdomen.

In some women, pregnancies cause the abdominal skin and muscles to become loose and flabby. In other women and in men, excessive weight gain followed by weight reduction leaves a layer of loose excessive skin and stretched-out, thin musculature. Abdominoplasty is designed to correct these conditions. Hernias are also corrected.

Some patients think abdominoplasty is a weight-loss technique. This is not so. Although the procedure removes some fat, it is not a substitute for a healthy diet or sensible exercise. Patients should be at normal or near-normal weight before surgery.

Complete abdominoplasty is performed for those patients requiring maximum correction. A horizontal incision is made low on the abdomen at the level of the pubic hair. The abdominal musculature is tightened with stitches, and any hernias or weaknesses are repaired. The umbilicus (belly button) is usually circumscribed during the operation. It remains in the same position on the abdominal wall but is brought out through a new skin opening.

In some patients requiring lesser corrections a limited procedure is performed (modified or miniabdominoplasty). There is no scar around the umbilicus, and other scars are shorter.

At the time of your consultation, I will inform you whether you are a candidate for a complete or limited abdominoplasty.

Combined Procedures   Abdominoplasty may be combined with intra-abdominal procedures such as tubal ligation or with cosmetic operations on other parts of the body such as breast or facial surgery. Liposuction of the hips and other areas is commonly performed with abdominoplasty.

Anesthesia   Complete abdominoplasties require general anesthesia given by an expert anesthesiologist who charges separately for his services. Limited abdominoplasties can be done under local anesthesia.

Duration of Operation   Operating time is 1 to 3 hours depending on the scope of the procedure.

Hospitalization vs. Ambulatory Surgery
Complete abdominoplasty requires hospitalization. The patient is admitted the morning of hospitalization. Discharge is 3 days after surgery.

More limited abdominoplasties can be done on an ambulatory basis. The patient reports to the hospital or office in the morning and remains for 4 hours after surgery. Ambulatory patients who live more than 1 hour away must stay overnight in Manhattan after surgery. If you desire, we will recommend a nearby hotel.

You will need to have a friend or relative accompany you when you leave, remain with you overnight, and accompany you when you return to the office the morning after surgery. If a relative or friend is not available to you, we will recommend a nurse.

During your consultation I will tell you if surgery will require an overnight stay at the hospital.

After Surgery   Patients having complete abdominoplasty remain in bed until the next morning. A urinary catheter will be placed during your operation while you are asleep and remain for 1 or 2 days after surgery. Patients having more limited abdominoplasties do not have a urinary catheter. You can expect some pain in the incision, but this is alleviated with medication and gradually subsides as you begin to walk. A narrow bandage is removed the day after surgery, and you may shower. All stitches are internal and self-dissolving.

Physical Activity After Surgery/Return to Work   Most people return to their usual activities and to work 2 weeks after the operation. Strenuous sports, however, are prohibited for 2 months.

Photographs Photographs, which do not include the face, are important aids in planning and performing the surgery and become a permanent part of your patient record. They are taken before and after surgery.

Scars Following full abdominoplasty, you can expect a horizontal scar low on the abdomen and a circular scar within the umbilicus. More limited abdominoplasties do not require a scar around the umbilicus. In some patients a different type or location of scar may be necessary because of individual anatomic variations. If this is so in your case, I will inform you at the time of your consultation. Although occasional findings at operation dictate that the scar be somewhat longer or in a different position than planned before surgery, I will make every effort to keep the scar as short and inconspicuous as possible.

The scars tend to fade with time and are usually not troublesome. Nevertheless, you should be aware that all scars are permanent, and their width, height, and color are not totally predictable.

Pregnancy If you plan to have children in the future, you should not have an abdominoplasty as the entire abdomen will stretch considerably with pregnancy. Wait until you have completed your family.

Diminished Sensibility As with any surgical procedure, small nerves to the skin are interrupted during abdominoplasty. Portions of your abdomen will feel numb or have less than full feeling. Sensibility returns over several months, but some diminished feeling may last indefinitely.

Swelling Swelling of the abdomen is normal following surgery. During the first week your clothes may fit you more tightly, and you may weigh more than before. The swelling subsides starting the second week after surgery, but some lower abdominal fullness persists. You may expect to see about 50% of your total contour improvement at 2 weeks and about 75% at 1 month. It usually takes an additional 2 months for the last bit of swelling to recede. Occasional patients may see continued improvement up to 6 months after surgery, but changes beyond 3 months are usually subtle.

Complications The most common complication is hematoma, or a collection of blood under the skin of the abdomen. This occurs in approximately 5% of patients and may necessitate returning the patient to the operating room to remove the blood.

Infection or wound healing problems, including loss of skin and excessive scarring, occur less frequently in my experience. Other serious or even life-threatening complications are possible. Pulmonary thromboembolism (blood clot traveling to the lungs) has been reported in a recent survey of plastic surgeons as occurring with an incidence of 1 in 400. Obesity is the most frequent associated predisposing factor. I do not offer this operation to obese patients, and I have never seen this complication in my personal practice.

I mention the above not to alarm or frighten you since my own experience with this operation has been favorable, and the vast majority of patients are satisfied. I am, however, compelled to give you full information on side effects, undesirable sequelae, and complications no matter how remote their possibility.

Cigarette Smoking If you smoke, the likelihood of wound healing problems and other complications increases. Smokers must *stop smoking completely* at least 2 weeks prior to surgery. "Cutting down" is not enough. Complete cessation of smoking is mandatory.

• • •

Should you not understand any of the foregoing, or should you want more information, please ask. Occasional questions will arise after you have left the office. Feel free to call for additional information. If necessary, a second visit can be scheduled. Find out all you need to know. I wish all patients to be fully informed.

Operative Technique

General anesthesia is used most frequently, but an epidural can be given if the patient requests it. Small volumes confined to the lower abdomen can be treated under local anesthesia. With both general and epidural anesthesia, large volumes of lidocaine with epinephrine are infiltrated 10 minutes prior to beginning suction.

I generally use a 3.7 mm Mercedes Type cannula, although smaller and larger sizes are suitable, depending on fat volumes. A long cannula (30 cm) permits creation of slight lateral and midline furrows to mimic the longitudinal depressions of the semilunar line and linea alba. If only the lower abdomen is to be treated, a 20 cm cannula suffices. Smaller diameter cannulas are useful for the area around the umbilicus since the scarring of the umbilicus and the fibrous tissue associated with periumbilical perforators make this fat more resistant to extraction. A 1.8 or 2.4 mm cannula placed through the pubic incisions aids in removal of this more tenacious fat. Volumes suctioned from the abdomen range from 100 to 1000 cc. Aspiration of more than 1000 cc generally means that the patient is seriously overweight and would be better served by a diet and exercise regimen.

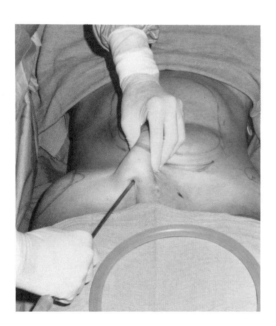
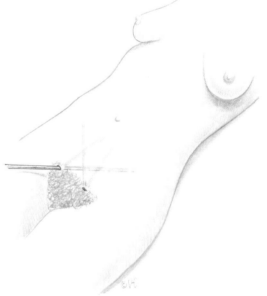

Suctioning is started through the right pubic incision with the patient in the supine position. Lifting the skin around the access incision makes it easier to find the correct plane next to the musculofascia. Fat is suctioned at as deep a level as possible, keeping the cannula close to the fascia.

As in almost all anatomic areas, the use of more than one access incision creates a mesh undermining and provides a smoother contour. Initially the entire lower abdomen is treated through the right pubic incision; about half the expected volume is removed from this incision. The remainder of the expected volume to be suctioned is removed from the left pubic access incision, again treating the entire lower abdomen.

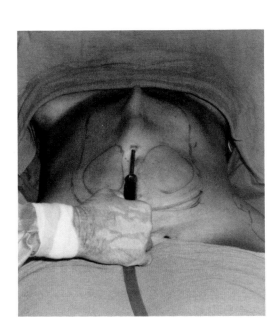 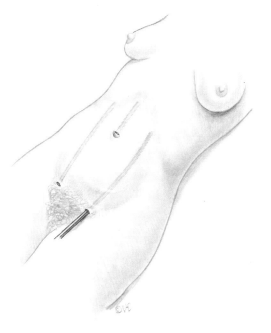

If the upper abdomen requires treatment, it can be approached either from the umbilical and inframammary incisions or with longer cannulas inserted through the pubic incisions. Mesh undermining and controlled volume contouring are used as in the lower abdomen.

Controlled suction at the midline close to the skin will produce a vertical longitudinal depression similar to the normal anatomic depression over the linea alba.

Upper abdominal fat has more fibrous tissue and is more difficult to extract than fat below the umbilicus. Unless the subcutaneous layer in the upper abdomen is notably thickened, liposuction will produce only limited improvement. If the hips and flanks are to be treated in conjunction with abdominal liposuction, the patient is rolled to the side.

Abdominal scars should be approached with care. Although abdominal perforations with cannulas are rare,[71] those that have occurred have been associated with preexisting abdominal scars (personal communication from several surgeons). During the final phase of suctioning small cannulas should be used to "feather" the edges of the treated areas and smooth any residual lumps. No visible or palpable irregularities or steps should be left.

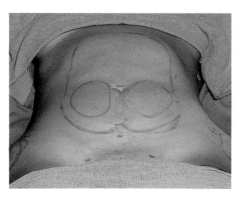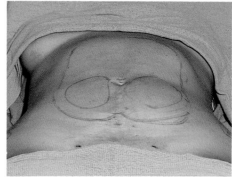

When suctioning is finished, abdominal contour should be reduced as in this patient who is shown before and after suctioning of the right side only. Skin and subcutaneous tissue thickness should be at least 1 cm (2 cm when pinched together). The exact thickness is not as important as the difference in thickness before and after suctioning. Comparing the thickness of abdominal skin and skin of an adjacent area is also helpful.

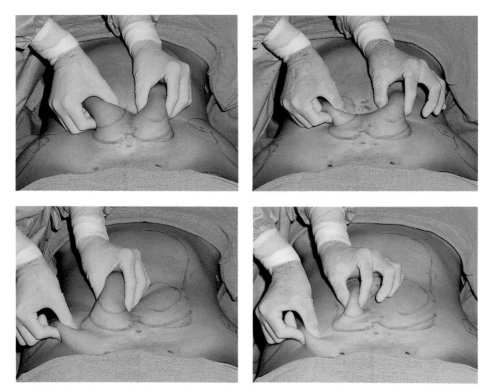

Upper left: Pinch thickness of abdomen before suction. *Upper right:* The pinch test after suction of one side only. *Lower left:* The pinch test in the abdomen before suction compared to pinch thickness of an adjacent area. *Lower right:* Pinch thickness after suction. Thinner patients will have a thinner residual subcutaneous layer than heavier patients.

Quantitative assessment and accurate volumetric measurement of fat also help refine results.

Postoperative Care and Recovery

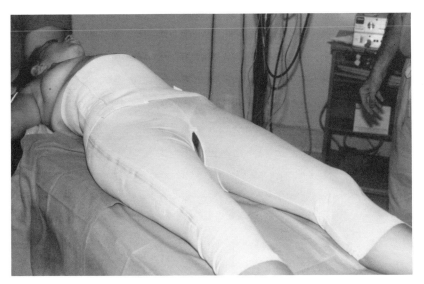
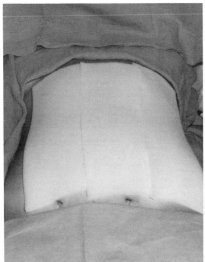

For women, medical-grade compressive garments for the torso and lower extremities (Polli garments) are most comfortable since they don't ride up and can be worn for several weeks after surgery. They also compress the hips, thighs, and knees if these have been treated. If only the abdomen is treated, the all-in-one garments are unnecessary, and simple application of a layer of adherent foam sponge (Reston) will provide sufficient compression.

For men, a large athletic supporter is useful. It covers most of the lower abdomen, and the cup and straps keep it from riding up. The upper abdomen is covered with a binder. Adherent foam sponge is generally not a good option for men since their hair makes application difficult and removal painful.

Although the postoperative course for abdominal suction is similar to that for other areas, several differences deserve mention. Patients may experience more postoperative pain in the abdomen than in other anatomic areas, probably from irritation of the underlying musculoaponeurosis, which is aggravated every time the patient breathes deeply, sits up, or otherwise uses the abdominal musculature.

The large number of perforating vessels between the fascia and subcutaneous tissues causes more intense bleeding, particularly in the lower abdomen, and blood and other fluid may dissect into the soft tissues of the genitalia, causing extensive swelling and discoloration.

Reduction in swelling, resolution of bruising, and return to daily activities follows a time course similar to that after liposuction of other areas. Most patients may return to full activities other than sports within 4 days. More vigorous activity is resumed gradually after the first week, with resumption of sports activities 3 to 4 weeks after surgery.

Results

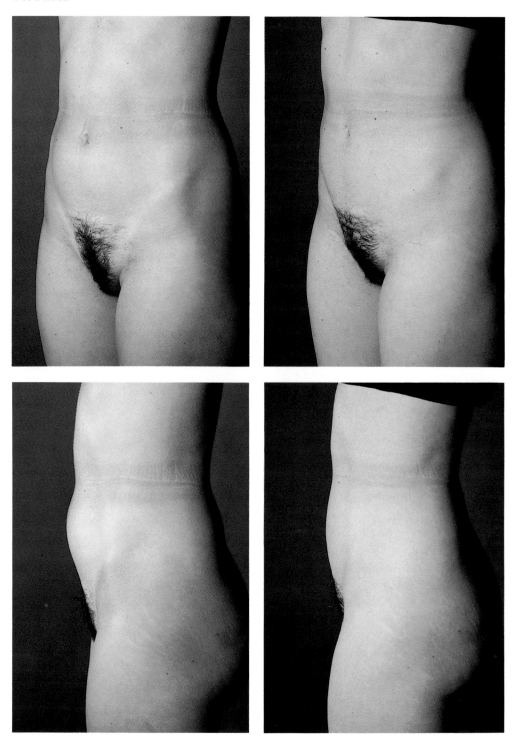

This 31-year-old, 5-foot 2-inch, 100-pound woman is shown before and 6 months after suction of 150 cc from the anterior abdomen. Removal of relatively small volumes can produce dramatic results in women with small frames. A smooth, convex lower abdomen is critical to achieving a pleasing contour.

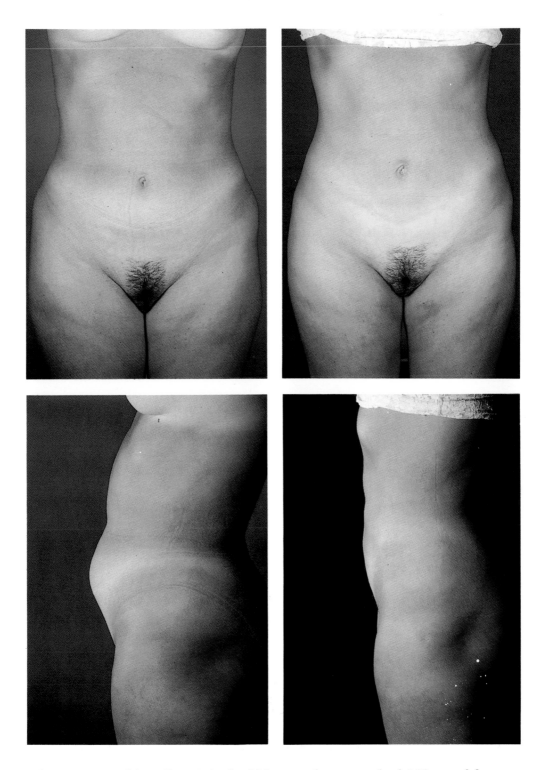

This 43-year-old, 5-foot 2-inch, 120-pound woman had 250 cc of fat suctioned from the anterior abdomen. Her hips and lateral thighs were also treated. Six months after surgery abdominal fullness is reduced, the skin is smooth, and the upper and lower abdomen have a normal round contour.

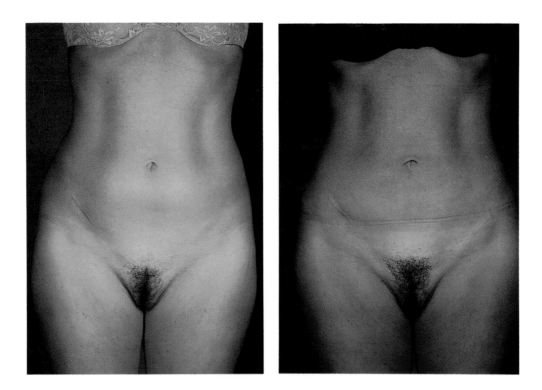

This 42-year-old, 5-foot 6-inch, 120-pound woman had 200 cc of fat suctioned from the lower abdomen. Removing less fat would have preserved a more rounded appearance. The result is also marred by localized overresection that has caused a surface depression slightly below and to the right of the umbilicus.

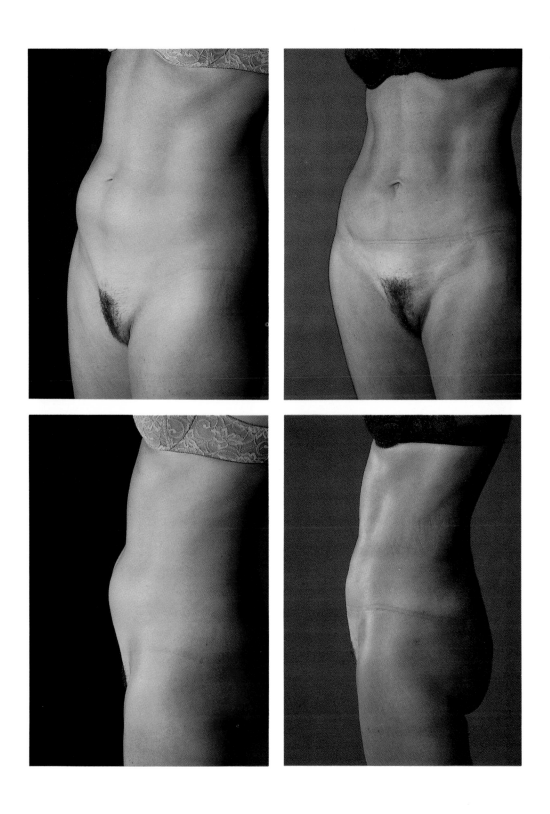

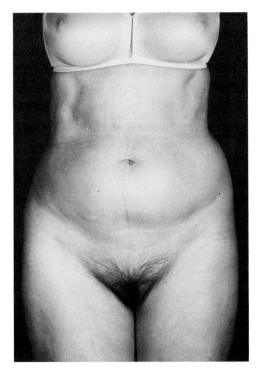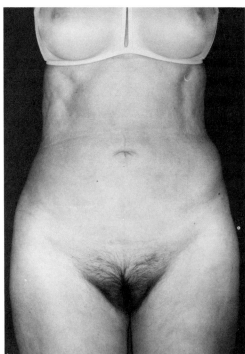

This 59-year-old patient, who was 5 feet 6 inches tall and weighed 128 pounds wanted the flattest possible abdomen and was willing to accept the inevitable surface irregularity. Removal of 550 cc from the abdomen left an unnaturally flat lower abdomen 6 months after surgery. I also treated the hips and medial thighs.

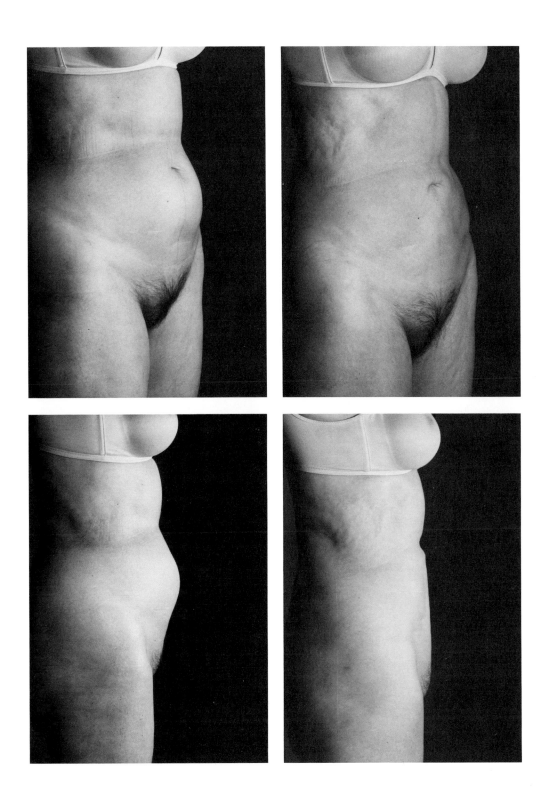

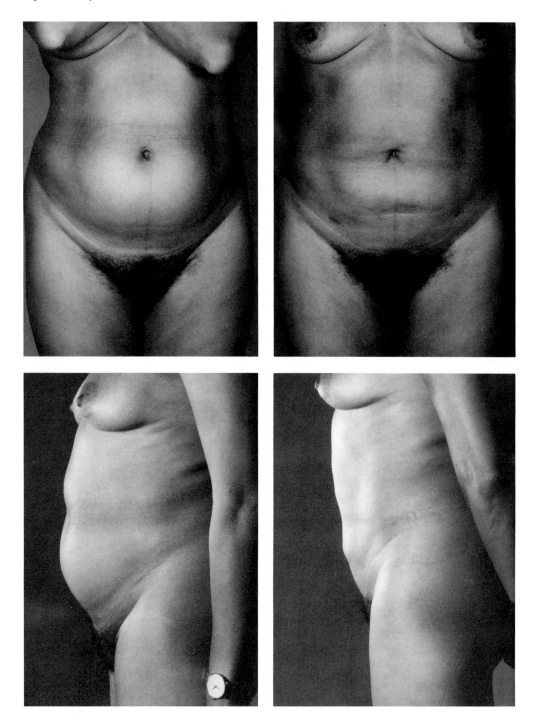

At 5 feet 7 inches and 142 pounds this woman was only slightly overweight, but she carried most of her excess fat in the anterior abdominal subcutaneous compartment. She had minimal laxity of abdominal skin and musculature. Eight months after removal of 750 cc from the abdomen and flanks the abdominal volume is reduced, the skin is smooth, and surface features are normal. Results are equivalent or better than could have been achieved with abdominoplasty. This patient was operated on before I began using access incisions hidden in pubic hair.

COMPLETE ABDOMINOPLASTY WITH TRANSLOCATION OF THE UMBILICUS

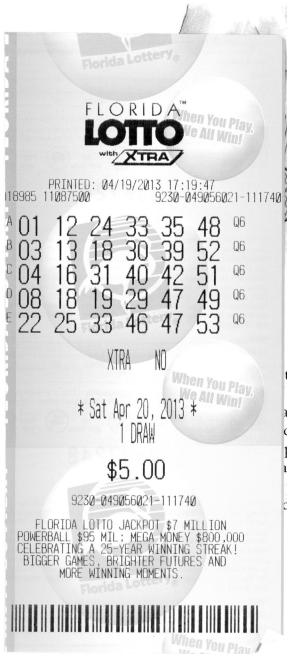

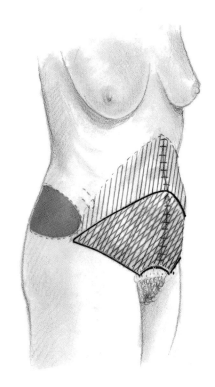

transverse incision is used to achieve wide under-
the abdominal skin and to remove the abundant
a). A hallmark of the procedure is circumscription
cus to release its tethering effect and relocation of
position in the undermined skin flap. Musculofas-
ated by suture plication from xiphoid to pubis.
present. Adjunctive hip suction is routine, but
upper abdomen increases the risk of necrosis and

Markings

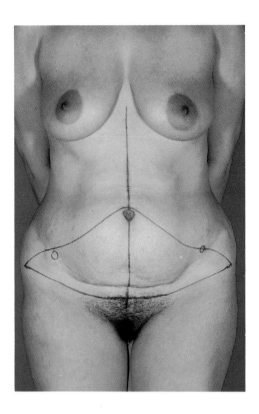

The abdominal midline is marked from the xiphoid to 3 cm below the pubic hairline with the patient standing. The anterior superior iliac spines are outlined with circles. The patient is placed supine for the remainder of the markings, which may be performed after induction of anesthesia. A low transverse incision is drawn with its central portion 1 cm inside the pubic hairline and its lateral segments curving gently upward roughly parallel to the crural fold. The exact position, direction, and length of the incision varies depending on the patient's anatomy.

Lines are drawn from the midline just above the umbilicus to the lateral extremes of the planned low transverse incision. These lines denote the proposed limit of skin removal. They are marked while the patient is supine so as not to overestimate the amount of skin excision. The lengths of the upper lines should equal the lengths of the lower lines to ensure a smooth final closure without "shirring" or dog ears. A circle 1.5 to 2.0 cm in diameter is drawn around the umbilicus.

Operative Technique

General anesthesia is used. The patient is placed supine on the operating table with a foot rest in place to prevent sliding down when the back is elevated. After induction of anesthesia, the top 3 cm of pubic hair is shaved, and a Foley catheter is inserted to monitor urine output and facilitate nursing care in the first 24 hours after surgery.

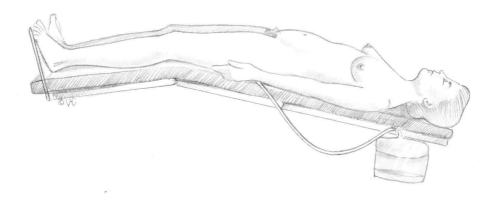

A slight Trendelenburg position with knees flexed is used for flap dissection.

Preliminary Suction of Hip/Flank Area

Suctioning of the iliac crest area is indicated to reduce excess fat in many patients. Skin excision of the lower abdomen with upper flap advancement and closure tends to produce lateral bunching of skin and subcutaneous tissue over the iliac crest. Preliminary suctioning of fat in this area will reduce or in some cases eliminate posterolateral bulging. Suctioning is performed through stab incisions in the lateral portion of the planned lower abdominal incision by rolling the patient. If a second posterolateral access incision is needed, the patient can be easily rolled over to make this site accessible.

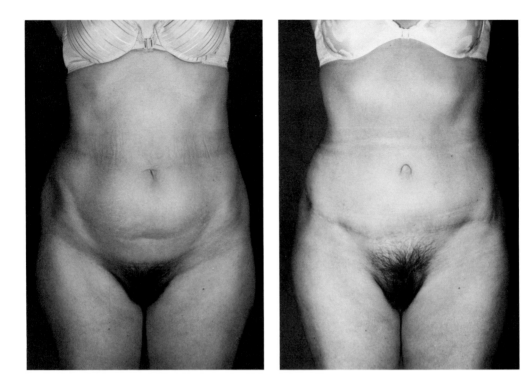

This 49-year-old woman had moderate fullness of the hips; abdominoplasty would have accentuated this bulge. I suctioned 150 cc from each hip
as well as 300 cc from each outer thigh at the time of abdominoplasty. Hip
fullness was reduced 12 months after surgery. The asymmetric scar was
secondary to uneven skin excision.

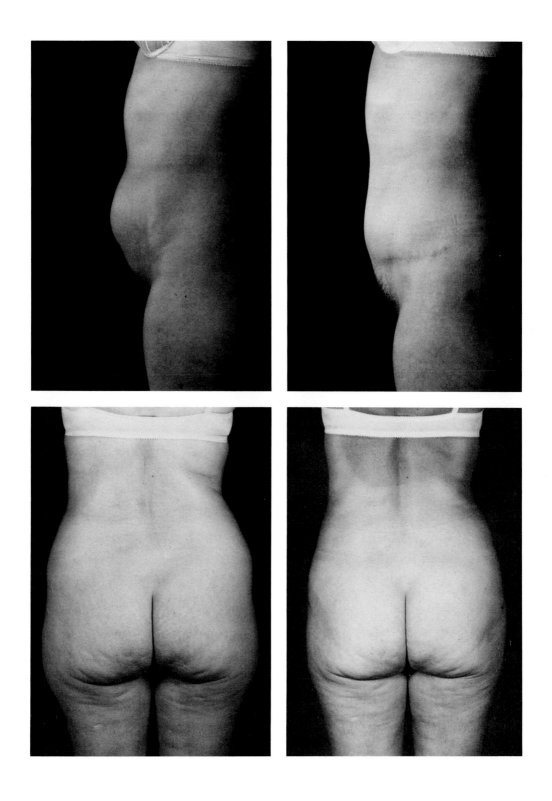

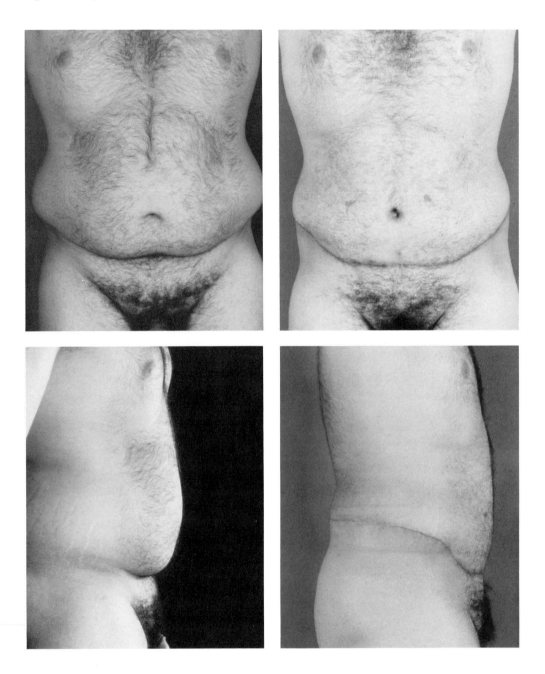

If excessive skin is present, the abdominoplasty excision should be extended laterally over the iliac crest. This 27-year-old physician had lost 60 pounds during his internship. Excessive fullness of the hips required extension of the abdominoplasty excision. Suctioning of the flank without skin excision would have left residual lateral skin bulk. Postoperative photographs were taken at 6 weeks; the patient then moved to another state and no other follow-up visits were made.

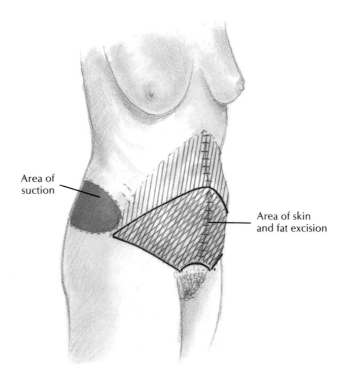

Area of
suction

Area of skin
and fat excision

Suctioning the hip area does not jeopardize flap blood supply, but suctioning of the central proximal flap places the very important superficial superior epigastric artery and its branches at risk. Suctioning the upper lateral flap near the external oblique's slips of origin may damage superficial branches of the lower intercostals. I do not suction these areas when raising an abdominoplasty flap to the xiphoid and costal margin, particularly if the flap may be closed under tension.

If flap elevation is limited, liposuction may be used in areas where flaps have not been elevated. The extent of liposuction should be inversely proportional to the extent of flap elevation. Teimourian and Gotkin[73] treat overweight patients with combined abdominoplasty and aggressive liposuction but limit elevation of the abdominoplasty flap to 5 cm above the umbilicus.

Flap Elevation

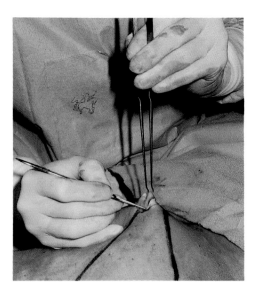

The umbilicus is pulled out with two skin hooks and circumscribed with a No. 15 scalpel blade. Metzenbaum scissors are used to free the umbilical stalk from the surrounding fat down to the aponeurosis. No fat is left on the stalk. A low transverse incision is made, and the superficial inferior epigastric and superficial circumflex iliac vessels are isolated and cauterized. If the vessels are very large, they are tied off.

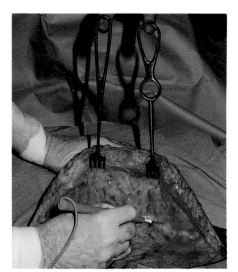 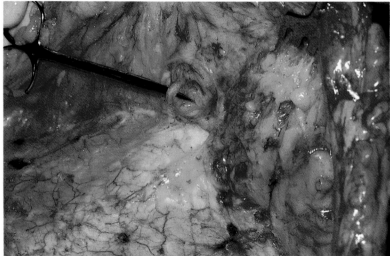

The flap is elevated to the umbilicus using a cutting cautery. The innominate fascia (fascia of Gallaudet) is left undisturbed on the musculoaponeurosis. Leaving the fascia on the aponeurosis reduces bleeding by preserving the plexus of small vessels just deep to the innominate fascia. Perforators are identified and coagulated before they are divided. The tip of the scissor is behind a perforator that is passing from fascia to flap.

As dissection approaches the umbilicus, I protect the umbilical stalk with one hand and continue dissecting around and above the stalk.

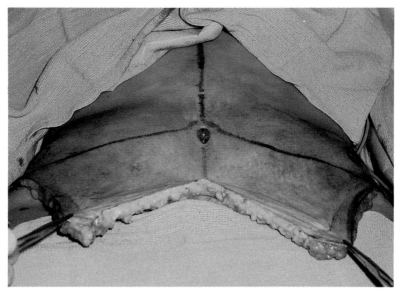

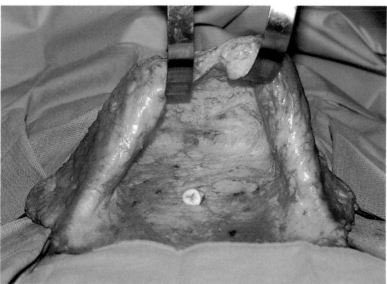

Exposure can be improved by pulling down the flap and dividing it in the midline as far as possible (the distance depends on how much flap the surgeon is certain he will excise). Partial division of the flap gives better exposure and facilitates dissection as the flap is elevated to the xiphoid and costal margin.

Musculoaponeurotic Repair

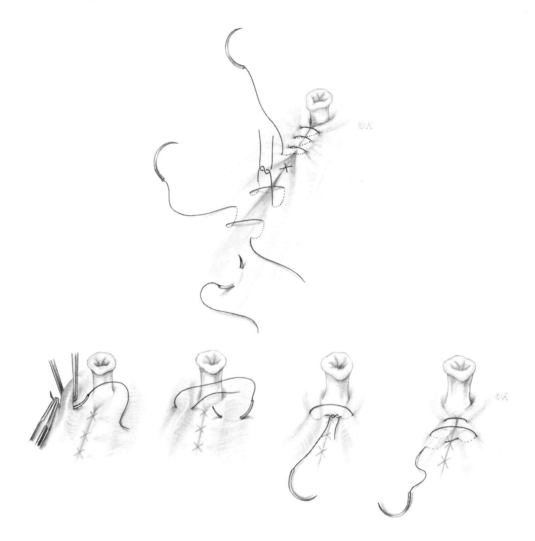

When flap undermining is complete, the musculoaponeurosis is tightened. Interrupted figure-of-eight sutures of 2-0 braided nylon (Neurolon; Ethicon, Somerville, N.J.) are placed from xiphoid to pubis to imbricate the fascia and close any diastasis. Suturing begins at the xiphoid and extends the entire length of the abdomen. Failure to imbricate the upper abdomen will predictably leave a bulge in this area. A second and third layer of continuous running suture is placed over the first if necessary. Although the additional sutures may rotate the rectus abdominis muscles inward, function is not affected.[74]

Transverse waistline plication[75] and elevation and advancement of external oblique flaps[68] have been advocated to increase waist cinching and muscle tautness. I rarely use these maneuvers since I find they add very little to the central plication. Psillakis[76] has reported removal of lower costal cartilages to cinch the torso and reduce conspicuous lower rib cage asymmetries. I have not tried this technique.

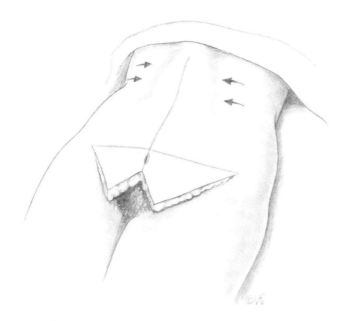

Musculoaponeurotic tightening draws the skin and subcutaneous tissues medially and may produce central skin bulging and lateral dimpling, which should be released by further dissection and superolateral freeing of the flap.

Removing Excess Skin and Subcutaneous Tissue

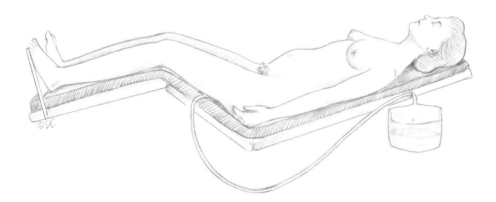

After the musculoaponeurosis has been tightened, the operating table is put in maximal flex position. Then the back is elevated as much as needed to reduce skin tension so that all of the skin below the umbilicus can be excised. Waist flexion may be only slight if the skin is very redundant or close to 90 degrees if necessary.

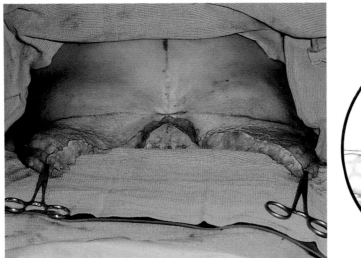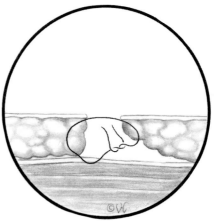

The skin flap is pulled down over the pubis and divided in the midline to above the old umbilical aperture. A temporary suture joins the central portion of the flap to the pubis. This suture also is secured to the musculo-fascia to prevent excessive upward migration of the escutcheon.

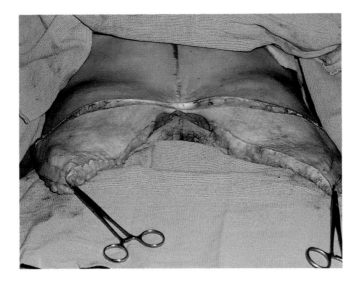

The excision follows the markings made at the beginning of the operation. If indicated, skin is excised above the original markings.

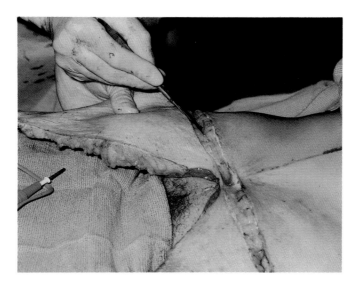

The wound edges are beveled to remove excess fat. The beveling may be carried well up into the flap in heavier patients.

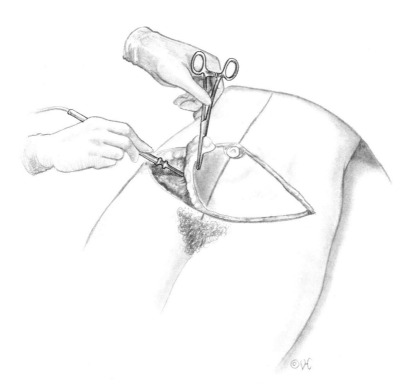

If the surgeon is certain that the entire ellipse of skin below the umbilicus can be removed, this segment may be excised at the beginning of the operation before dissecting the upper flap.

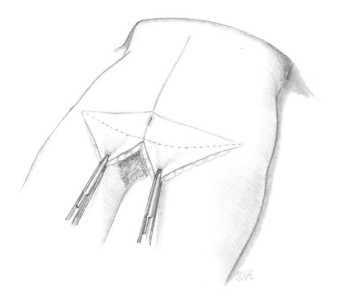

Almost all women who have borne children have sufficient abdominal laxity to permit excision of the skin between the umbilicus and the pubic hairline. On the uncommon occasion that all of the skin cannot be excised, the flap is pulled down as far as possible without creating undue tension, and the midline is divided to the limit of planned flap excision.

With the two halves of the flap kept on equal tension, straight lines are drawn from the top of the midline incision to the lateral ends of the low transverse incision (the previous markings are used as a guide for maintaining symmetry), and excess flap is excised. The old umbilical aperture remains in the midline and is closed vertically at the end of the operation.

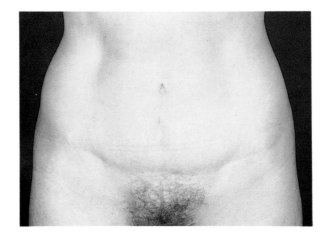

In some patients the bottom but not the top of the old umbilical aperture reaches to the pubis, and closure is converted to an inverted T with a short vertical arm. The midline portion of the scar is rarely a significant cosmetic problem.

Positioning the New Umbilical Site

With the flap still secured to the pubis, the patient is temporarily taken out of the waist-flexed position for accurate positioning of the new umbilical opening.

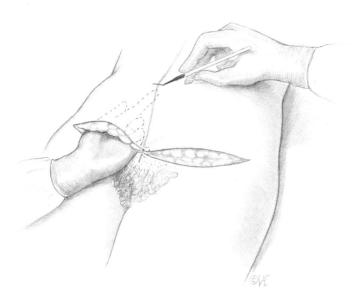

I place my hand under the flap to palpate the umbilicus and push against the flap at the umbilical position. The new umbilical position is marked on the skin at the midline. The umbilicus should sit approximately at the level of the top of the iliac crests.[77]

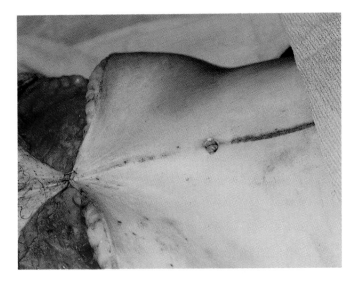

A 12 mm transverse opening centered on the midline is made at this point. Skin tension will transform this slit into an oval or round shape.

Defatting the Flap

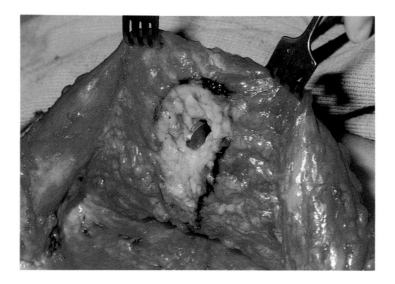

The central suture is released, and the flap is turned up so its undersurface can be defatted. An ellipse is marked in ink on the fat around the umbilicus. The ellipse extends from the umbilicus 6 cm in a superior direction and 3 cm laterally and inferiorly. The fat around the umbilicus is excised with scissors, tapering the excision into the remainder of the flap. An instrument has been placed through the umbilicus to indicate its position on the flap. Additional fat may be removed in the midline up to the xiphoid, creating a gentle midline furrow when the flap is replaced. Alternatively, in the very thin patient, midline scoring of the fat to the dermis will release fascial support so that the fat falls away from the midline, also creating a furrow. Defatting around the umbilicus assists in recreating the umbilical depression. The upper midline depression mimics a normal and desirable feature of the youthful abdomen. Additional defatting of the lower flap may be performed as necessary.

Closure

The operative field is irrigated with saline solution to remove fat particles and other debris. Jackson–Pratt suction drains are placed in the lower abdomen and brought out through stab incisions in the pubic hair.

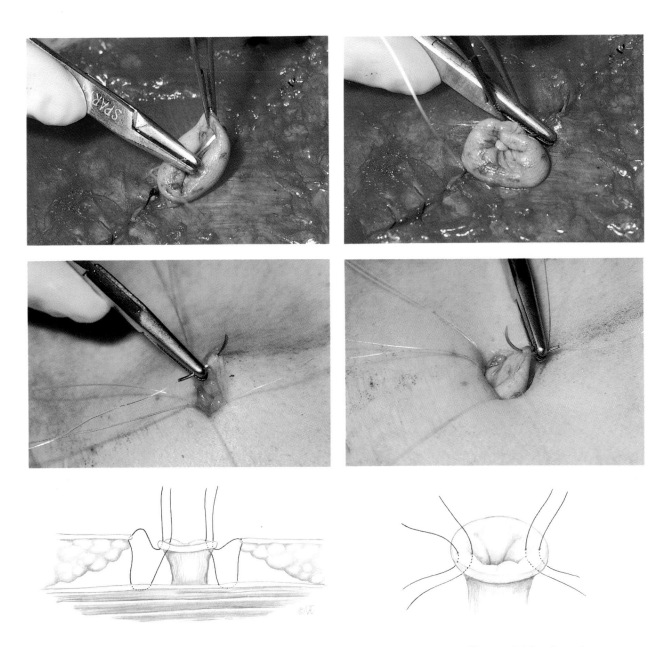

A 3-0 polydioxanone suture (PDS; Ethicon Inc., Somerville, N.J.) is placed through the umbilical skin at 12 o'clock and through the fascia just above the umbilicus. Three similar sutures are placed at 3, 6, and 9 o'clock. The needles are led through the new umbilical opening to the skin surface and then sutured through the dermis of the umbilical aperture and back through the umbilical skin as half-buried vertical mattress sutures. The sutures are left long and clamped to the drapes. They will be tied at the end of the operation.

The table is flexed to facilitate closure, and the midline of the flap is again sutured to the midline of the pubis with a single buried 2-0 braided nylon suture (Neurolon) placed through all layers of the subcutaneous fascia and catching the musculofascia.

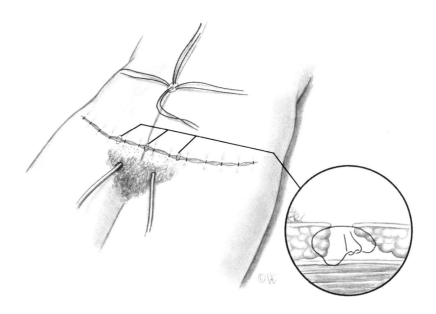

Skin staples are used to position the lateral portions of the flap so that there are no dog ears or folds. If there is great disparity in length between the upper and lower flaps, the incision is extended laterally as far as necessary to remove the excess.

Once the flap is correctly positioned for closure, two additional deep Neurolon sutures are placed at either lateral end of the pubic hairline similar to the one in the midline, also catching the musculoaponeurosis. The remainder of the deep closure is accomplished with interrupted 0 chromic sutures through the superficial fascia. The skin is closed with intracuticular running 3-0 PDS.

Umbilicoplasty

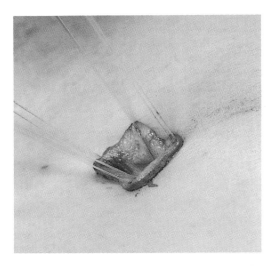 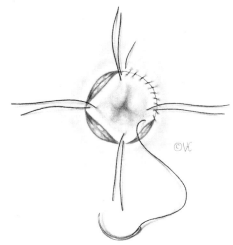

Pulling up on the previously placed umbilical sutures aligns the umbilical stalk with the new aperture in the flap.

A running 4-0 plain suture is used to approximate umbilical skin to the flap, after which the 3-0 PDS sutures are tied.

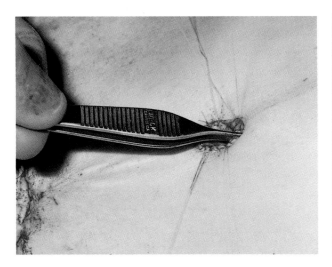 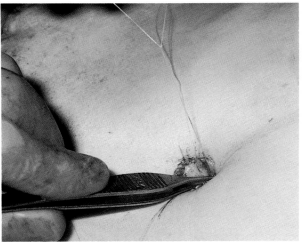

The assistant uses a forceps to grasp the umbilicus and the adjacent flap and presses the tissues to the deep fascia while the surgeon ties the PDS sutures. Securing the surrounding skin to the fascial level recreates the umbilical depression.

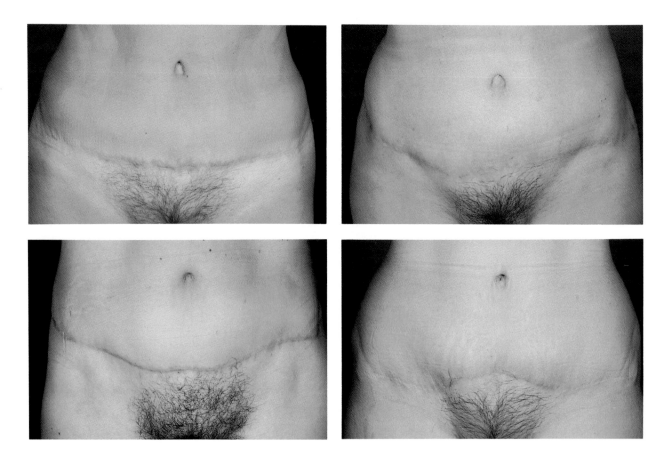

Other methods of creating a natural-looking umbilicus have been described,[78-80] but I find the simple technique outlined here gives predictable and pleasing results.

A light dressing is placed on the low transverse suture line, but the umbilicus is left exposed.

Postoperative Care and Recovery

The patient is extubated while still deeply anesthetized to prevent bucking or coughing. A strong Valsalva maneuver could disrupt the musculofascial plication. A stretcher is not used for transport to the recovery room. Instead, the patient's bed, made up in a semi-Fowler position, is brought to the operating room, and the patient is transferred from the operating room table to the bed directly. She is always kept in a flexed position. She will stay in her bed while in the recovery area and during transport to her room.

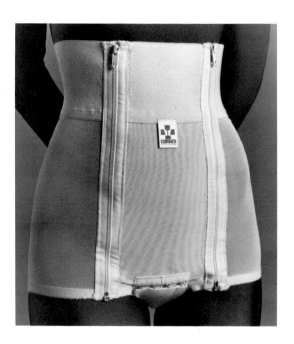

The next morning the Foley and intravenous catheters are removed. An abdominal binder (Caromed) is placed over the lower abdomen during ambulation. When the patient is in bed, I prefer to leave the flap exposed for observation and to avoid unnecessary compression. A light diet is begun and advanced as tolerated. The head of the bed is gradually lowered each day. By the time the patient leaves the hospital, the bed is usually adjusted to 30 degrees or less.

The patient is discharged on the third postoperative day and occasionally earlier. At home the patient sleeps with head and knees elevated on pillows for about a week. Patients should wait 2 weeks before resuming sedentary work. Vigorous sports are prohibited for 2 months.

Results

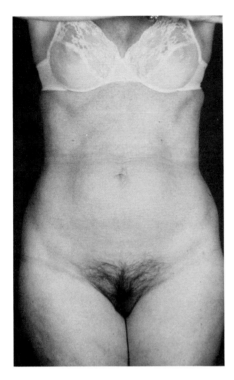 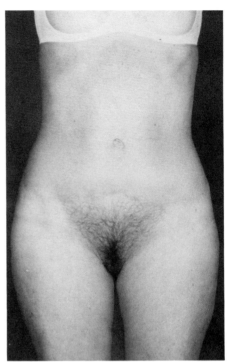

This 46-year-old mother of three gained 45 pounds during each pregnancy. She was 5 feet 6 inches tall and weighed 129 pounds at consultation. Her concerns centered around abdominal protuberance and skin laxity, particularly the slight wrinkling above the umbilicus. She also sought thigh reduction. She wore a size 6 to 8 in blouses and jackets but needed a size 10 to 12 for skirts and some dresses.

Abdominoplasty was performed simultaneously with liposuction of the hips, lateral thighs, medial thighs, and knees (total volume 1200 cc). Sixteen months after surgery abdominal contour is reduced and waist suppression is restored. The overall result is a smaller, more youthful abdomen with normal, rounded contours. She is able to fit into size 8 skirts and dresses. The umbilicus is larger than ideal because the new aperture was cut at 18 mm instead of 12 to 14 mm, a seemingly trivial difference but enough to be noticeable.

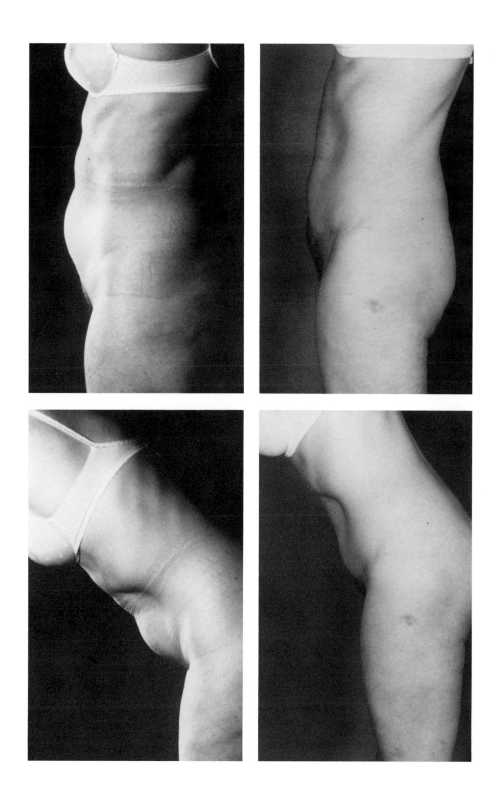

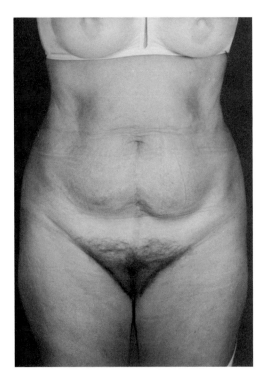 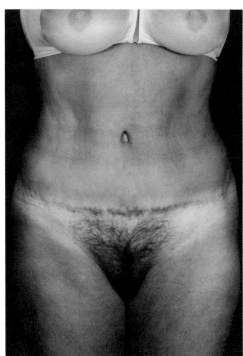

Indications for complete abdominoplasty in this 54-year-old woman included extremely lax abdominal skin, a low midline scar, and moderate excess of subcutaneous fat. The waist was narrowed by plication of the diastasis recti. Postoperative views were taken 12 months after surgery.

Contour improvement is excellent. The central portion of the scar was widened and the erythema persisted even beyond 24 months, but the patient readily accepted the suboptimal scar as a necessary consequence of the surgery.

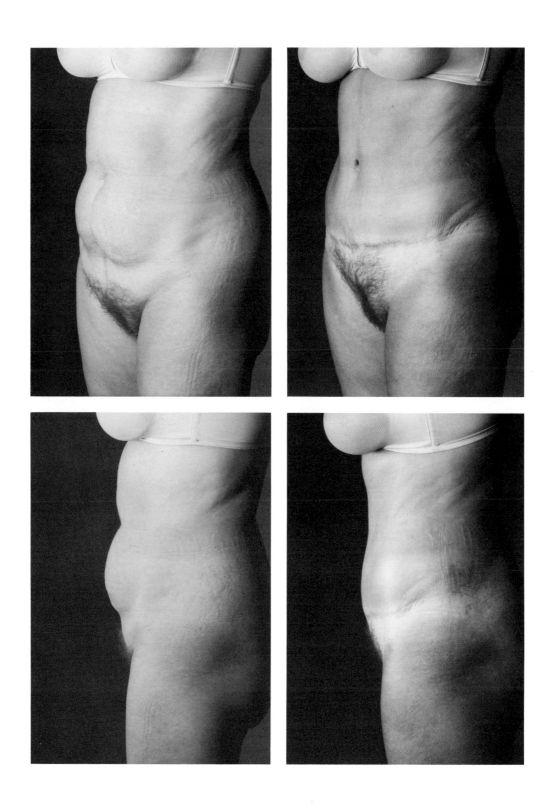

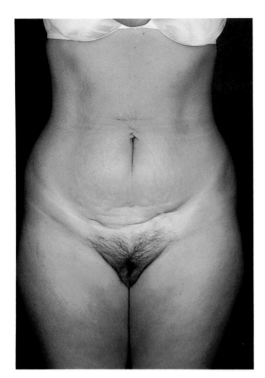 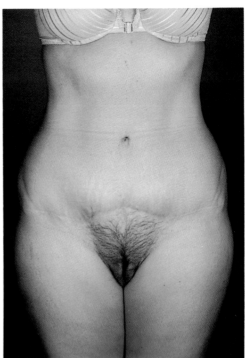

This 45-year-old woman, who was 5 feet 4 inches tall and weighed 125 pounds, had striated skin hanging over a low, transverse scar. She is pictured 12 months after complete abdominoplasty with a modified W incision and aspiration of fat from the hips and outer thighs. Central plication of the diastasis narrowed the waist. The upper midline depression was accentuated by liposuction.

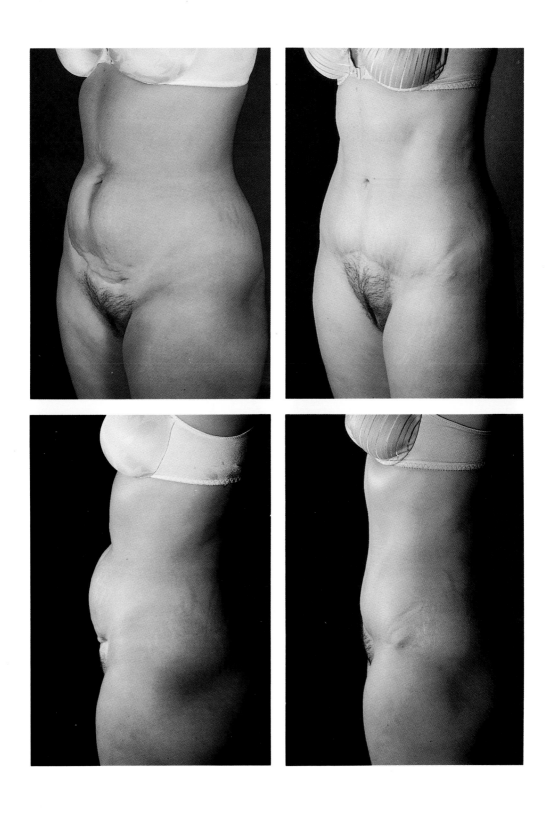

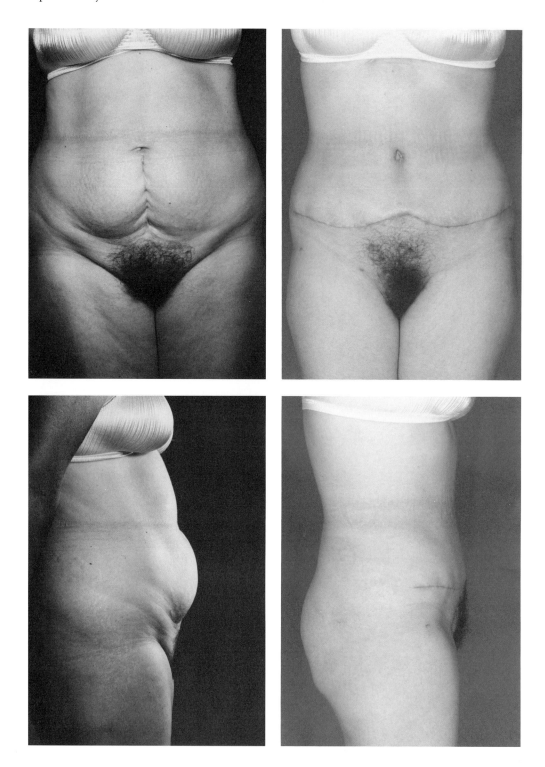

This 46-year-old, 5-foot 2-inch, 131-pound woman had had two children by cesarean section. She found the appearance of her lower abdomen distasteful, particularly the depressed vertical scar. Six weeks following complete abdominoplasty and liposuction of 150 cc from each hip, contour was reduced in both the lower and upper abdomen despite postoperative swelling. Her waist was narrowed by midline plication.

During dissection of the upper flap I divided the right superficial superior epigastric artery. At the conclusion of the operation the right side of the flap was pale and there was little bleeding from the cut edge. I therefore decided not to increase tension on the flap by anchoring it to the fascia next to the pubis. Instead, the escutcheon was permitted to elevate slightly. The distal right side of the flap was pale and dusky for a few hours after surgery but recovered without skin loss or other untoward event.

COMPLETE ABDOMINOPLASTY WITHOUT UMBILICAL TRANSLOCATION (MODIFIED ABDOMINOPLASTY)

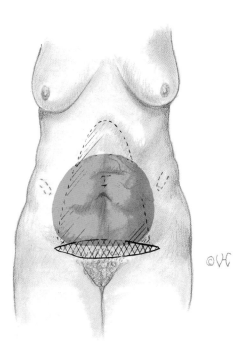

This operation permits fascial tightening above and below the umbilicus and removal of a limited amount of lower abdominal skin. The amount of skin removal is restricted since the umbilicus is not translocated. A low transverse incision 1 cm inside the pubic hairline extends laterally no farther than the anterior superior iliac spines. The umbilicus is not circumscribed and may or may not be disinserted with the flap. Fascial plication is performed above and below the umbilicus. Excess fat may or may not be present.

Markings

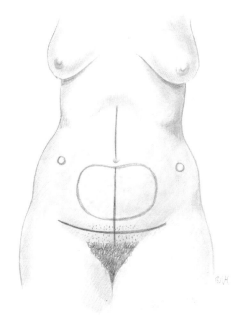

Areas to be suctioned and the anterior abdominal midline are marked with the patient standing. The lower line of incision is marked with the patient supine and is usually a gentle curve parallel to the natural skin creases 1 cm inside the top of the pubic hairline and extending laterally as far as a line dropped vertically from the anterior superior iliac spines. Alternatively, a W-type incision[42] can be used to keep the lateral ends of the scar high, which allows the patient to wear high-cut bathing suits.

Operative Technique

It is possible to use local anesthesia combined with dissociative techniques,[43] but I find general anesthesia efficient, safe, and predictable. Infiltration of dilute lidocaine with epinephrine solution is used for all patients.

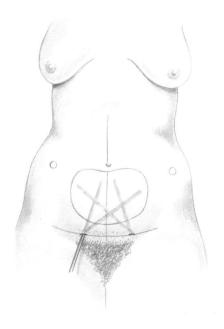

Preliminary suctioning is used as indicated. Since flap elevation is more limited than in standard abdominoplasty, suctioning may be performed more aggressively. Nevertheless, it is important to be as atraumatic as possible, particularly in the area in which the flap will be raised. The suction tip is kept close to the fascia both to avoid irregularities of the skin surface and to protect the subdermal circulation.

Flap Elevation and Fascial Repair

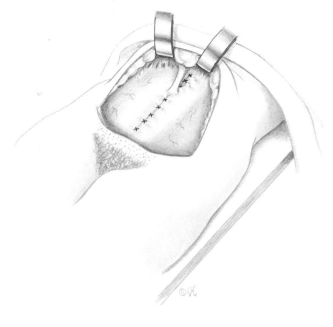

After the preliminary suctioning is completed, the incision is opened to the musculoaponeurosis and the flap raised to the umbilicus and above, leaving the base of the umbilicus intact. Fascial laxity is repaired by plicating the diastasis recti as in complete abdominoplasty. Long Deaver retractors facilitate dissection and placement of sutures above the umbilicus.

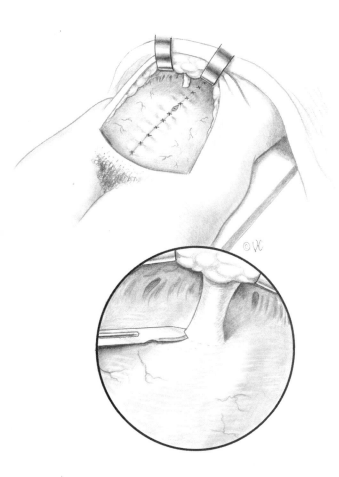

If greater exposure is required, the umbilical stalk can be cut at its base and unimpeded undermining continued to the costal margin.[68] Brisk bleeding from the umbilical artery remnant is frequently encountered and should be controlled with cautery. A previous umbilical scar contraindicates amputation of the umbilical stalk. The increased exposure permits facile imbrication of the entire length of midline fascia from xiphoid to pubis. The fascial defect secondary to dividing the umbilicus should always be repaired.

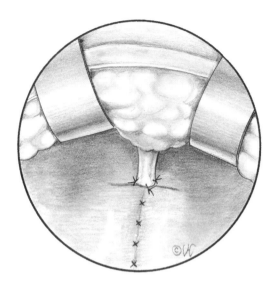

At the conclusion of the procedure the umbilicus is sutured back to the midline with 3-0 chromic sutures at its original position or slightly lower if additional skin needs to be excised. The line of fascial plication may not always be coincident with the anatomic midline, particularly if there is scoliosis. The umbilical suture should be placed with care and the position of the umbilicus checked with reference to surface landmarks before closing the skin. Alternatively, the umbilical stalk can "free float," but this technique can result in a flattened, featureless scar instead of the desired depression.

Only minimal laxities of the upper abdominal skin can be corrected without lowering the umbilicus to an unsightly position. Bozola and Psillakis[68] warn against lowering the umbilicus to less than 14 cm above the pubis, whereas Matarasso[2] states that it should not be lowered more than 2 to 3 cm and no less than 10 cm above the pubic hairline.

My approach is based on the observation that the umbilicus looks best when it is at its natural location slightly below the narrowest point of the torso at the level of the highest point of the iliac crest.[77] Significant deviations from this normal location in relation to known anatomic landmarks will draw the eye to an abnormal and unattractive displacement. Although I do not hesitate to divide the insertion of the umbilicus to facilitate exposure to the upper abdomen, I rarely lower it.

Skin Excision and Closure

Following fascial repair and suturing of the umbilical stalk (when it has been divided), flat suction drains are placed under the flap and brought out through stab incisions in the pubic hair. The table is then flexed to 150 degrees to facilitate closure.

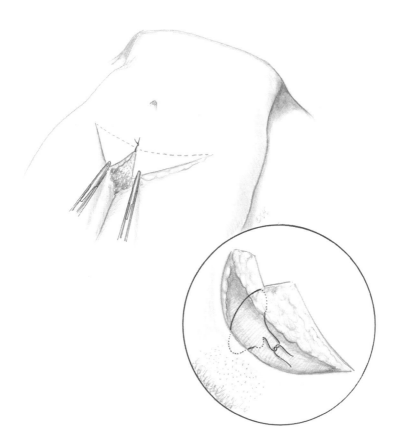

The flap is pulled down over the incision and the investing fascia with minimal tension and then split in the midline, at which point it is sutured to the lower incision with a single 2-0 Neurolon suture as in standard abdominoplasty. The two halves of the excess flap are excised, and the wound is closed in layers.

Postoperative Care and Recovery

A light dressing is applied for 24 hours. The patient is kept in the semi-Fowler position with 30 degrees of head elevation for 24 hours; elevation is then gradually reduced. Drains are removed after 24 hours. An abdominal compression garment is worn for 2 weeks to ensure flap adherence.

Patients usually return home the day after surgery, although occasional patients will require 48 hours of postoperative care in the hospital. Bed rest at home is advised for the rest of the week. Patients may get up for meals and to go to the bathroom. Depending on the extent of skin undermining and aponeurotic plication, patients return to sedentary activities 1 to 2 weeks after surgery. Sports are prohibited for 2 months.

Although modified abdominoplasty is less physiologically disruptive than complete abdominoplasty, resting at home for a minimum of 1 week is a critical part of the postoperative regimen. Early resumption of activities will result in an increased incidence of seromas.

Results

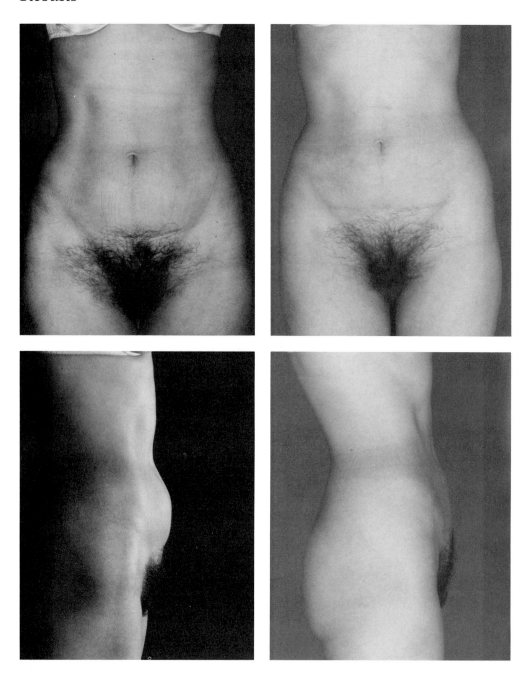

This 34-year-old, 5-foot 7-inch, 124-pound woman wanted the size of her abdomen and thighs reduced. She had undergone hysterectomy 2 years previously. Liposuction was performed on the abdomen, thighs, and knees (less than 100 cc removed from the abdomen). Through the low transverse hysterectomy incision a skin-fat flap was elevated to 10 cm above the umbilicus, which was left in situ. The midline was plicated with a single row of interrupted sutures above the umbilicus and a double row below. No excess skin was removed. She is seen 18 months after surgery.

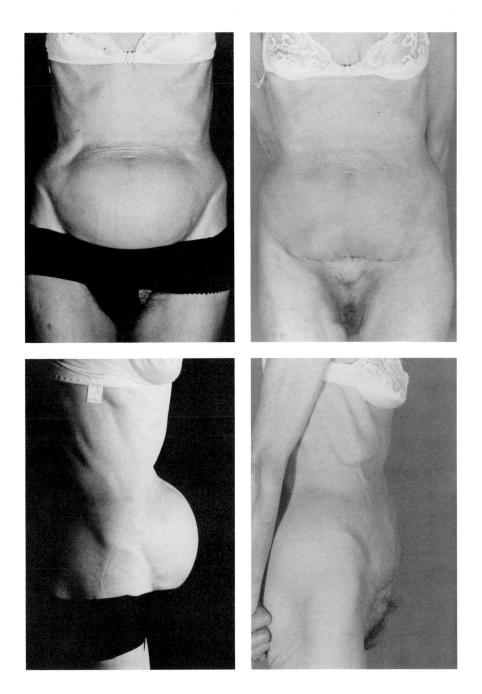

This 58-year-old, 5-foot 2-inch, 93-pound woman sought treatment for severe lower abdominal protrusion resulting from musculofascial relaxation and slight lumbar lordosis. Most of her garments had to be custom-tailored because she could not fit into the standard clothes sizes. She had almost no subcutaneous fat. She smoked two packs of cigarettes a day. Although preoperative pulmonary function tests showed adequate reserve, I limited her procedure to a modified abdominoplasty under epidural anesthesia because of her inability to stop smoking. I left the umbilical stalk in situ and placed three plication sutures above the umbilicus. The procedure resulted in a significant improvement and greater flexibility in choice of clothing. She is shown before and 2 weeks after surgery.

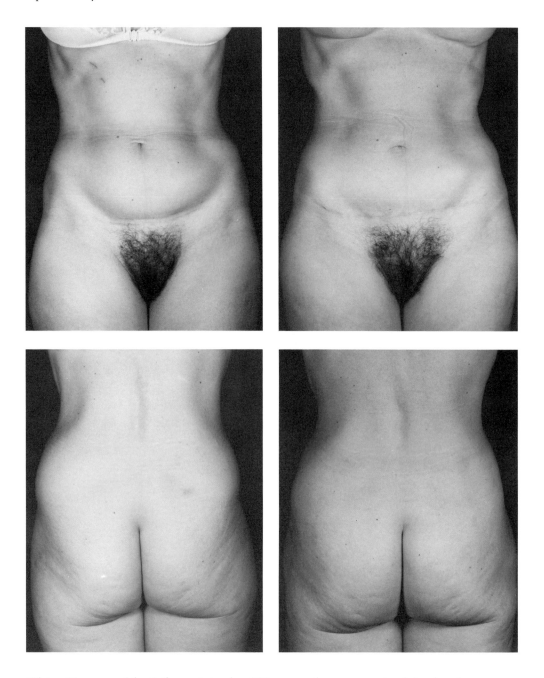

This 49-year-old, 5-foot 6-inch, 122-pound woman had had a hysterectomy after having two children. She had a subcutaneous fat thickness of less than 2 cm. Her abdominal protuberance was largely due to lax skin and musculature. She requested as flat an abdomen as possible and wished to be rid of even the minimal skin laxity evidenced by the slight wrinkling directly above the umbilicus.

She is seen 11 months after complete abdominoplasty, liposuction of 200 cc from the anterior abdomen, elevation of a skin–fat flap to the xiphoid (the umbilicus was disinserted), and plication of the midline above and below

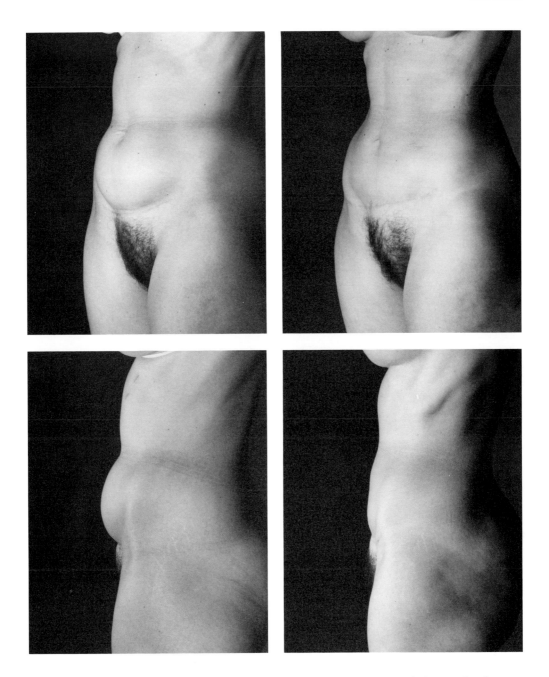

the umbilicus. A 6 cm wide ellipse of skin was removed from the lower abdomen, and the umbilicus was reinserted 2 cm below its former site.

The goals of a flat abdomen and tight skin have been achieved. The slight lowering of the umbilicus is not an aesthetic handicap (the skin impression of the elastic top of the patient's panty hose delineates the waist and the increase in distance from waist to umbilicus after surgery). Liposuction of the hips reduced protuberance in this area. A relatively narrow waist was maintained by the cinching effect of the midline plication. The lengthening of the scar was necessitated by removal of lower abdominal skin without creating dog ears.

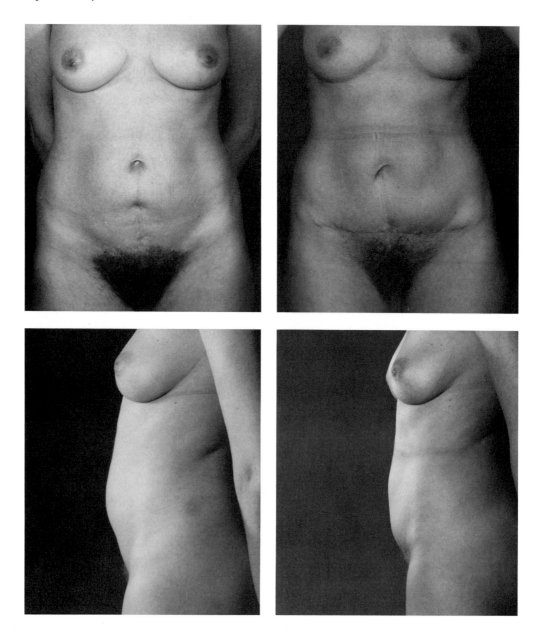

This 41-year-old woman had borne two children by cesarean section. Her protuberant abdomen was due almost entirely to musculofascial relaxation with moderate skin laxity and minimal excess subcutaneous fat. A long-standing umbilical hernia was 2 cm in diameter.

I performed a modified abdominoplasty with liposuction of the anterior abdominal wall. The umbilicus was disinserted to afford more complete exposure and the hernia repaired. The umbilicus was reattached approximately 2 cm below its original site, and a 4 cm ellipse of skin was removed from the lower edge of the flap. Eight months later abdominal contour is improved, and most of the vertical scar is eliminated.

The result is marred by inferolateral malplacement of the umbilicus. A secondary procedure could centralize the umbilicus but would not elevate it. The patient has refused reoperation.

LOWER ABDOMINOPLASTY (MINIABDOMINOPLASTY)

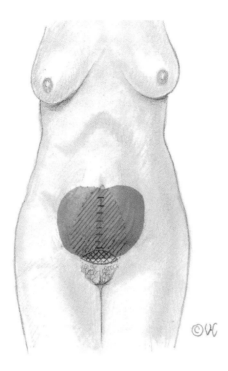

This operation produces a low transverse scar hidden within the pubic hairline. Because of the short transverse length of the scar, only very small amounts of skin can be removed in the vertical dimension (3 to 4 cm). Associated fat removal can be performed by suction or open excision. I find its indications limited and use it infrequently.

Markings

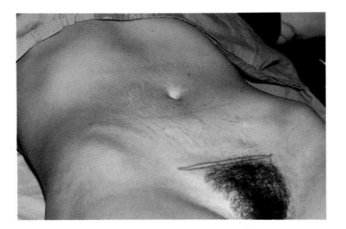

Areas for liposuction are marked with the patient in the standing position. With the patient supine a low transverse incision is drawn 1 cm below the pubic hairline. The lateral extent of the incision usually does not extend beyond the natural pubic hairline.

Operative Technique

Since the operative field is limited to the area below the umbilicus, local infiltration of anesthesia is suitable. General anesthesia may be used at the discretion of the surgeon.

If suction is needed, it is performed first, as in modified abdominoplasty.

Flap Elevation and Skin Excision

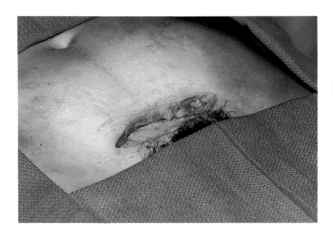 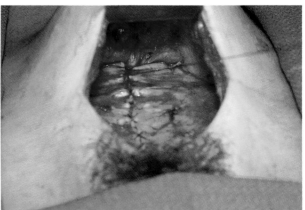

After suctioning is completed, the skin and subcutaneous tissue of the lower abdomen are elevated to the umbilicus. The musculofascia is tightened with a series of imbricating sutures of 2-0 braided Neurolon. The excess skin is then excised from the flap, as in modified abdominoplasty. Flat suction drains are placed through stab wounds in the pubic hair and the wound is closed in layers.

Postoperative Care and Recovery

A light dressing is placed on the wound. If the patient is ambulatory, an abdominal binder is placed over the lower abdomen. The abdominal binder should not be too tight to avoid possible vascular compromise of the flap. Drains are removed at 24 hours. To promote flap adherence, patients are instructed to remain in bed for 3 days except for meals and using the bathroom. They remain at home for 1 week. Sports are prohibited for 2 months to ensure the integrity of the muscle repair.

Results

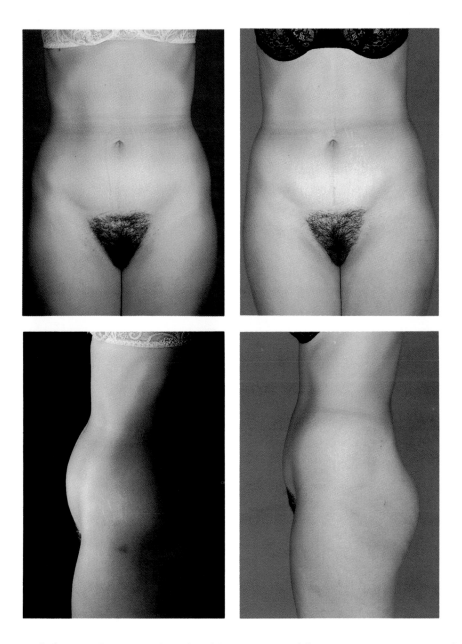

Lower abdominal protrusion in this 35-year-old woman was primarily a function of musculofascial laxity. Contributing to the fullness was a small amount of excess subcutaneous fat and a postural forward pelvic thrust. A transverse scar in the upper pubic hair was from a previous tuboplasty. Surgery consisted of liposuction of 100 cc from the lower abdomen, a double-layer plication of the diastasis recti from umbilicus to pubis, and excision of a 3 cm wide ellipse of skin, including the old suprapubic scar. Thirteen months after surgery the abdomen is less protuberant but still retains a normal rounded convexity. The patient requested additional surgery to produce a totally flat abdomen. Since the subcutaneous fat layer was already quite thin and since further fascial tightening would not correct her posture, no further procedures were done.

ABDOMINAL SURGERY AFTER MAJOR WEIGHT LOSS

These patients often require several operations to remove excess tissue from areas in addition to the abdomen, and an overall program should be developed to plan the nature and timing of each procedure before the first operation is begun. If enough excess skin is present to create intertrigo, skin infections, skin breakdown, or inflammatory conditions should be controlled. A 2- to 3-week period of intensive washing and attention to skin hygiene may be necessary prior to surgery.

Blood loss may be significant because of the extent of the procedure, and preparations for autologous transfusion are prudent, particularly if multiple procedures are to be performed.

Markings

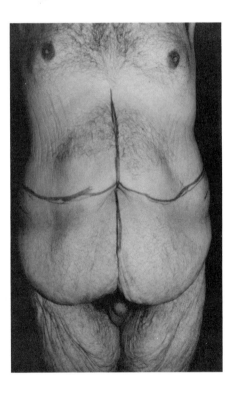 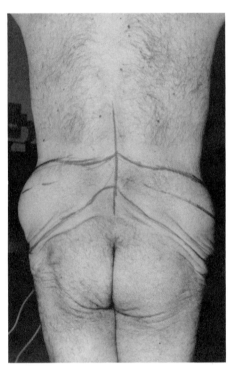

Planning of abdominoplasty incisions should also take into consideration the likelihood of excisions from adjacent areas. Markings are made with the patient standing and should include all the excess skin and subcutaneous tissues. It is not critical to remove the last centimeter of excess, and a difficult closure under tension should be avoided. Incisions are designed for optimal removal of excess skin and may be a combination of transverse and vertical. If significant excess fat is present, surgery usually consists of en bloc resection with little or no skin undermining.

Operative Technique

Anesthesia is induced and the patient intubated on a stretcher next to the operating table. The patient is then placed prone on the table (see Chapter 3, p. 50).

First, the posterior excess is removed up to the midaxillary line. The level of dissection is between the superficial and deep layers of the superficial fascia. The deep fat is left in situ. As the dissection proceeds to the anterior abdomen, the posterior deep fat layer ends and the level of dissection will be the external oblique muscle aponeurosis. After the back is closed, the patient is turned supine, reprepped and draped, and the anterior excess removed in a manner similar to complete abdominoplasty except that flap dissection may be limited. Fascia plication and skin closure are as described for complete abdominoplasty.

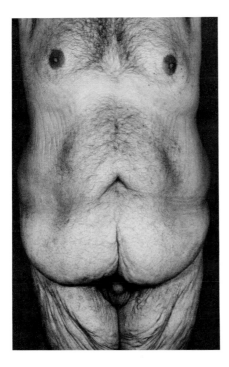 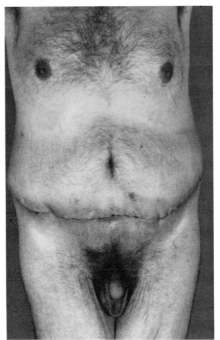

This 37-year-old man had lost 160 pounds and maintained a stable weight of 185 pounds for 5 years. He is shown before and 2 weeks after circumferential abdominoplasty. The excised specimen weighed 10 pounds.

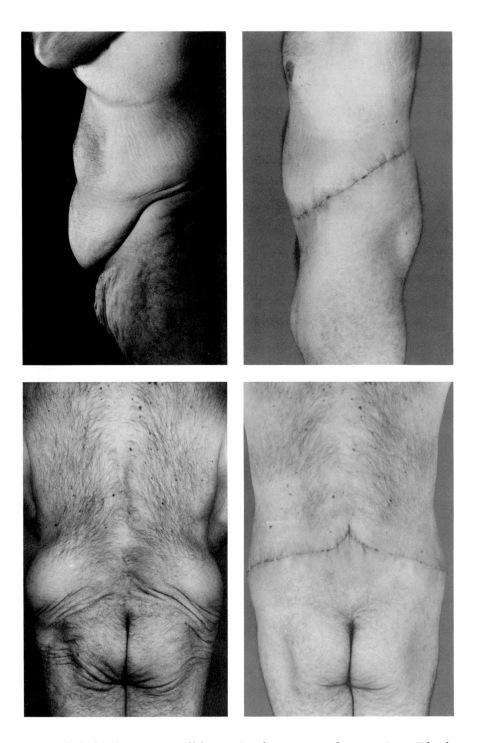

Excess medial thigh tissues will be excised at a second operation. The lateral thigh and buttock excess has been improved, however, by the flank and back excisions.

COMBINED PROCEDURES
Abdominoplasty Combined With Liposuction of Distant Areas

Abdominoplasty is commonly combined with suction of distant areas such as the thighs or knees. I generally perform liposuction first, turning the patient side to side as necessary. Following completion of suction, the patient is returned to the supine position, a Foley catheter is placed, and the abdomen is prepped again for abdominoplasty.

If large volumes (usually >1000 cc) are to be suctioned in conjunction with abdominoplasty, the patient predonates autologous blood.

Abdominoplasty Combined With Cosmetic Procedures Other Than Liposuction

Abdominoplasty is commonly combined with other cosmetic operations, most frequently breast reduction or augmentation.[35,72,81-83] Face lifts and other operations are also done simultaneously.[72]

The breast reduction or other ancillary procedure is usually performed first, and as one operative team closes the breasts or other area, the primary surgeon performs the abdominoplasty. Cardoso de Castro and Daher[81] reported a series of 30 breast reductions combined with abdominoplasty in which the complete operation usually required less than 3 hours.

Abdominoplasty Combined With Intra-Abdominal or Major Pelvic Procedures

Although Voss, Sharp, and Scott[84] showed an increased incidence of pulmonary embolism in patients undergoing abdominoplasty combined with a major pelvic procedure, other studies have not supported their findings.[38,67,72,85,86]

Grazer[35] recommended that the intra-abdominal or pelvic procedure be done first and that the abdominoplasty be postponed if the patient lost more than 300 ml of blood or if the plastic surgeon believed that the second procedure should not be done. Hester et al.[72] found that the incidence of pulmonary embolus was significantly increased in obese patients who had combined procedures.

Patient selection for combined procedures (cosmetic, intra-abdominal, or major pelvic) should be particularly stringent. Patients should be in excellent health, relatively young, not obese, and not represent "extreme" cases. Because the probability of these patients needing transfusion is increased, most should be prepared for autologous transfusion.

COMPLICATIONS
Liposuction

The most feared complication of abdominal liposuction is penetration of the abdominal wall by the cannula and injury to a viscus or solid organ. This complication, although rare, usually occurs in association with a preexisting abdominal scar and is probably secondary to scar-induced misdirection of the cannula. Prevention involves gentle technique and particular care when suctioning a scarred abdomen.

If the mishap is recognized or suspected during surgery, intraoperative surgical consultation is indicated; the investigation and treatment should be carried out under the direction of the general surgeon before the patient is awakened. If the plastic surgeon is unaware of the penetration at surgery, a high index of suspicion is needed to recognize it in the postoperative period. Unusual pain and signs of peritoneal irritation are the most likely clues. Again, prompt surgical consultation with appropriate investigation and laparotomy, if indicated, can prevent an unpleasant complication from becoming a catastrophe.

Although swelling and bruising are more intense on the abdomen than elsewhere, expanding hematomas are rare. No case has occurred in my personal practice. Swelling and bruising of the genitalia are not a complication but rather an expected sequela of which the patient should be informed in advance.

Irregularities and asymmetries can occur in the abdomen as in other areas, but a problem unique to the abdomen is irregularities due to residual fat around the umbilicus. The fat in this area is more difficult to remove because of increased fibrous tissue and the scarring associated with the umbilicus. There is also a tendency for increased folds because of the tethering effect of the umbilicus. Removal of periumbilical fat with smaller cannulas will minimize occurrence of this unsightly sequela.

Abdominoplasty

Grazer and Goldwyn[70] in 1977 and Teimourian and Rogers[71] in 1989 published surveys of all plastic surgeons in the United States and Canada concerning complications in abdominoplasty. The former report included 10,490 abdominoplasties and the latter 25,562. These two studies give an excellent overview of abdominoplasty complications. In addition, several surgeons have looked critically at abdominoplasty complications in their own personal series,[37,44,59,69,86-88] whereas others have specifically examined complications when abdominoplasty was combined with other procedures.[27,35,67,72,85] These studies provide useful supplementary information regarding the prevalence of complications, their prevention, and their treatment.

Deaths

Grazer and Goldwyn[70] and Teimourian and Rogers[71] reported mortality rates of 0.16% (162/100,000) and 0.04% (41/100,000), respectively. Looked at another way, in the 1977 survey, 1 in 617 operations resulted in the death of the patient, whereas by 1989, only 1 in 2324 operations resulted in a mortality.

Although neither of these studies examined risk factors in patients who died compared to those who survived, both series revealed pulmonary thromboembolism as a leading cause of death. Six of 17 deaths in the earlier study and 6 of 11 deaths in the later study were attributed to pulmonary thromboembolism.

Much higher death rates have been reported for belt lipectomy (2 deaths, both from pulmonary embolism, in 150 operations)[87] and in operations performed mostly for obesity (2 deaths, 1 from pulmonary thromboembolism, in 65 operations).[89] On the other hand, experienced surgeons have reported large personal series of operations, in excess of 500 procedures each,[72,90,91] without a mortality.

Thus abdominoplasty has a significant and measurable associated mortality, with death rates in individual series varying widely. In my opinion, eliminating high-risk patients (the obese or those with major cardiovascular, pulmonary, or other organ system impairment) will reduce the risk of death. Rigorous patient selection is probably the single most important step in performing consistently safe abdominoplasty.

Pulmonary Embolus

Pulmonary embolus is the most frequent serious complication and the most common cause of death following abdominoplasty. Grazer and Goldwyn[70] reported a 0.81% (810/100,000) and Teimourian and Rogers[71] a 0.25% (248/100,000) incidence of thromboembolism. Between 1 in 8[70] and 1 in 10[71] episodes of thromboembolism resulted in death. Of all deaths, 35%[70] to 55%[71] were from pulmonary embolism.

Hester et al.[72] drew attention to the fact that obesity predisposes to pulmonary embolism. Other etiologic factors associated with thromboembolism include disorders of clotting, cancer, advanced age, sepsis, immobilization, dehydration with venous stasis, and prior thromboembolism.[92]

Administration of intravenous alcohol has been advocated for prophylaxis of pulmonary thromboembolism and pulmonary fat embolism in abdominoplasty patients,[85,93] but there have been no controlled trials to validate its efficacy. Low-dose heparin has been proved to reduce the incidence of pulmonary thromboembolism,[92,94,95] but its use has been associated with significant bleeding episodes.[96] Patients who have had a previous thromboembolic episode are at increased risk, and the surgeon may want to give low doses of heparin if he decides to proceed.

My personal approach to this problem is not to perform cosmetic abdominoplasty on high-risk patients, particularly those who are obese, frail, or elderly, to keep all patients well hydrated during surgery and immediately thereafter, and to mobilize patients rapidly after surgery.

Respiratory Decompensation

Musculofascial plication decreases intra-abdominal volume by pushing abdominal contents against the diaphragm, which impedes diaphragmatic excursion and reduces respiratory reserve.[88,97] Patients with preexisting conditions that compromise pulmonary function (the obese, smokers, and those with chronic lung disease) are at increased risk of developing postoperative acute respiratory decompensation.

Bellero et al.[88] recommended preoperative pulmonary function tests on all patients suspected of having decreased pulmonary reserve. If pulmonary function was significantly reduced and could not be improved by a vigorous preoperative course of physical therapy, they canceled surgery.

The final common pathway of most deaths following abdominoplasty has been respiratory decompensation. Patient selection for abdominoplasty should include a critical evaluation of respiratory function in those suspected of having preexisting respiratory compromise.

Skin Necrosis

Grazer and Goldwyn[70] reported skin loss to be one of the four most frequent complications following abdominoplasty but did not give its exact incidence. Teimourian and Rogers[71] reported an incidence of 0.86% (858/ 100,000) "major skin loss." Skin loss in other series has ranged from 0.5% to 2.5% of operations.[37,86]

Distal flap necrosis is more likely if there are transverse upper abdominal scars. Elbaz and Flaguel,[59] however, have shown radiographically that scars after 1 year have significant blood flow across the cicatrix. The older the scar, the less likely it is to contribute to flap necrosis.

Converting a low transverse incision into an inverted T increases the incidence of flap necrosis by interfering with crossover blood supply in the distal flap.[59,60] Closure under excessive tension and rough handling of the proximal flap can also cause flap necrosis as well as excessive suction of the proximal flap and immediately adjacent areas.

An unrecognized and undrained major hematoma or flap infection can also result in distal flap necrosis.

Perhaps the most common preventable cause of flap necrosis is cigarette smoking.[98] All patients should stop smoking completely for 2 weeks before and 2 weeks after abdominoplasty.

Flap necrosis is heralded by a dead white appearance of the skin with no capillary filling when the skin is depressed and released. The white color progresses to bluish purple and then to black over several days. Immediate release of the flap in the first few hours after surgery may reduce the area of eventual necrosis. Once the necrosis is established, however, the wound should be treated conservatively with debridement of only that tissue which is definitely necrotic. Conservative treatment generally results in a better late appearance than aggressive debridement and skin grafting.

Wound Dehiscence

Grazer and Goldwyn[70] reported a 5.4% incidence of wound dehiscence. Predisposing causes are closure under excessive tension, failure to keep the patient in a hip-flexed position after surgery, and inadequate number or strength of sutures in the deep and subcutaneous closures.

Wound Infection

Grazer and Goldwyn[70] reported a 7.3% incidence of wound infection after abdominoplasty. Most infections are minor and manifested by redness around the umbilicus or the lower abdominal closure. Cultures of any discharge should be taken and appropriate antibiotics given. The majority of infections will resolve with antibiotic treatment.

Severe infections or abscess formation requires open drainage, which is best performed in the operating room under general anesthesia. In the case of an abscess the undersurface of the flap should be thoroughly explored to find occult loculations of pus. After the pus is drained and the abscess cavity irrigated, drains should be placed and enough of the wound left open to ensure adequate continued dependent drainage. The wound can be allowed to heal by secondary intention.

Hematomas

Grazer and Goldwyn[70] reported a hematoma incidence of 6.0%. Considering only those collections requiring drainage, others have reported lower incidences: 1.33%,[59] 3% (includes seromas and hematomas),[37] and 3.8% (includes hematomas and "serosanguineous fluid" that required drainage).[91]

Small hematomas are usually resorbed without requiring treatment. Large or expanding hematomas are most commonly caused by bleeding from the superficial inferior epigastric or superficial circumflex iliac artery in the lower flap or from a large perforator on the fascia.

Meticulous hemostasis during the operation will minimize the incidence of hematomas. The inferior epigastric and superficial circumflex iliac vessels should be individually identified and cauterized (or ligated if they are very large). When the excess tissue is cut from the upper flap, the vessels should again be sought out and cauterized. As the flap is raised, a filmy layer of fascia should be left on the musculoaponeurosis. This practice reduces bleeding from the plexus of vessels lying on the aponeurosis and also permits individual identification and cauterization of perforating vessels as they emerge from the fascia. If the vessels retract beneath the aponeurosis and continue to bleed, hemostasis is much less certain and requires figure-of-eight oversewing of the area.

The abdomen should be observed frequently in the first few hours after surgery, during which time most hematomas occur. I prefer not to apply a binder or any other occlusive dressing so that the lower abdomen is available for inspection. Hematomas are heralded by lower abdominal swelling. The distal flap may become bluish from venous congestion or, more ominous, white from arterial compromise.

When a large hematoma is discovered in the immediate postoperative period, sutures should be released at the bedside to provide immediate drainage and relieve pressure on the flap. The patient is returned to the operating room and given a general anesthetic. The hematoma is completely evacuated and bleeders controlled. Persistent bleeding, especially from multiple sites, suggests a clotting disorder and should be investigated and treated appropriately.

Hematomas discovered after the first 48 hours are usually smaller and stable and can be drained at the bedside. If in doubt as to adequacy of drainage or if continued bleeding is suspected, it is always best to return the patient to the operating room where a thorough inspection of the operative site can be carried out with the patient asleep and pain-free.

Seromas

Seromas occur frequently, particularly after modified or miniabdominoplasty. An incidence of 15% has been reported,[44] but I suspect the true incidence is higher, particularly since many of the smaller ones go undetected and are resorbed spontaneously. Pitanguy[32] believes that immediate postoperative compression with a plaster of Paris abdominal mold weighted with a sandbag will prevent seromas. He keeps the mold in place for 48 hours. Suction drains probably reduce the incidence of seromas, but their efficacy has not been proved.

Most large seromas become manifest at the first postoperative office visit as a ballottable swelling in the lower abdomen. They are treated by aspiration under sterile conditions with 18-gauge needles on 50 ml syringes. A needle placed through the lower abdominal skin causes no pain since this area remains hypesthetic for several months after surgery. Treatment usually has to be repeated every 3 to 4 days with gradually decreasing volumes aspirated until the seroma is small enough for the remaining fluid to be resorbed. Complete resolution may require 2 to 4 weeks.

Occasional seromas persist and become organized into pseudobursae. If they cause noticeable swelling, they can be excised through the original incision. Reoperation should be delayed for 6 months after the original surgery. CT or MRI helps confirm the diagnosis prior to secondary surgery.

The operation consists of complete excision of the bursa through the original incision. The excision should be performed with electrocautery to minimize bleeding. The wound is closed over multiple suction drains. An abdominal binder is placed as soon as flap viability is certain and before the patient begins to ambulate. The patient is cautioned to rest at home for at least 1 week after the surgery. Julliard[99] advises suturing the undersurface of the flap to the musculoaponeurosis to ensure adherence and prevent recurrence, but I have not found this maneuver necessary.

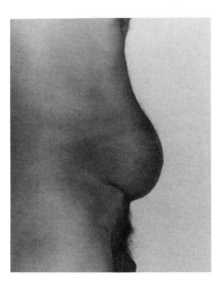

This 37-year-old man underwent modified abdominoplasty and was discharged after 48 hours in the hospital. The day after leaving the hospital he took a brisk half-mile walk. Within hours, his abdomen distended.

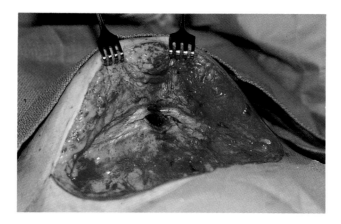

I aspirated large volumes of serosanguineous fluid on multiple occasions over the next few weeks, but his abdomen never resumed its initial postoperative state. Six months after surgery I excised a large calcified pseudobursa. He remained at home and curtailed activities for 1 week after the second surgery and the seroma did not recur. In retrospect, it would have been better to have returned the patient to the operating room for more complete drainage in the early postoperative period.

Seromas are easier to prevent than treat. Many form because of failure of early flap adherence secondary to patient overactivity. Consequently, I confine the patient to bed for 72 hours (except for meals, using the bathroom, and ambulation in the hospital hallway). I also insist the patient remain at home to rest for a full week after surgery even if she has had only a limited abdominoplasty. Since instituting the above regimen I have not had to treat a postoperative seroma.

Umbilical Deformities

In complete abdominoplasty with umbilical circumscription, if the midline has been marked accurately with indelible ink, both on the upper flap and on the pubis below the hairline, placing the new umbilical site in the midline should be relatively straightforward. If malplacement occurs during translocation, it is difficult if not impossible to correct without additional scarring. When the umbilicus remains attached to the skin flap but is disinserted at the base, replacement at the midline requires careful checking of position relative to surface landmarks.

Umbilical stenosis is usually a late result of infection. It can also occur from overaggressive resection of periumbilical fat from the flap surrounding the new umbilical aperture, particularly in an obese patient or if there is excessive tension on the periumbilical skin from sutures tacked to the fascia and the skin.

Necrosis and complete loss of the umbilicus can also result from vascular compromise or infection. Excessive defatting of the umbilical stalk is not a cause of vascular compromise since the umbilicus has its own blood supply through the central umbilical skin.[100] Repair of a significant umbilical hernia can, however, obliterate the central blood supply, and if the patient has had a previous umbilical herniorrhaphy or if one is done simultaneously with abdominoplasty, the umbilicus may be at risk.

A stenosed or obliterated umbilicus is a significant aesthetic handicap. Several methods of neoumbilicoplasty have been described to create a semblance of the normal umbilical scar.[101-104]

Deformities of the Low Transverse Scar

Hypertrophic scars can be treated with injections of triamcinolone acetonide (Kenalog), but most will improve without any treatment. It may take 2 years or longer for full scar maturation, and patients should be discouraged from scar revision before that time. After 2 years there will be little change in the scar. Moreover, the inflammatory process in the surrounding tissues has abated, the tissues are looser, and a scar revision may be performed with greater facility and more likelihood of success.

Wrinkling or folding of the skin above the scar and dog ears at the ends of the scar are a consequence of disparity in length of closure lines in the upper and lower flaps. They are avoided by carefully measuring the planned excision lines to ensure that they are of near equal length. Minor disparities can be corrected by careful closure and aligning the wound edges with staples in a trial closure so that any disparity is distributed evenly along the suture line. If a major disparity exists, it is preferable to take out a dog ear at the lateral end of the incision and extend the wound upward, downward, or straight out, depending on what is needed. Patients are generally accepting of a lateral scar extension but are intolerant of wrinkles and folds above the scar.

Excessive elevation of the scar and the pubic escutcheon are avoided by attaching the flap to the musculoaponeurosis with key sutures of nonabsorbable material (see p. 274).

If more tissue is removed from one side of the flap than the other, the final scar will be elevated on the side from which the extra tissue was excised. Careful preoperative marking and precise utilization of these markings at the time of skin excision should eliminate this complication.

Numbness

The lateral femoral cutaneous nerve emerges from the abdomen and lies superficial to the deep fascia 1 cm medial to the anterior superior iliac spine en route to the anterolateral aspect of the upper thigh. The nerve is at risk during abdominoplasty. Should it be cut, the patient will have a distressing and permanent loss of sensation on the upper anterolateral aspect of the proximal thigh.

Leaving a filmy layer of fascia and some of the fat on the musculoaponeurosis at the lateral aspect of the incision around the anterior superior iliac spine will protect the nerve. If the nerve is divided and the problem is recognized at surgery, the nerve should be repaired under magnification.

All patients will have loss of sensibility of the skin over the lower abdominal flap. The intensity of the hyperesthesia abates with time, but full return of preoperative sensibility does not occur.

Bulging of the Epigastrum

When the surgeon has not plicated the upper portion of the diastasis, the upper musculoaponeurosis continues to bulge. Also, if the upper abdominal skin is not adequately undermined over the lower thorax and xiphoid, plication of the diastasis will cause a midline bunching of the skin and subcutaneous fat. Complete plication of the midline diastasis and adequate undermining will avoid this problem.

─────────────── REFERENCES ───────────────

1. Lewis CM. Early experience of aspirative lipoplasty of the abdomen. Aesthetic Plast Surg 11:33-40, 1987.
2. Matarasso A. Abdominolipoplasty. Clin Plast Surg 16:289-303, 1989.
3. Pitanguy I. Body contour. Am J Cosmetic Surg 4:283-298, 1987.
4. Demars and Marx (1890). Cited in Elbaz JS, Flaguel G. Plastic Surgery of the Abdomen (translated by WT Keavy). New York: Masson USA, 1979, p 42.
5. Kelly HA. Report of gynecological cases. Johns Hopkins Hosp Bull 10:196-197, 1899.
6. Kelly HA. Excision of fat of the abdominal wall—Lipectomy. Surg Gynecol Obstet 10:239-234, 1910.
7. Desjardin A. Lipectomy for extreme obesity. Paris Chir 3:466-484, 1911.
8. Jolly R. Die Operation des Fettbauches (abdominoplasty). Berl Klin Wochenschr 48:1317-1318, 1911.
9. Schepelmann E. Bauchdeckenplastik mit besonderer Berucksichtigung des Hangebauches. Beitr Klin Chir 3:372-399, 1918.
10. Flesch-Thebesius M, Weinsheimer K. Die Operation des Hangebauches. Chirurgie 3:841-846, 1931.
11. Passot R. Chirurgie Esthétique Pure. Paris: G. Doin, 1931, pp 261-267.
12. Babcock WW. A Textbook of Surgery for Students and Physicians, 2nd ed. Philadelphia: WB Saunders, 1935.
13. Thorek M. Plastic reconstruction of the female breast and abdomen. Am J Surg 43:268-278, 1939.
14. Somalo M. Dermolipectomía abdominal. In Anales del Primer Congreso Latino-Americanos de Cirujanos Plásticos, vol 2. São Paulo: 1941, p 2104.
15. Foged J. Operative treatment of abdominal obesity, especially pendulous abdomen. Br J Plast Surg 1:274-283, 1949.
16. Jackson J, Steeper J. Operative excision of giant panniculus adiposus. J Int Coll Surg 15:85-88, 1951.
17. Moore HG, Harkens HN. The surgical correction of panniculus adiposus abdominis. Surgery 34:728-734, 1953.
18. Galtier M. Surgical therapy of obesity of the abdominal wall with ptosis. Mem Acad Chir 81:341-344, 1955.
19. Galtier M. L'obésité de la paroi abdominale avec ptose. Presse Med 70:135-136, 1962.

20. Allansmith R. An excision of abdominal fat apron. AMA Arch Surg 80:327-332, 1960.
21. González-Ulloa M. Belt lipectomy. Br J Plast Surg 13:179-188, 1960.
22. Fernández JC. Dermolipectomía vertical del abdomen. Semin Med 120:431-432, 1962.
23. Belin RP, Stone NH, Fischer RP, Scott WR. Improved technique of panniculectomy. Surgery 59:222-225, 1966.
24. Castanares S, Goethel JA. Abdominal lipectomy: A modification in technique. Plast Reconstr Surg 40:378-383, 1967.
25. Kamper MJ, Galloway DV, Ashley F. Abdominal panniculectomy after massive weight loss. Plast Reconstr Surg 50:441-446, 1972.
26. McGraw LH. Surgical rehabilitation after massive weight reduction. Plast Reconstr Surg 53:349-352, 1974.
27. Savage RC. Abdominoplasty combined with other surgical procedures. Plast Reconstr Surg 70:437-443, 1982.
28. Zook EG. The massive weight loss patient. Clin Plast Surg 2:456-466, 1975.
29. Schepelmann E. Die Erhaltung des Nabels bei Hangebauchoperationen. Zentrabl Gynakol 48:2289-2290, 1924.
30. Vernon G. Umbilical transplantation upward and abdominal contouring in lipectomy. Am J Surg 94:490-492, 1957.
31. Callia WEP. Dermolipectomía abdominal. Centro de Cinematografía Carlo Erba. São Paulo: 1965, p 1.
32. Pitanguy I. Abdominal lipectomy: An approach to it through an analysis of 300 consecutive cases. Plast Reconstr Surg 40:384-391, 1967.
33. Serson D. Planeamiento geométrico ladero lipectomía abdominal. Rev Esp Cir Plast 4:37, 1971.
34. Baker TJ, Gordon HL, Mosienko P. A template (pattern) method of abdominal lipectomy. Aesthetic Plast Surg 1:167-176, 1977.
35. Grazer FM. Abdominoplasty. Plast Reconstr Surg 51:617-623, 1973.
36. Pitanguy I. Surgical reduction of the abdomen, thighs and buttocks. Surg Clin N Am 51:476-479, 1971.
37. Regnault P. Abdominoplasty by the W technique. Plast Reconstr Surg 55:265-274, 1975.
38. Grazer FM, Klingbeil JR. Body Image: A Surgical Perspective. St. Louis: CV Mosby, 1980.
39. Planas J. The "vest over pants" abdominoplasty. Plast Reconstr Surg 61:694-700, 1978.
40. Elbaz JS. Abdominal plastic surgery: Horseshoe technique. Ann Chir Plast 19:155-158, 1974.
41. Glicenstein J. Les difficultés du traitement chirurgical des dermodystrophies abdominales. Ann Chir 20:147-155, 1975.
42. Greminger RF. The mini-abdominoplasty. Plast Reconstr Surg 79:356-365, 1983.
43. Wilkinson TS, Schwartz BE. Individual modifications in body contour surgery: The "limited" abdominoplasty. Plast Reconstr Surg 77:779-784, 1986.
44. Cardoso de Castro C, Cupello MB, Cintra H. Limited incisions in abdominoplasty. Ann Plast Surg 19:436-447, 1987.
45. Grauer WO, Moss AA, Cann CE, Goldberg HI. Quantification of body fat distribution in the abdomen using computed tomography. Am J Clin Nutr 39:631-637, 1984.
46. Krotkiewski M, Björntorp P, Sjöstrom L, Smith U. Impact of obesity on metabolism in men and women: Importance of regional adipose tissue distribution. J Clin Invest 72:1150-1162, 1983.
47. Hollinshead WH. Anatomy for Surgeons, vol 2. New York: Hoeber, 1956.
48. Aitken AB. Note on the insertion of the rectus abdominis muscle. Glasgow Med J 77-78:171-172, 1912.
49. Anson BJ, McVay CB. The anatomy of the inguinal and hypogastric regions of the abdominal wall. Anat Rec 70:211-225, 1938.

50. Chouke KS. The constitution of the sheath of the rectus abdominis muscle. Anat Rec 61:341-349, 1934.

51. Cullen TS, Brödel M. Lesions of the rectus abdominis muscle simulating an acute intra-abdominal condition: I. Anatomy of the rectus muscle. Bull Johns Hopkins Hosp 61:295-348, 1937.

52. McVay CB, Anson BJ. Composition of the rectus sheath. Anat Rec 77:213-225, 1940.

53. Elbaz JS, Dardour JC. Anatomy and physiology of the arteries and veins of the abdominal wall. In Marchac D, ed. Transactions of the Sixth International Congress of Plastic Surgeons. Paris: Masson, 1975, p 561.

54. Bedran HA, El-Helaly MS, Safe I. The lateral intercostal neurovascular free flap. Plast Reconstr Surg 73:17-26, 1984.

55. Bishop WE, Carr BW, Anson BJ, Ashley FL. The parietal intermuscular plexus of the thoracic nerves. Quart Bull Northwestern Univ Med School 17-18:209-216, 1943.

56. Boyd JB, Taylor GI, Corlett R. The vascular territories of the superior epigastric and deep inferior epigastric systems. Plast Reconstr Surg 73:1-16, 1984.

57. Brown RG, Vasconez LO, Jurkiewicz MJ. Transverse abdominal flaps and the deep epigastric arcade. Plast Reconstr Surg 55:416-421, 1975.

58. Daniel RK, Kerrigan CL, Gard DA. The great potential of the intercostal flap for torso reconstruction. Plast Reconstr Surg 61:653-665, 1978.

59. Elbaz JS, Flaguel G. Plastic Surgery of the Abdomen (translated by WT Keavy). New York: Masson USA, 1979.

60. Huger WE. The anatomic rationale for abdominal lipectomy. Am Surg 45:612-617, 1979.

61. Manchot C. The Cutaneous Arteries of the Human Body (translated by J Ristic and WD Morain). New York: Springer-Verlag, 1983.

62. Milloy FJ, Anson BJ, McAfee DK. The rectus abdominis muscle and the epigastric arteries. Surg Gynecol Obstet 110:293-302, 1960.

63. Salmon M. Artères de la peau: Etude anatomique et chirurgicale. Paris: Masson, 1936.

64. Taylor GI. Discussion of Hester TR, Nahai F, Beegle PE, Bostwick J III. Blood supply of the abdomen revisited, with emphasis on the superficial inferior epigastric artery. Plast Reconstr Surg 74:667-700, 1984.

65. Taylor GI, Daniel RK. The anatomy of several free flap donor sites. Plast Reconstr Surg 56:243-253, 1973.

66. Ferner H, ed. Pernkopf Atlas of Topographical and Applied Human Anatomy, vol 2. Baltimore: Urban & Schwarzenberg, 1980.

67. Freedom J. Abdominoplasty with celiotomy: Evaluation and technique. Int Surg 68:75-77, 1983.

68. Bozola AR, Psillakis JM. Abdominoplasty: A new concept and classification for treatment. Plast Reconstr Surg 82:983-993, 1988.

69. de Souza Pinto EB, de Almaida AEF, Knudsen AM, de Andrade SMFS, de Medeiros JC. A new methodology in abdominal aesthetic surgery. Aesthetic Plast Surg 11:213-222, 1987.

70. Grazer FM, Goldwyn RM. Abdominoplasty assessed by survey with emphasis on complications. Plast Reconstr Surg 59:513-517, 1977.

71. Teimourian B, Rogers WB. A national survey of complications associated with suction lipectomy: A comparative study. Plast Reconstr Surg 84:628-631, 1989.

72. Hester TR Jr, Baird W, Bostwick J III, Nahai F, Cukic J. Abdominoplasty combined with other major surgical procedures: Safe or sorry? Plast Reconstr Surg 83:997-1004, 1989.

73. Teimourian B, Gotkin RH. Contouring of the midtrunk in overweight patients. Aesthetic Plast Surg 13:145-153, 1989.

74. Toranto IR. The relief of low back pain. The WARP abdominoplasty: A preliminary report. Plast Reconstr Surg 85:545-555, 1990.

75. Jackson IT, Downie PA. Abdominoplasty—The waistline stitch and other refinements. Plast Reconstr Surg 61:180-183, 1978.

76. Psillakis JM. Plastic surgery of the abdomen with improvement in the body contour: Physiopathology and treatment of the aponeurotic musculature. Clin Plast Surg 11:455–477, 1984.

77. Dubou R, Ousterhout DK. Placement of the umbilicus in an abdominoplasty. Plast Reconstr Surg 61:291–293, 1978.

78. Avelar J. Abdominoplasty—Systematization of a technique without external umbilical scar. Aesthetic Plast Surg 2:141–151, 1978.

79. Freeman BS, Wiene DR. Abdominoplasty with special attention to construction of the umbilicus: Technique and complications. Aesthetic Plast Surg 2:65–74, 1978.

80. Juri J, Juri C, Raiden G. Reconstruction of the umbilicus in abdominoplasty. Plast Reconstr Surg 63:580–582, 1979.

81. Cardoso de Castro C, Daher M. Simultaneous reduction mammaplasty and abdominoplasty. Plast Reconstr Surg 61:36–39, 1978.

82. Hinderer UT. The dermolipectomy approach for augmentation mammaplasty. Clin Plast Surg 2:359–369, 1975.

83. Planas J. Introduction of breast implants through the abdominal route. Plast Reconstr Surg 57:434–437, 1976.

84. Voss SC, Sharp HC, Scott JR. Abdominoplasty combined with gynecologic surgical procedures. Obstet Gynecol 67:181–186, 1986.

85. Perry AW. Abdominoplasty combined with total abdominal hysterectomy. Ann Plast Surg 16:121–122, 1986.

86. Avelar J. Abdominoplasty: Technical refinement and analysis of 130 cases in 8 years' follow-up. Aesthetic Plast Surg 7:205–212, 1983.

87. Vilain R, Dubousset J. Technique et indications de la lipectomie circulaire: 150 observations. Ann Chir 18:289, 1964.

88. Bellero V, et al. Abdominoplasty: Physiorespiratory, surgical, aesthetic problems. Riv Ital Chir Plast 5:417, 1973 (abstracted in Plast Reconstr Surg 56:356, 1975).

89. Vandenbussche F, Meresse V, Debaere PA, Vandevorde J, Lagoche G. Abdominal lipectomy: Morphological indications and choice of operative technique. In Transactions of the Sixth International Congress of Plastic Reconstructive Surgeons. Paris: Masson, 1976.

90. Grazer FM. Personal communication, 1990.

91. Pitanguy I. Aesthetic Plastic Surgery of the Head and Body. New York: Springer-Verlag, 1981.

92. Roberts HR, Adel S, Bernstein EF. Prevention of venous thrombosis and pulmonary embolism: Consensus conference. JAMA 256:744–749, 1986.

93. Matthews WA. Discussion of pulmonary complications following abdominal lipectomy. Plast Reconstr Surg 71:816–817, 1983.

94. Kakkar VV, Field ES, Nicolaides AN, Flute PT, Wessler S, Yin ET. Low doses of heparin in prevention of deep-vein thrombosis. Lancet 2:669–671, 1971.

95. Kakkar VV, Corrigan T, Spindler J, Flossard DP, Flute PT, Crellin RQ, Wessler S. Efficacy of low doses of heparin in prevention of deep-vein thrombosis after major surgery. Lancet 2:101–106, 1972.

96. Pachter HL, Riles TS. Low dose heparin: Bleeding and wound complications in the surgical patient. Ann Surg 186:669–674, 1977.

97. Hunter GR, Crapo RO, Broadbent TR, Woolf RM. Pulmonary complications following abdominal lipectomy. Plast Reconstr Surg 71:809–813, 1983.

98. Aston SJ. Abdominoplasty. In Rees TD, ed. Aesthetic Plastic Surgery, vol 2. Philadelphia: WB Saunders, 1980, pp 1007–1038.

99. Julliard A. Les grands épanchements permanents dans la lipectomie antérieure [Huge permanent effusions in anterior lipectomy]. Ann Chir Plast 21:267–270, 1976.

100. Cullen TS. Embryology, Anatomy and Diseases of the Umbilicus. Philadelphia: WB Saunders, 1916.

101. Baroudi R. Umbilicoplasty. Clin Plast Surg 2:431–448, 1975.

102. Guerrerosantos J, Dicksheet S, Carrillo C, Sandoval M. Umbilical reconstruction with secondary abdominoplasty. Ann Plast Surg 5:139–144, 1980.

103. Kirianoff TG. Making a new umbilicus when none exists. Plast Reconstr Surg 61:603–604, 1978.

104. Grazer FM, Klingbeil JR, Regnault P, Planas J R. Colloquium: Abdominoplasty. Ann Plast Surg 2:242–243, 1979.

——— SUGGESTED READINGS ———

Anson BJ, McVay CB. Inguinal hernia I. The anatomy of the region. Surg Gynecol Obstet 66:186–191, 1938.

Appiani E. Muscular plastic for aesthetic conformation of abdominal girdle. Ann Plast Surg 13:97–106, 1984.

Arem AJ, Kischer CW. Analysis of striae. Plast Reconstr Surg 65:22–29, 1980.

Aston SJ, Pickerell KL. Reconstructive surgery of the abdominal wall. In Converse JM, ed. Reconstructive Plastic Surgery, 2nd ed, vol 7. Philadelphia: WB Saunders, 1977.

Avelar J. Fat suction versus abdominoplasty. Aesthetic Plast Surg 9:265–276, 1985.

Babcock WW. The correction of the obese and relaxed abdominal wall with especial reference to the use of buried silver chain. Am J Obstet 74:596–611, 1916.

Baron HC. The surgical treatment of panniculus adiposus abdominis. GP 20:130–133, 1960.

Baroudi R, Keppke EM, Tozzi Netto F. Abdominoplasty. Plast Reconstr Surg 54:161–168, 1974.

Barsky AJ, Kahn S. Principles and Practice of Plastic Surgery. New York: McGraw-Hill, 1964, pp 543–546.

Borges AF. Reconstruction of the umbilicus. Br J Plast Surg 28:75–76, 1975.

Callia WEP. Uma plastica para o cirurgiao geral. Med Hosp [São Paulo] 1:40, 1967.

Cardosa de Castro C. Abdominoplastias. Rotina J Bras Med 30:103, 1976.

Carreirao S, Correa WE, Carvalho Dias L, Pitanguy I. Treatment of abdominal wall eventration associated with abdominoplasty techniques. Aesthetic Plast Surg 8:173–179, 1984.

Carvalho CGS, Baroudi R, Keppke EM. Anatomical and technical refinements for abdominoplasty. Aesthetic Plast Surg 1:217–228, 1977.

Clarkson P. Lipodystrophies. Plast Reconstr Surg 37:499–503, 1966.

Coffey RC. Plastic surgery of the abdominal wall. Surg Gynecol Obstet 10:90–93, 1910.

Dufourmentel C, Mouly R. Chirurgie Plastique. Paris: Flammarion, 1959, pp 381–389.

Dufourmentel C. Chirurgie réparatrice et corrective. Paris: Masson, 1939.

Elbaz JS, Dardour JC, Ricbourg B. Vascularisation artérielle de la paroi abdominale. Ann Chir Plast 20:19–29, 1975.

Faivre J. L'ombolic dans la chirurgie esthétique de l'abdomen. In Précis de Chirurgie Esthétique. Paris: Maloine, 1976, p 137.

Fernández JC, Correa Itturaspe M. Lipectomía del abdomen. Bol Trab Soc Argent Cir 22:591, 1961.

Fischl RA. Vertical abdominoplasty. Plast Reconstr Surg 51:139–143, 1973.

Floras C, Davis PKB. Complications and long term results following abdominoplasty: A retrospective study. Br J Plast Surg 44:190–194, 1991.

Gillies H, Millard DR Jr. The Principles and Art of Plastic Surgery, vol 2. Boston: Little, Brown, 1957, pp 291–420.

González-Ulloa M. Abdominal wall disfigurement. Ann Plast Surg 4:357–369, 1980.

González-Ulloa M. Circular lipectomy with transposition of the umbilicus and apo-neurolytic technic. Cirurgia 27:394–409, 1959.

Grazer FM, Klingbeil JR. Abdominoplasty. In Courtiss EH, ed. Aesthetic Surgery: Trouble, How To Avoid It and How To Treat It. St. Louis: CV Mosby, 1978.

Grazer FM, Matthews WA. Invited comments re article on perioperative warfarin therapy in combined abdominal lipectomy and intraabdominal gynecological surgical procedures. Ann Plast Surg 25:42–43, 1990.

Guerrerosantos J, Spaillat L, Morales F, Dicksheet S. Some problems and solutions in abdominoplasties. Aesthetic Plast Surg 4:227-237, 1980.

Hakme F. Abdominoplasty: Peri- and supraumbilical lipectomy. Aesthetic Plast Surg 7:213-220, 1983.

Henle JFG. Handbuch der gesasslehre des Menschen. In Handbuch der systematischen Anatomie des Menschen. Vivweg Braunschweig 1869.

Hester TR, Nahai F, Beegle PE, Bostwick J III. Blood supply of the abdomen revisited, with emphasis on the superficial inferior epigastric artery. Plast Reconstr Surg 74:657-670, 1984.

Hunter GR, Barney MF, Crapo RO, Broadbent TR. Perioperative warfarin therapy in combined abdominal lipectomy and intraabdominal gynecological surgical procedures. Ann Plast Surg 25:36-41, 1990.

Lagache G, Vandenbussche F. Indications, contre indications et résultats de la technique de Callia dans le traitement des ptoses cutanées abdominales avec ou sans surcharge graisseuse. Ann Chir Plast 16:37-50, 1971.

Larkin CN. Lipectomy for abdominal fat. Conn M J 14:706-709, 1950.

Lewis JR. Atlas of Aesthetic Plastic Surgery. Boston: Little, Brown, 1973.

Lewis JR. Midabdominoplasty. Aesthetic Plast Surg 3:195-199, 1979.

Malbec EF. Técnica de lipectomía. Prensa Med Argent 35:1251-1254, 1948.

Masson JK. Lipectomy: The surgical removal of excess fat. Postgrad Med 32:481-488, 1962.

Masterson JP. Necrosis of the abdominal wall following operations. Aust N Z J Surg 37:183-187, 1967.

May H. Reconstructive and Reparative Surgery, Philadelphia: FA Davis, 1947, pp 392-395.

Mitz V, Elbaz JS, Vilde F. Etude des fibres élastiques dermiques au cours d'opérations plastiques du tronc. Ann Chir Plast 20:31-35, 1975.

Nahai F, Brown RG, Vasconez LO. Blood supply to the abdominal wall as related to planning abdominal incisions. Am Surg 42:691-695, 1976.

Palmer B, Hallberg D, Backman L. Skin reduction plasties following intestinal shunt operations for treatment of obesity. Scand J Plast Reconstr Surg 9:47-52, 1975.

Pick JW, Anson BJ, Ashley FL. The origin of the obturator artery. Am J Anat 70:317-343, 1942.

Pitanguy I. Thigh lift and abdominal lipectomy. In Goldwyn RM, ed. Unfavorable Results in Plastic Surgery—Avoidance and Treatment. Boston: Little, Brown, 1972, p 387.

Psillakis JM. Abdominoplasty: Some ideas to improve results. Aesthetic Plast Surg 2:205, 1978.

Psillakis JM, Appiani EA, de la Plaza R. Color Atlas of Aesthetic Surgery of the Abdomen. New York: Thieme, 1991.

Rao VVS. Augmentation mammaplasty and abdominoplasty in one stage. Plast Reconstr Surg 43:148-151, 1969.

Rebello C, Franco T. Abdomotomies. Clin Plast Surg 2:411-429, 1975.

Regnault P. The history of abdominal dermolipectomy. Aesthetic Plast Surg 2:113-123, 1978.

Regnault P. Lipectomy. In Grabb WC, Smith JW, eds. Plastic Surgery, 3rd ed. Boston: Little, Brown, 1979, p 838.

Reich J. The surgical improvement in appearance of the female body. Med J Aust 2:767, 1974.

Ryan RF. Which patient needs the abdominoplasty? Plast Reconstr Surg 82:437-443, 1982.

Smith L. Excision of panniculus adiposus. J Med Assoc GA 28:193-196, 1939.

Taylor GI, Watterston PA, Zelt RG. The vascular anatomy of the anterior abdominal wall: The basis for flap design. Perspect Plast Surg 5(1):1-28, 1991.

Thorek P. Anatomy in Surgery. Philadelphia: JB Lippincott, 1951, pp 363-397.

Toranto IR. Resolution of back pain with the wide abdominal rectus plication abdominoplasty. Plast Reconstr Surg 81:777-779, 1988.

Weinhold S. Bauchdeckenplastik. Zentralbl Gynaekol 38:1332-1338, 1909.

Chapter 10

HIPS AND FLANKS

The hips and flanks are treated frequently in both women and men. "Hips" refers to that area in a woman which is directly over the iliac crests. "Flanks" refers to that area in a man which is superoposterior to the iliac crest. There is anatomic and gender overlap, but, typically, the hips are problematic for women and the flanks for men.

In men the excess fat is commonly referred to as "love handles" or a "spare tire" and is often the presenting complaint. In women the hips are rarely the primary reason for consultation but are frequently treated in conjunction with the abdomen or lateral thighs.

HISTORY

In the 1960s and 1970s Schrudde pioneered fat removal through small incisions. His work was confined to the thighs and lower legs, and he made no mention of treatment of the hips or flanks.[1,2] By the late 1970s surgeons began to treat the hips, and Teimourian and Fisher,[3] in reporting their first 54 cases, mentioned seven instances of "flank curettage," all in association with abdominoplasty. Kesselring[4] treated the hips in less than 8% of his first 105 cases, but almost 30% of Illouz's operations involved the hips.[5] Fournier and Otteni[6] and Courtiss[7] also described successful treatment of this area. Currently 45% of liposuction operations in my practice involve the hips, and almost all abdominoplasties include adjunctive hip suctioning.[8]

In the last 3 years there has been a renewed interest in direct surgical excision of flank tissue.[9-12] Baroudi[9,10] and Baroudi and Moraes[11] viewed flank excision as a natural extension of abdominoplasty and medial thigh lifts, whereas Lockwood[12] emphasized the benefits of flank excision in improving thigh and buttock contour and eliminating "cellulite" (see Chapter 11, Thighs and Buttocks).

AESTHETIC AND ANATOMIC CONSIDERATIONS

Although general aesthetic and anatomic considerations are discussed in Chapter 11, the anatomy of the subcutaneous fat in the hips and flanks deserves additional comment. In this region the subcutaneous fat is divided into two well-defined layers: superficial and deep. The superficial fat is encased in the superficial fascial system (SFS).[13] The SFS comprises several interconnected membranous sheets of fascia, providing structural support to the fat and overlying skin. The superficial fat is a light yellow color and densely structured. The deep fat compartment contains less structured fat with fewer fascial elements. It is slightly darker and more orange in color.

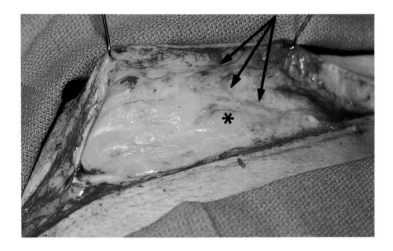

The white membranous SFS (arrows) lies superficial to the darker deep fat (asterisk) seen emerging through the cut fascia.

The SFS sends connecting fascial elements to the deep muscle fascia in certain well-defined regions to form *zones of adherence*. These zones of adherence define the boundaries and extent of the deep fat compartments.

Gender Differences

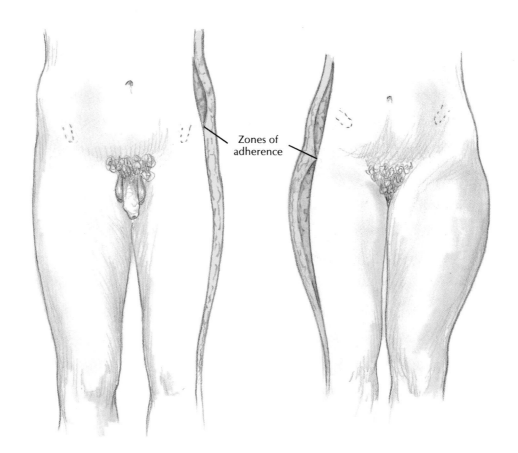

Zones of
adherence

The inferior boundary of the deep fat compartment differs in men and women. In men the inferior zone of adherence is along the iliac crest, confining the deep fat to the area cephalad to the iliac crest. In women the zone of adherence is more inferior, localizing the deep fat pocket to the area overlying the iliac crest. Note also the more prominent lateral thigh deep fat compartment in women.

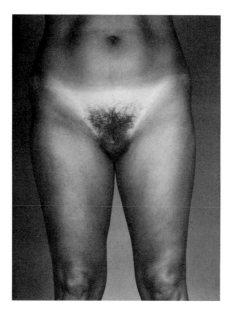 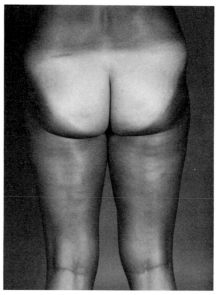

In women of normal weight, excess fat over the hips is generally well localized and confined to the lateral iliac crest area. Even overweight women tend to deposit most of their excess hip fat laterally. This 44-year-old woman was 5 feet 5 inches tall and weighed 142 pounds, 25 pounds more than her usual 117 pounds. Despite her weight gain, most of the hip excess is confined to the lateral iliac crest.

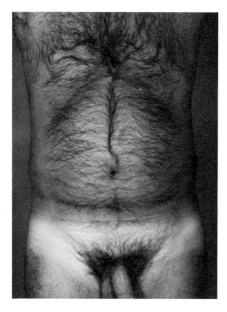 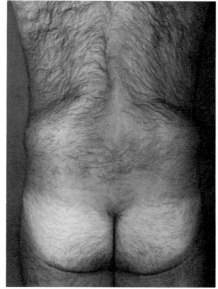

This man had also gained weight and was well above his youthful ideal. Typical of men, however, the excess fat is deposited in a more cephalad position and tends to extend around to the back as a roll.

TREATMENT OPTIONS

Liposuction is the treatment of choice for patients of both sexes who have localized excess subcutaneous fat without redundant skin. Nevertheless, patients with only moderate skin laxity who also have excess fat can obtain contour reduction from liposuction alone. Severe skin laxity requires direct excision of skin and subcutaneous tissues. These excisions are almost always performed in conjunction with abdominoplasty or thigh lift (see pp. 262, 298-300 for flank excision with abdominoplasty and pp. 392-401 for flank excision with thigh lift). When the skin is loose, suction volume should be reduced so as not to accentuate hanging skin.

PREOPERATIVE EVALUATION AND COUNSELING
Physical Examination

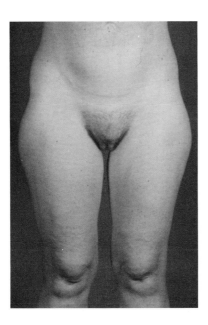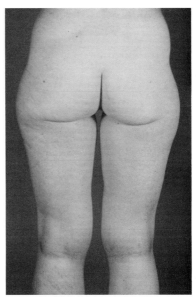

Assessment of posture is particularly important. Skeletal abnormalities may cause significant side-to-side asymmetries. In this patient the right hip protrudes more than the left, but the excess fat is not the cause of the asymmetry. The fullness of the right hip and greater trochanter results from scoliosis.

Preoperative volumetric assessments are an additional aid in operative planning. Although most hip asymmetries are secondary to scoliosis, differential volume removal can sometimes compensate for skeletal asymmetries and should be noted in the plan at the initial physical examination. Preoperative asymmetry should be pointed out and the patient informed that while every attempt will be made to compensate differences, perfect symmetry is usually not possible.

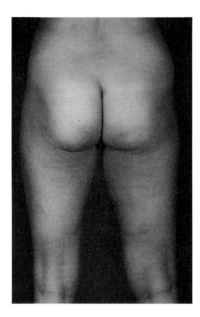 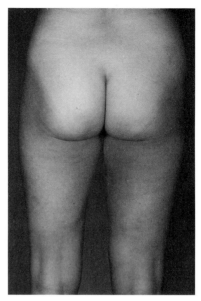

This woman's right hip fullness was partially attributable to skeletal asymmetry, but she also had a significant soft tissue differential volume. In fact, the entire right torso and lower extremity were larger than the left. There was no evidence of vascular malformation. I removed 100 cc from the right hip as well as tissue from both thighs and the right knee. I did not treat the left hip or left knee. Six months after surgery symmetry was improved, but she was not fully satisfied with her appearance, particularly the asymmetry. Therefore I removed an additional 50 cc from the right hip and smaller amounts from the medial thighs. Since she did not return for a follow-up visit, photographs following the second procedure are not available.

The pinch test plus lifting the skin will distinguish bulging due to excess fat vs. bulging from excess skin.

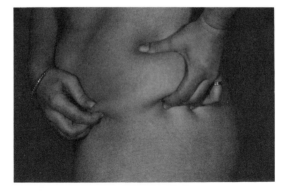

In most candidates for liposuction a 4 to 5 cm thickness of skin can be pinched between the index finger and thumb, but a 3 cm pinch thickness can also contain enough fat for successful contour reduction. The difference in pinch thickness between the hip and an adjacent area that does not need treatment is more important than absolute measured thickness.

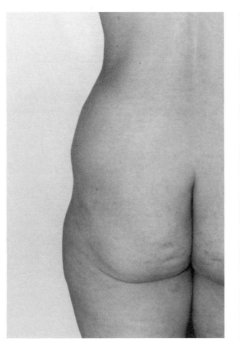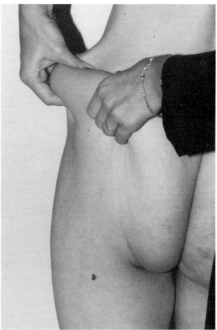

Lifting the skin will demonstrate skin laxity and help select those patients who are candidates for hip/flank excision.

Defining Patient Goals

Although most women want volume reduction of the hips, a significant number of patients prefer to retain a moderate fullness. They see hip roundness as an important secondary sexual characteristic. "It makes me look more feminine" or "I want *some* hips" are common expressions during the initial interview and examination. A slight fullness to the hips is also seen as accentuating waist definition.

For women, fit of clothes and appearance in clothing are usually the paramount reasons for liposuction, with appearance in a bathing suit or nude an important secondary consideration. In men the major aesthetic goal is to decrease the circumference of the lower torso and accentuate the breadth of the shoulders. Appearance in clothes is also the principal concern. Men complain of inability to wear form-fitting sports clothes. They view a roll hanging over the belt as a sign of physical flabbiness and loss of youthful vigor.

Informed Consent

Informed consent for hip liposuction does not differ from informed consent for other areas and is discussed on pp. 5-7 and 17-19. Informed consent for hip and flank excisions is discussed on pp. 361-363.

LIPOSUCTION
Markings

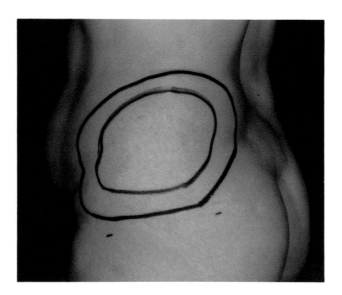

The patient is marked while standing. Protuberant areas and access incisions are outlined. Generally two access incisions are sufficient. They are placed inferior to and at either end of the protuberant areas. If the hip/flank roll is extensive, particularly if it approaches the midline in the back, additional access incisions are used. Keeping the incisions inferior to the protuberant areas is generally convenient for cannula manipulation and also leaves scars that can be readily covered by most bathing attire.

Operative Technique

In women, if only the hips are treated, local anesthesia is sufficient. In men, because the flank area is usually more extensive and the subcutaneous tissue more fibrous, general anesthesia is preferred. Treatment of multiple areas in patients of either sex is performed under general or regional anesthesia.

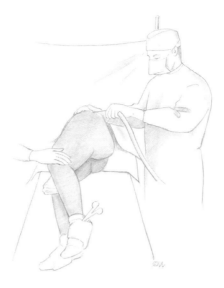

I prefer to have the patient placed in the lateral decubitus position; this position puts the hip/flank area in the most convenient and accessible location. If the prone position is used, access to the more anterior segments is limited. If liposuction of the hips is combined with abdominoplasty, I treat the patient in the supine position and roll her slightly to reach more posterior areas.

The average volume removed is 100 to 200 cc per side in women and slightly more in men; however, volumes may range from 50 to 300 cc. I use Mercedes Type cannulas with diameters of 3.0 to 6.0 mm, the exact size depending on the volume to be removed.

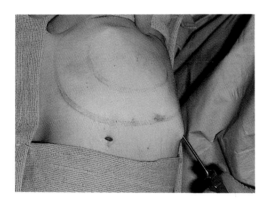
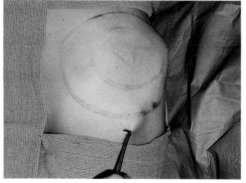

Ten minutes after infiltration of local anesthetic approximately half of the expected volume is removed from the first access incision. The second access incision is used to remove the remainder of the fat, creating a meshwork pattern of tunnels. Contour and pinch thickness are checked frequently as the end point is approached.

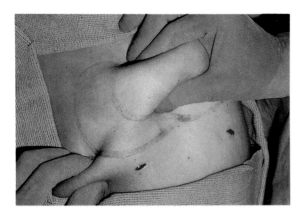 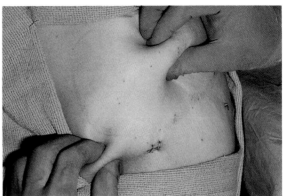

A final pinch test of 2 cm of fat between the fingers is generally the minimal desirable thickness, but comparison of pinch thicknesses between the hip and a nontreated adjacent area is the most important aid in determining the end point. On the left, pinch thickness over the hip prior to liposuction is compared to pinch thickness over the adjacent groin. On the right, pinch thickness over the hip has decreased after liposuction and is more comparable to pinch thickness over the groin.

In women the fat is usually directly over the iliac crest and aspiration is straightforward. In men the involved area is usually larger and the volume greater. The supporting fascial framework is better developed, more extensive, and stronger than in women. Consequently, more physical effort is required to extract fat, and bleeding may be more extensive.

Volumetrics is an important adjunctive aid. After the first side is completed, the exact volume is noted so that an identical volume can be removed from the opposite side. Differential volumes are removed as appropriate to compensate for asymmetries.

At the conclusion of surgery incision sites are stapled, and the area is covered with an adherent layer of foam sponge or compressive garment.

Results

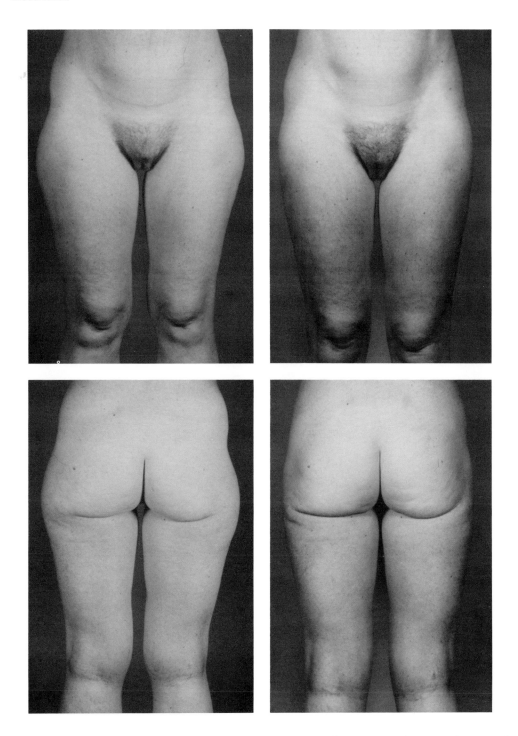

This woman was 5 feet 6 inches tall and weighed 122 pounds. A volume of 75 cc was removed from each hip. The knees and lateral and medial thighs were also treated. She is shown 7 months after liposuction. Persistent fullness over the right hip is skeletal in origin.

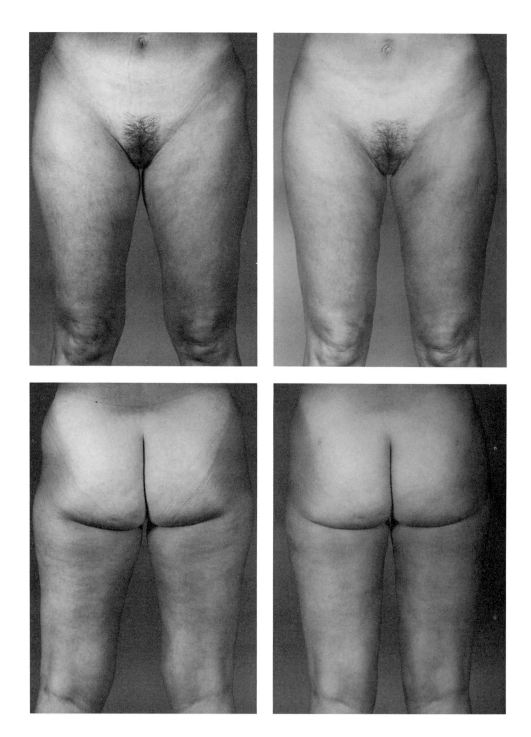

This 5-foot 2-inch, 120-pound patient is shown 5 months after removal of 100 cc from each hip plus treatment of her abdomen, thighs, and knees. The protrusive fullness at her hips was due almost entirely to fat and was very well localized, permitting a significant reduction with rather small volume removal. Since the situation in the subtrochanteric region was the same, I was able to achieve a rather smooth curve from hip to thigh.

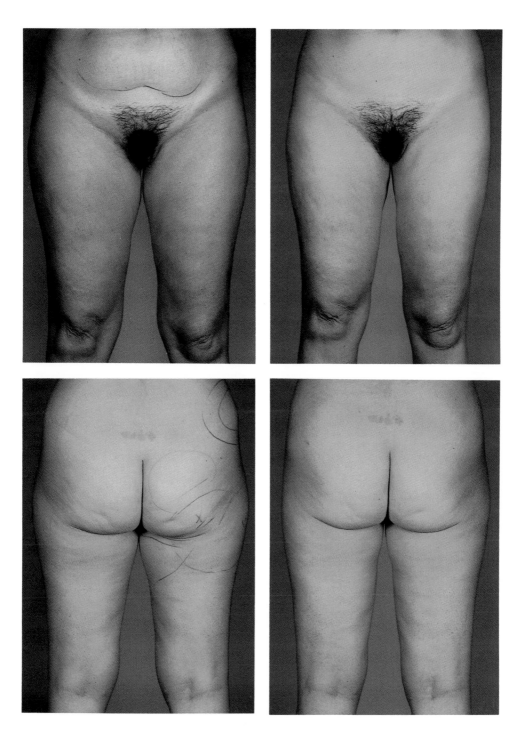

This 46-year-old woman, who was 5 feet 5 inches and weighed 135 pounds, had a 100 cc volume removed from each hip as well as liposuction of the abdomen, thighs, and knees. She is shown 6 months after surgery. Her fat was not quite as well localized as the previous patient, and she was moderately overweight. Therefore some residual fullness was unavoidable. Nevertheless, liposuction achieved significant reduction.

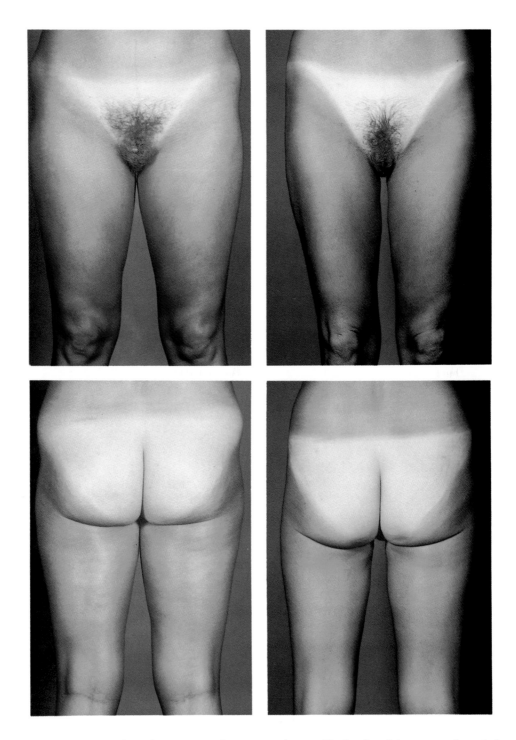

This 41-year-old, who was 5 feet 5 inches tall, had a history of weight fluctuation varying from 115 to 142 pounds. At consultation she weighed 142 pounds. She related that even when her weight was its lowest her hips were too full. I removed 150 cc from each hip and also treated her thighs, knees, and abdomen. She is shown 10 months after liposuction and weight loss of 25 pounds. Liposuction and weight loss complemented each other. The proximal medial thigh depression could be improved with additional liposuction of the adjacent distal area.

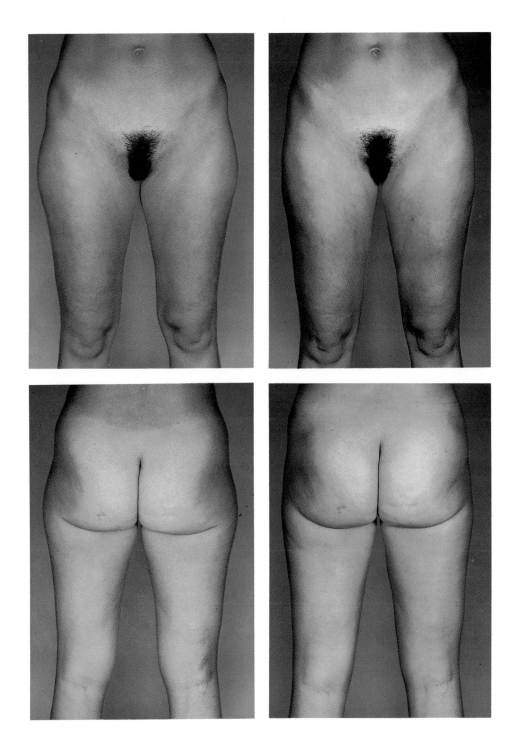

This 31-year-old woman, who was 5 feet 6 inches tall and weighed 118 pounds, had 100 cc of fat suctioned from each hip. Her thighs and knees were also treated. Seven months after surgery her hips are reduced in bulk despite a weight gain of 10 pounds.

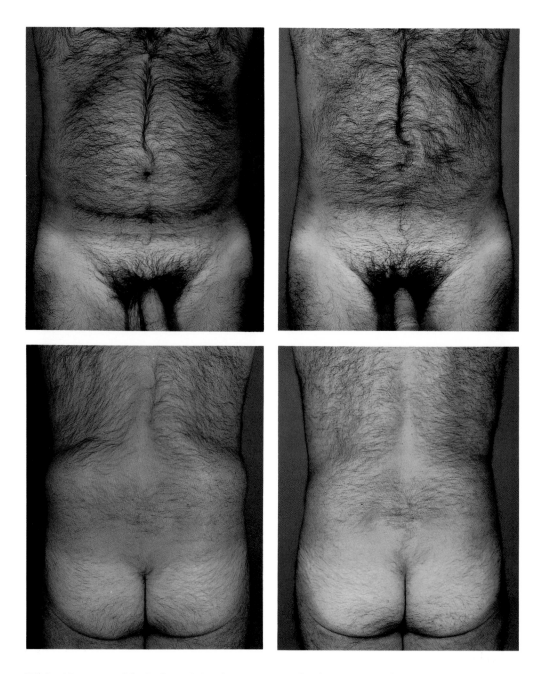

This 48-year-old, 5-foot 9-inch man weighed 165 pounds, 27 pounds more than his weight at age 18. As in most men, the excess fat was concentrated in his anterior abdomen and flanks. Liposuction of 250 cc from each flank dramatically reduced his "spare tire." His anterior abdomen was also treated.

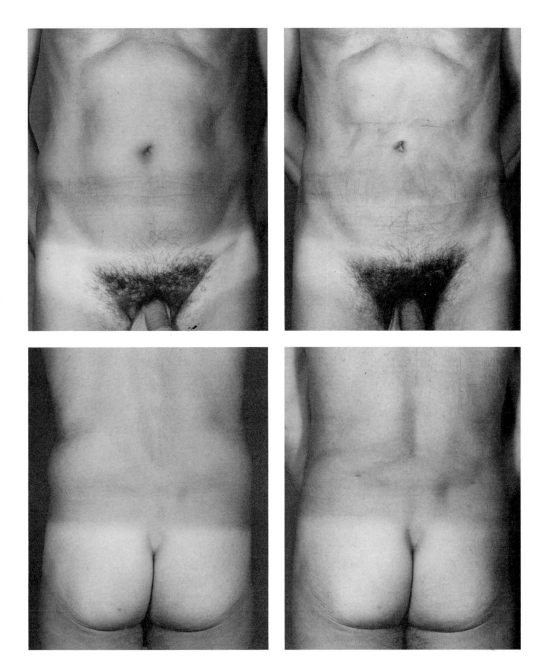

This 46-year-old, 6-foot man was 15 pounds over his ideal weight of 175 pounds. Excess fat localized on the anterior abdomen and hip/flank area extended around the trunk as a posterior roll. A total of 300 cc was removed from each flank, and his abdomen was also treated. He is shown 4 months after surgery.

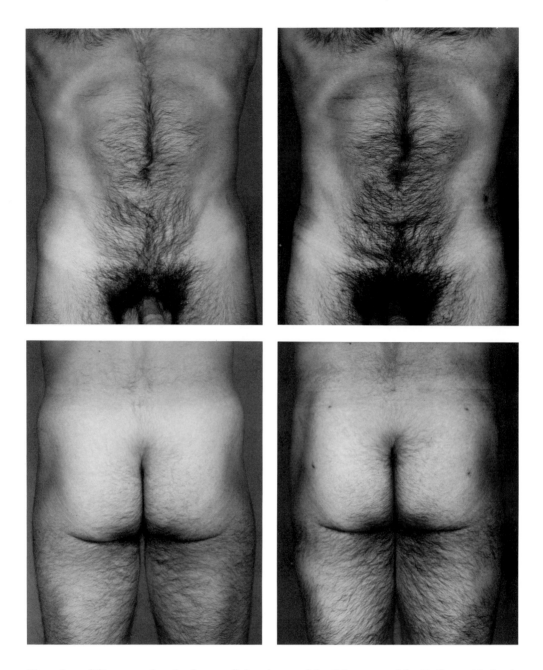

Despite diligent physical conditioning, this 36-year-old, 5-foot 10-inch man retained a small, but persistent fullness of the flanks at a weight of 158 pounds. He is shown 6 months after liposuction of 100 cc from each flank. Diminution in contour was maintained despite a 10-pound weight gain. The abdomen and outer thighs were also treated. The hyperpigmented, hypertrophic scar over the left anterior iliac crest gradually faded in intensity but was always more noticeable than other scars. I suspect that excessive trauma during surgery was the culprit.

Postoperative Care

If only the hips have been treated, no garment is necessary since the area is usually covered with a layer of adherent foam sponge for a few days. An abdominal binder made by any of a number of manufacturers can also be used. When multiple areas have been treated, an all-in-one garment (Polli) that covers the area from the knees to the upper abdomen must be purchased before surgery.

If only the hips have been treated, patients may return to all activities except sports within 48 to 72 hours. Soreness, although present, is generally not severe enough to inhibit daily functioning. Sports may be resumed in 2 weeks. If multiple areas are treated, recovery follows the course described on pp. 68-70.

COMPLICATIONS AND UNAESTHETIC RESULTS

Serious medical complications are rare when only the hips/flanks are treated. This area is also very forgiving of technical errors. Because the deep fat compartment is well developed and easily accessible, significant contour changes can be achieved with removal of deep fat only. In most patients the superficial fat remains largely undisturbed, making surface depressions and other irregularities uncommon. For the same reasons, this area infrequently requires secondary surgery. When secondary surgery is performed, it is usually for correction of side-to-side asymmetry.

──────────── REFERENCES ────────────

1. Schrudde J. Lipexeresis as a means of eliminating local adiposity. Aesthetic Plast Surg 4:215-226, 1980.
2. Schrudde J. Suction curettage for body contouring. Clin Plast Surg 11:445-456, 1984.
3. Teimourian B, Fisher JB. Suction curettage to remove excess fat for body contouring. Plast Reconstr Surg 68:50-58, 1981.
4. Kesselring UK. Regional fat aspiration for body contouring. Plast Reconstr Surg 72:610-619, 1983.
5. Illouz Y-G. Body contouring by lipolysis: A 5-year experience with over 3,000 cases. Plast Reconstr Surg 72:593-597, 1983.
6. Fournier PF, Otteni FM. Lipodissection in body sculpturing: The dry procedure. Plast Reconstr Surg 72:598-609, 1983.
7. Courtiss EH. Suction lipectomy: A retrospective analysis of 100 patients. Plast Reconstr Surg 73:780-794, 1984.
8. Pitman GH, Holzer J. Safe suction: Fluid replacement and blood loss parameters. Perspect Plast Surg 5(1):79-89, 1991.
9. Baroudi R. Body contour surgery. Clin Plast Surg 16:263-277, 1989.
10. Baroudi R. Flankplasty. In Hetter GP, ed. Lipoplasty: The Theory and Practice of Blunt Suction Lipectomy. Boston: Little, Brown, 1990, pp 399-416.
11. Baroudi R, Moraes M. Philosophy, technical principles, selection, and indications in body contouring surgery. Aesthetic Plast Surg 15:1-18, 1991.
12. Lockwood TE. Transverse flank/thigh/buttock lift with superficial fascial suspension. Plast Reconstr Surg 87:1019-1027, 1991.
13. Lockwood TE. Superficial fascial system (SFS) of the trunk and extremities: A new concept. Plast Reconstr Surg 87:1009-1018, 1991.

Chapter 11

THIGHS AND BUTTOCKS

More liposuction procedures are performed on the thighs and buttocks than any other area of the body. The plethora of beautiful young women with perfectly smooth thighs and small, firm buttocks seen on TV and the movie screen and found in advertisements in popular magazines serve as a constant reminder to the average woman that she somehow doesn't approach the ideal. It is not surprising that women seek surgery to achieve an idealized form that few normally have beyond their teenage years. Liposuction has proved particularly attractive and has all but replaced thigh and buttock lifts, which are now reserved for patients with exceptionally lax skin who are willing to accept the associated scarring.

HISTORY

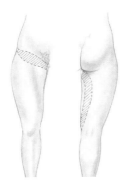

Lewis' operation (1957)

R.P. Posse[1] is credited with performing the first plastic surgery operation on the lower limbs. In 1957 J.R. Lewis[2-4] reported an operation in which he treated medial thigh excess due to massive weight loss with a combined one-stage vertical and horizontal skin excision. The resultant scar was an inverted L with a horizontal component in the groin and a vertical limb extending down the posteromedial aspect of the thigh.

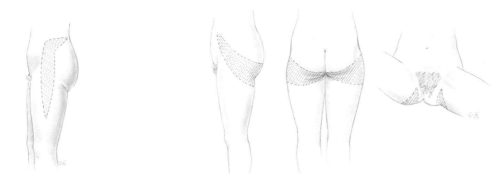

Farina's operation (1960)   Pitanguy's operation (1964)

Three years later Farina et al.[5,6] described a lateral thigh and buttock lift. They excised a vertical strip of skin and fat from the lateral aspect of the buttock and thigh. The vertical excision was joined to a horizontal wedge along the iliac crest. Final closure was an inverted L.

In 1964 Pitanguy[7,8] fired the imagination of plastic surgeons and the lay public with his description of an operation for what he termed "trochanteric lipodystrophy." His procedure, designed for simultaneous treatment of the buttocks, lateral thighs, and medial thighs, was performed through a near circumferential incision around the upper thigh and buttock. The resulting scar could be concealed by a bathing suit or shorts. Although Pitanguy's initial report tendered few details, subsequent articles provided a fuller explanation of his technique and results.[9-11]

In 1975 Hoffman and Simon[12] reported their experience with Pitanguy's operation. Their results on the outer thighs and buttocks were acceptable, but they found the operation "not satisfactory . . . for generally obese thighs or where medial redundancy [was] the presenting complaint." They stressed the significant morbidity and complication rate attending the procedure, in particular excessive scarring, asymmetry, and depressions.

Dissatisfied with conspicuous scars and gluteal depressions, several surgeons reported the use of inferiorly based buried dermal-fat flaps over the outer thigh and buttocks to prevent scar descent and/or an exaggerated gluteal depression. Delerm and Cirotteau,[13] Agris,[14] and Guerrerosantos[15] anchored the dermis to the underlying investing fascia. Teimourian and Adham[16] anchored the flap to the iliac crest periosteum as well as the fascia. Grazer and Klingbeil[17] tucked the inferior flap beneath the upper flap ("tuck and roll") without an anchoring stitch. Shaer[18] suggested a superiorly based dermal-fat flap to fill out the lateral gluteal depression.

Others emphasized sculpting techniques that left variable amounts of tissue in the area of excision and closed the inferior and superior flaps over a nonresected island of fat that might also include deepithelialized dermis, depending on how much bulk was desired.[11,17,19,20] For extra bulk the central tissue island could be plicated before closing the overlying flaps.[17,20] Attempts to prevent late scar descent in the medial thigh-groin area also produced a variety of deep tissue anchoring techniques.[21-25]

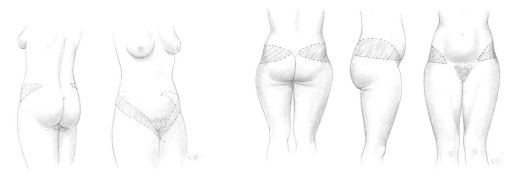

Baroudi's operation (1989)   Lockwood's operation (1991)

Baroudi[26,27] and Baroudi and Moraes[28] described a flank excision to slim and tighten the hip-flank area. By extending the excision in an antero-inferior direction into the inguinal and groin areas a simultaneous medial and lateral lift was created that produced "modest improvement of trochanteric and buttock regions."[26] Lockwood[29,30] reported a transverse flank excision to lift the entire flank, buttock, and lateral thigh area using the superficial fascial system (equivalent to Camper's and Scarpa's fascia) to anchor the deep closure. The resulting transverse scar was not visible in a bathing suit. Since tissue overlying the buttock was not resected, the problem of creating or worsening a gluteal depression was obviated. The transverse direction of the incision also preserved blood supply from superior gluteal artery perforators to the inferior flap.

Although the morbidity associated with thigh lift could be decreased by careful patient selection and refinement of technique, the long permanent scars remained the bêtes noires of these operations, and surgeons searched for other ways to contour the thighs and buttocks. Starting in 1964 Schrudde used curettes to remove fat from the lateral thighs through small incisions. His technique was published in German in 1977[31] and in English in 1980.[32] Other surgeons began to use suction to assist in removing fat through small incisions. Reports by the Fischers,[33] Kesselring and Meyer,[34] Illouz,[35-37] Teimourian and Fisher,[38] Fournier and Otteni,[39] Kesselring,[40] and Courtiss[41] attested to the rapid proliferation of information about suction-assisted fat removal and its equally rapid adoption as a new and effective method of treating excess fat in the thighs and elsewhere.

Combining liposuction with thigh lift, either synchronously or metachronously, has been the most recent step in the evolution of procedures for the thighs and buttocks, and several authors have described their philosophy and methods for combined procedures.[20,26,28,30,42,43]

AESTHETIC AND ANATOMIC CONSIDERATIONS

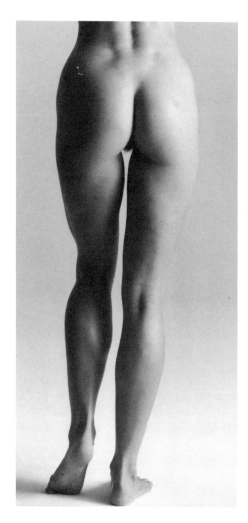

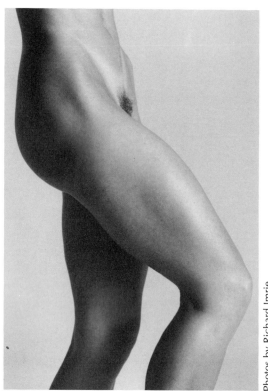

Photos by Richard Imrie

Popular culture and fashion dictate a particular idealized feminine form for the lower torso and upper thighs. Viewed from the front, a single smooth convex curve begins at the waist and extends downward over the iliac crest and greater trochanter before continuing to the knee. Viewed from the back, the same single smooth curve is sought even though most women have a more or less pronounced gluteal recess between the protuberant ilium and trochanter. The gluteal crease extends from the midline outward a variable distance, usually ending between one third and two thirds of the way to the lateral buttocks. The upper inner thighs meet briefly before separating en route to the knees. Viewed from the side, the normal lordotic curve sweeps gently onto the buttocks, which are maximally protuberant in their lower portion and join the thigh at an obtuse angle. Latin and African cultures idealize fuller buttocks with a more abrupt takeoff from the low back. Whatever the variations on the ideal, however, some gluteal fullness and rounding are universally perceived as youthful and desirable.

Musculoskeleton and Fat

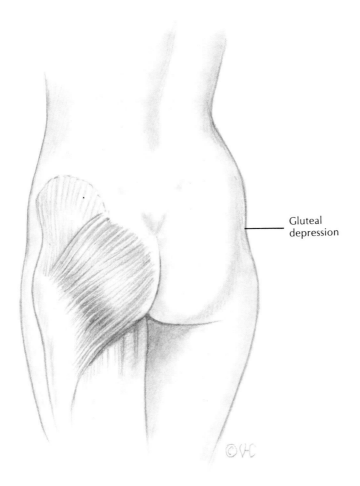

Gluteal
depression

The feminine skeleton flares at the iliac crest and again at the greater trochanter. The intervening space, called the gluteal depression, is a soft tissue recess filled, sometimes incompletely, by the gluteal muscle mass and fat. The subtrochanteric fat is particularly prominent, and a well-localized deep fat deposit overlays the lateral thigh caudal to the greater trochanter and posterior to the tensor fascia lata.

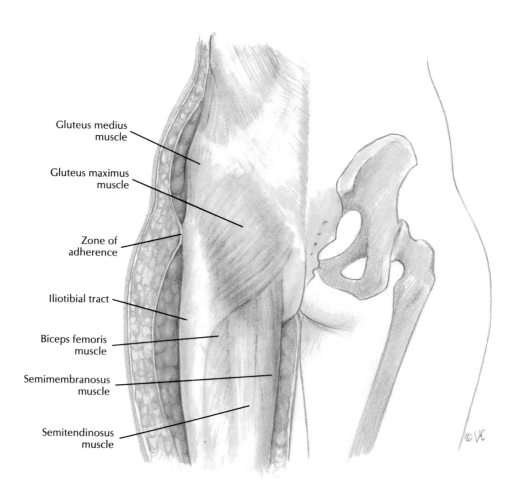

Gluteus medius
muscle

Gluteus maximus
muscle

Zone of
adherence

Iliotibial tract

Biceps femoris
muscle

Semimembranosus
muscle

Semitendinosus
muscle

The contour of the upper posterior thigh is largely determined by the muscle mass of the hamstrings, although some patients demonstrate a more or less prominent localized fat deposit parallel and just inferior to the gluteal crease. Buttock and thigh muscles are surrounded by the deep investing fascia (fascia lata) that condenses in the lateral thigh into a strong vertical band, the iliotibial tract.

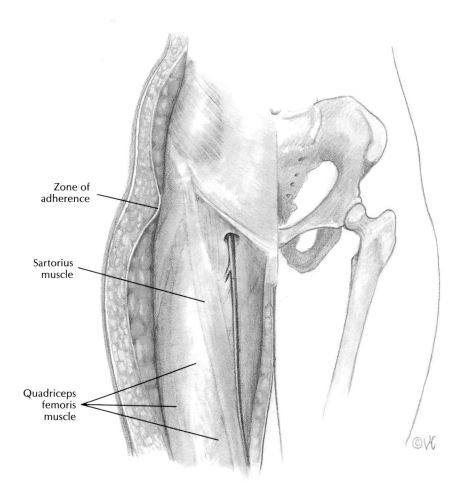

Zone of
adherence

Sartorius
muscle

Quadriceps
femoris
muscle

The quadriceps femoris muscle constitutes most of the upper anterior thigh bulk, over which the fat is rather evenly distributed when compared to the sharply localized deep fat overlying the upper lateral thigh.

"Zone of adherence" (see also p. 318) is Lockwood's term for an area along the deep or investing fascia where particularly strong and numerous attachments from the superficial fascia are found.[29] These attachments surround and define localized deep layers of subcutaneous fat.

Superficial Fascial System and Localized Deep Fat Deposits

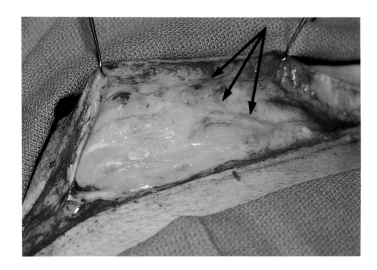

The superficial fascia covers the entire body surface but is particularly prominent in the lower trunk, buttocks, and upper thighs. In these areas the fat is divided into layers by one or more membranous fascial sheets (arrows), as seen running horizontally through the superficial fat in the flank area of this 36-year-old man.

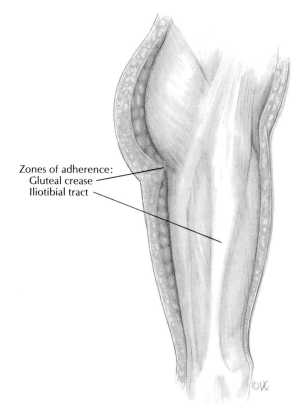

Zones of adherence:
Gluteal crease
Iliotibial tract

Additional vertical and oblique fascial elements connect the horizontal fascial layers to create a tightly structured framework of fat and fascia, which Lockwood called the superficial fascial system (SFS).[29] In the flanks, buttocks, and upper thighs the SFS overlays deeper, localized fat deposits[44] that are darker, more loosely structured, and contain fewer fascial supporting elements.

The SFS sends fascial elements through the deep fat deposits to attach to the underlying muscle investing fascia. These attachments are loose and permit the skin to glide easily over the muscle. In some areas, however, these deep fascial connections become prominent, condensing into more or less discrete bands or "zones of adherence"[29] and anchoring the skin to the deep fascia. Zones of adherence occur at the inguinal ligament, gluteal crease, iliotibial tract, and other areas. They frequently form the perimeter of localized fat deposits (e.g., subtrochanteric fat) and thus define the shape and localization of the deep subcutaneous fat.

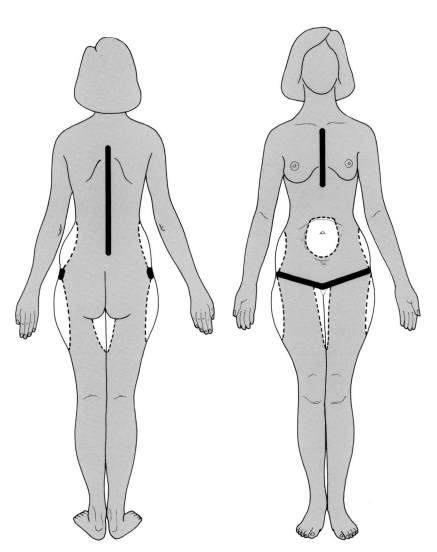

Diagram of SFS zones of adherence.
Black bands = most adherent; gray zones = adherent; white zones = least adherent.

Vascular Anatomy and Lymphatics

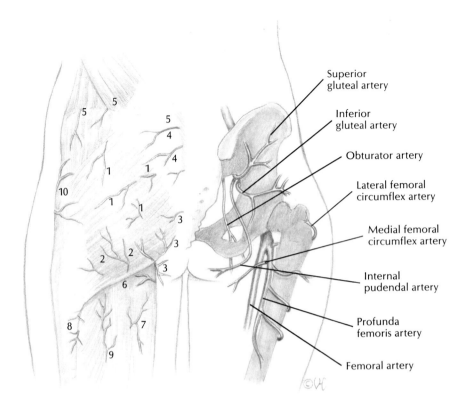

Cutaneous branches of:
1 = superior gluteal artery, 2 = inferior gluteal artery, 3 = internal pudendal artery, 4 = lateral sacral artery,
5 = iliolumbar and last lumbar arteries, 6 = obturator artery, 7 = medial femoral circumflex artery,
8 = profunda femoris artery, 9 = popliteal artery, 10 = lateral femoral circumflex artery

The dominant arterial supply to the skin of the buttocks is from musculo-cutaneous perforators of the inferior and superior gluteal arteries, partic-ularly the former, which is the most important cutaneous artery in the gluteal region.[45] The inferomedial aspect of this region receives collateral supply from the gluteal branch of the internal pudendal artery and from the cutaneous branches of the medial circumflex division of the profunda femo-ris artery. A branch from the fourth lumbar artery frequently supplies the skin over the anterosuperior border of the gluteus maximus. The superficial circumflex iliac artery may also reach the superolateral portions of the gluteal skin. Extensive subcutaneous anastomoses provide rich vasculariza-tion to the skin of this region, permitting extensive undermining without risk of skin necrosis.[46]

The posterior thigh skin is supplied from branches of the profunda femoris, in particular the lateral femoral circumflex artery supplying the upper lat-eral thigh over the vastus lateralis. Musculocutaneous branches from the first perforator supply the skin of the upper posteromedial thigh, anasto-mosing with inferior gluteal branches coming from above.

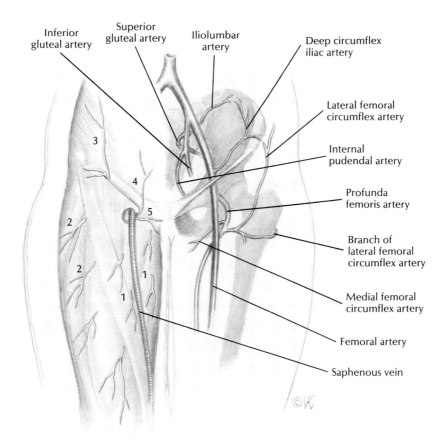

Inferior gluteal artery
Superior gluteal artery
Iliolumbar artery
Deep circumflex iliac artery
Lateral femoral circumflex artery
Internal pudendal artery
Profunda femoris artery
Branch of lateral femoral circumflex artery
Medial femoral circumflex artery
Femoral artery
Saphenous vein

1 = cutaneous branches of femoral artery, 2 = cutaneous branches of profunda femoris artery,
3 = superficial circumflex iliac artery, 4 = superficial inferior epigastric artery,
5 = superficial internal pudendal artery

Branches from the common and superficial femoral artery are dominant in the upper anteromedial thigh and groin region. Fanning out from the proximal femoral artery the triad of superficial inferior epigastric artery, superficial circumflex iliac artery, and superficial external pudendal artery supplies the lower trunk, upper thigh, and groin area with a rich anastomosing network of direct cutaneous arteries. Musculocutaneous perforators from the superficial femoral artery supply the more distal portion of upper thigh skin.

Venous drainage largely parallels the arterial supply with the conspicuous exception of the greater saphenous vein, which runs in the deep part of the superficial fascia on the medial aspect of the thigh before joining the femoral vein at the fossa ovalis. Much of the superficial lymphatic drainage of the medial lower extremity accompanies the saphenous vein before emptying into the subinguinal lymph nodes. The saphenous vein and its associated lymphatics should be preserved during medial thigh lift to prevent excessive postoperative swelling.

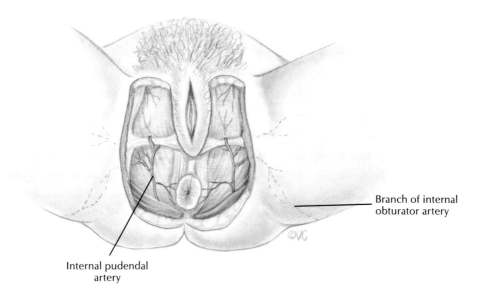

Branch of internal
obturator artery

Internal pudendal
artery

The skin of the genitofemoral sulcus and the genitalia are supplied by superficial branches of the internal pudendal artery, which anastomose with terminal branches of the external pudendal arteries in the anterior groin and with branches from the inferior gluteal artery and other vessels supplying the posterior thigh and groin.

Nerves

Buttock and upper thigh sensibility depends on nerve roots T12 to S3. The superior clunial nerves (cutaneous branches from dorsal rami of L1–3) supply the superior buttock. The medial buttock is supplied by the middle clunial nerves (cutaneous branches from dorsal rami S1–3), whereas the inferior buttock is supplied by the inferior clunial nerves that branch off the posterior femoral cutaneous nerve (S1–2) as it emerges from under the gluteus maximus to supply the skin of the posterior thigh. The lateral cutaneous branch of the iliohypogastric nerve supplies the area lateral to the buttock over the iliac crest; branches of the lateral femoral cutaneous nerve supply the skin inferolateral to the buttock. The posterior femoral cutaneous nerve also supplies the upper medial thigh and perineum via its perineal branches and the genitalia via the longest perineal branch, the inferior pudendal nerve.

The proximal anterior thigh is supplied by branches of the lateral femoral cutaneous nerve, genitofemoral nerve, ilioinguinal nerve, and a small inconstant branch of the obturator nerve. Significant numbness following thigh lifts is rare because of the considerable overlap of cutaneous nerves in this region.

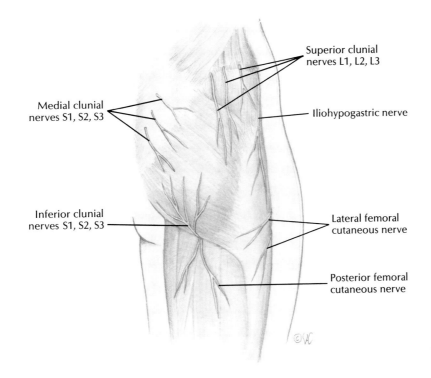

Superior clunial
nerves L1, L2, L3

Medial clunial
nerves S1, S2, S3

Iliohypogastric nerve

Inferior clunial
nerves S1, S2, S3

Lateral femoral
cutaneous nerve

Posterior femoral
cutaneous nerve

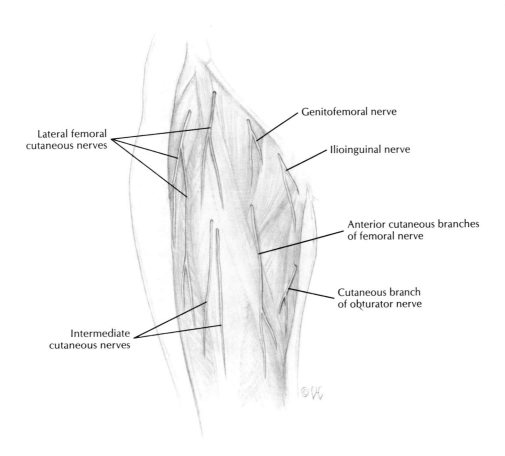

Lateral femoral
cutaneous nerves

Genitofemoral nerve

Ilioinguinal nerve

Anterior cutaneous branches
of femoral nerve

Cutaneous branch
of obturator nerve

Intermediate
cutaneous nerves

CLASSIFICATION AND TREATMENT OPTIONS

Patients requesting aesthetic contouring improvements in the thigh and buttock area can be divided into three groups.

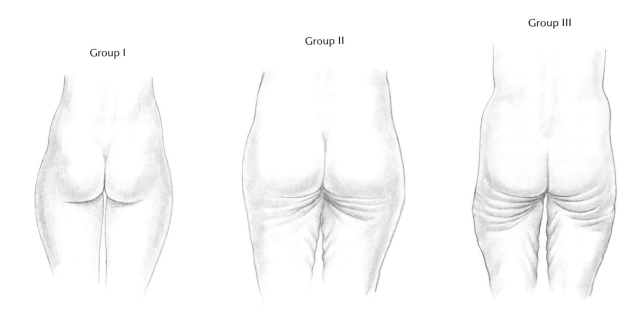

Patients in group I have well-localized excess fat with little or no skin laxity. They are generally less than 40 years of age. Optimal treatment for group I patients is liposuction.

Patients in group II have excess fat and varying degrees of skin laxity. The age range of these patients is most frequently 40 to 60 years old. Liposuction is the preferred treatment, although results may be compromised by the poor quality of skin. Those with greater degrees of skin laxity may also benefit from skin excision and lifting.

Patients in group III characteristically have little or no fat and severe skin laxity due to weight loss or age. They require skin excision and lifting for beneficial results. Generally little or no liposuction is indicated.

The overwhelming majority of patients seeking thigh and buttock treatment are categorized in groups I or II, and most will benefit from liposuction alone.

Patient Types
Thighs

Excessive fat in the lateral and medial thighs is the primary indication for liposuction. Fat deposits may be large or small in volume. If the fatty protuberance is well localized, the contour can be reduced.

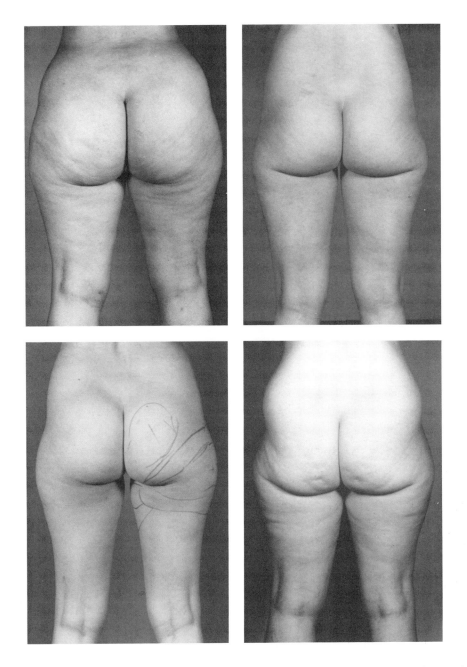

These four patients are of varying age, height, and weight. Their skin conditions range from tight and smooth to loose and irregular. They are all excellent candidates for liposuction because they have well-localized fat deposits in their medial and lateral thighs.

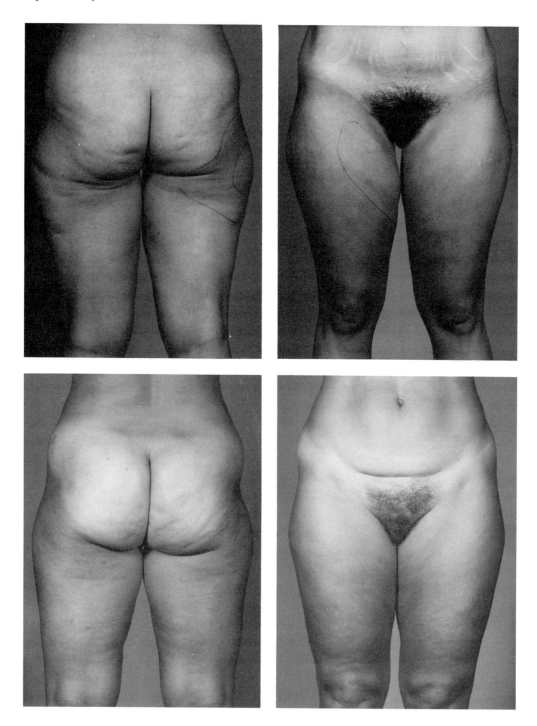

Patients with lax skin and relatively sparse or moderate fat deposits such as these two women should be considered for lateral and/or medial thigh lift. However, given the choice of a limited result with minimal scars or a maximally tightened skin envelope with long scars, most women will opt for liposuction, particularly if they are informed that a future thigh lift is not precluded.

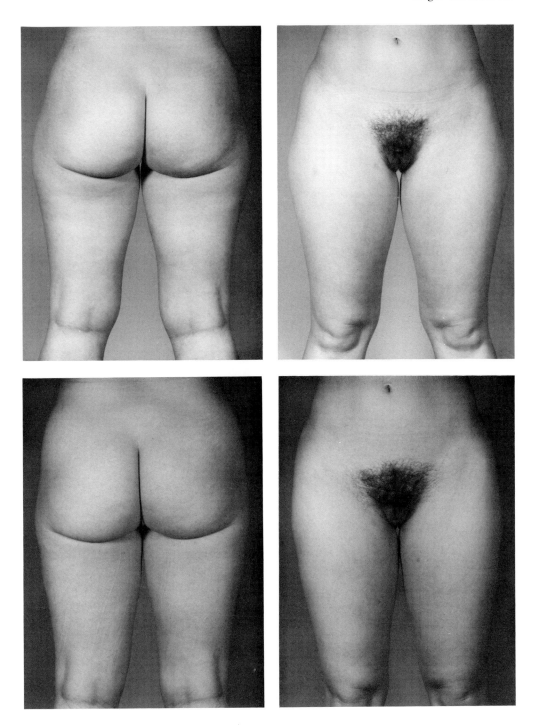

Patients with excessive anterior thigh bulk are frequently overweight and/or suffer from generalized fullness and bulkiness, so-called thunder thighs.[47] Although some of these patients are difficult to satisfy with liposuction alone, judicious anterior thigh fat removal in conjunction with circumferential treatment of the entire thigh can improve their appearance.

Buttocks

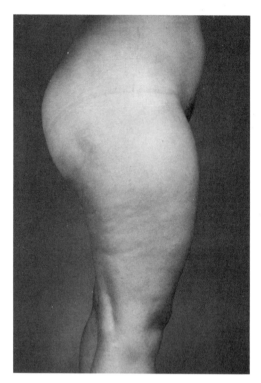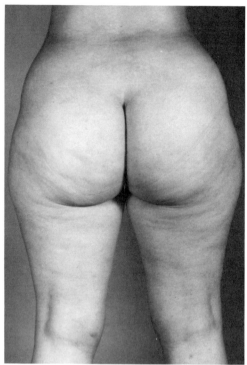

Patients with excessively full and protuberant buttocks (steatopygia) are candidates for liposuction. True steatopygia involves a pronounced fullness of the superior portion of the buttocks with a "shelving out" of this part of the anatomy and an increased anteroposterior girth secondary to excessive fat. Fat in the lower lateral portion of the buttocks is usually contiguous with lateral thigh fat and is treated with this area. Buttocks that are simply elongated will not respond to liposuction.

Laxity of the lower buttocks is most frequently a senile change (although it is sometimes seen in women in their thirties) or secondary to weight loss. Liposuction will only increase this deformity. Mild deformities can be corrected by excising a lenticular segment of skin and soft tissue with its long axis centered on the gluteal crease. The scar usually extends beyond the crease.

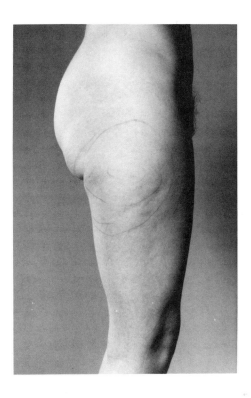

A secondary bulge below the gluteal crease is seen in some women, more commonly if they are overweight. This bulge can be reduced, but it usually cannot be totally eliminated. Moreover, liposuction of this subgluteal fat can reduce support for the buttock, causing increased sagging and overhanging of the lower buttock onto the upper posterior thigh.

The gluteal crease usually runs from the trochanteric area laterally to the junction of the medial one third and lateral two thirds of the buttocks. Some patients have little or no buttock crease and desire its elongation. Although this is technically possible,[43] I generally discourage patients seeking this change since a short buttock crease is a sign of youth and fitness.

PATIENT EVALUATION AND COUNSELING
Physical Examination

The physical examination is always performed with the patient fully disrobed and standing. Before starting the examination I ask the patient to point out areas of primary concern. She will usually put her hands on bulging areas and may add a verbal description of the emotional burden of her body disproportion. If the problem is skin laxity, she may pull up on the skin to show the desired degree of improvement. It is at this time, also, that the patient indicates the priority of her concerns. While the surgeon may notice first a striking fullness of the lateral thighs, the patient may be most concerned with buttock ptosis or a double roll in the lower buttock. The surgeon should listen and observe silently for a few moments so that he can properly direct his attention to those areas of paramount concern to the patient.

The thighs and buttocks are evaluated by inspection and palpation. Generalized skeletal abnormalities and asymmetries are noted first. Scoliosis will result in left-to-right differences in the heights of the iliac crests and greater trochanters, which in turn will cause asymmetries of the soft tissue profile. Lateral thigh asymmetries are more frequently due to scoliosis than to actual differences in volume of fat, and it is worthwhile to point this out to the patient at the time of the examination.

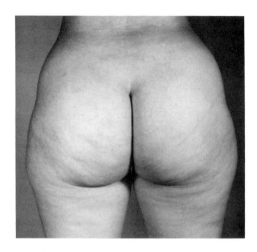

Note, for example, the slight elevation of the right iliac crest and greater trochanter with corresponding increased fullness of these areas.

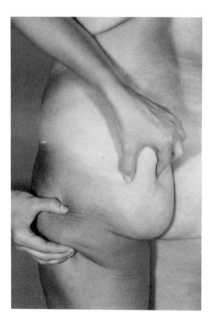
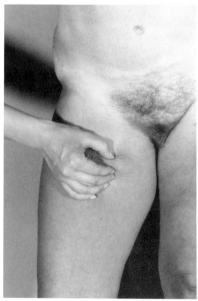

A pinch test is performed on the lateral thighs, buttocks, and medial thighs. As a rule, if a minimum of 4 to 5 cm can be pinched between the thumb and index finger over the lateral thigh, the patient will benefit from treatment. Patients who are otherwise quite thin and have disproportionate fat deposition in the lateral thighs may experience good results even if the fatty layer is thinner. The pinch test of buttock skin should demonstrate a similar thickness. The medial thighs have less fat, and a 3 cm thickness generally indicates liposuction will be beneficial.

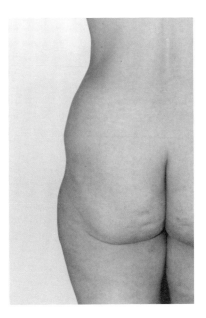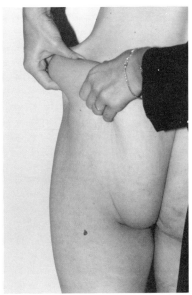

Lifting the tissues is another important maneuver. The surgeon should grasp the tissues over the hips and lift up to see the effect on the lateral thigh and buttock. If the fullness is due mostly to tissue laxity, the "lift test" will ablate buttock ptosis and diminish lateral thigh fullness, an indication for lateral thigh lift. The lift test should also be performed in the groin area to determine the degree of medial thigh laxity.

As the examination proceeds, the surgeon communicates his findings to the patient, informing her if she can reasonably expect a dramatic change from liposuction alone, if the results will be more limited, or if optimal improvement requires skin excision and lifting. The patient is given a mirror to examine each area for which treatment is recommended and to see for herself the thickness of the subcutaneous tissues and the effect on the thighs and buttocks when flank and buttock tissues are lifted.

Defining Patient Goals

Women often state that they want the lateral thighs totally "flat" and that, in particular, they want to be rid of the double bulge or "violin" deformity (fullness at the iliac crest area, fullness at the subtrochanteric area, and the intervening gluteal depression). Although a perfectly smooth, convex line along the lateral aspect of the thigh-hip area is seen in high fashion models and well-trained athletes, it is neither achievable nor desirable in every woman. In most patients a reduction of the double bulge is a more realistic goal than total elimination.

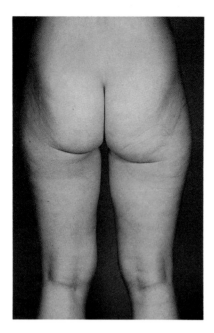 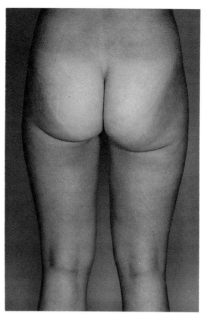

Removal of 250 cc from each outer thigh created the perfectly smooth contour this 5-foot 3-inch, 105-pound patient was seeking. Small amounts were also removed from the medial thighs and knees. Only a relatively subtle change was needed. This type of result is achieved in only a minority of patients. Most women will have some residual gluteal depression after surgery.

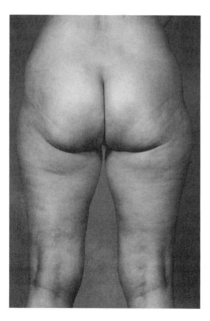 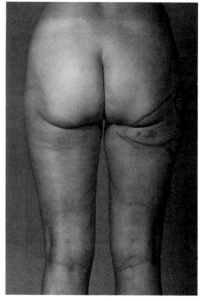

Removal of 350 cc from each outer thigh and 50 cc from each hip created a nearly smooth contour in this 5-foot 5-inch, 124-pound patient. She wanted still more tissue removed from the right lateral thigh and is shown marked for this secondary procedure in the postoperative view. An additional 100 cc was suctioned. She did not return for follow-up photographs.

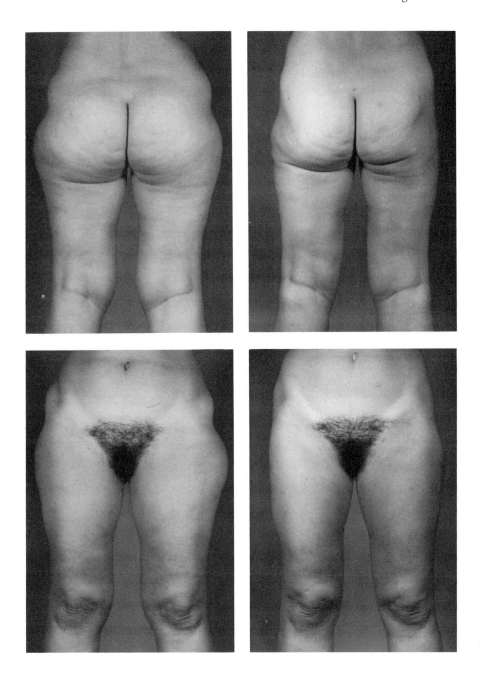

This 5-foot 6-inch, 155-pound patient had a more severe problem. Removal of 500 cc from each lateral thigh and 100 cc from each hip reduced the patient's bulk but did not create a single smooth curve from flank to thigh. The patient declined my offer of additional liposuction on the left lateral thigh, which would have produced a more symmetric appearance.

Patients may seek treatment because of difficulty fitting clothes. Not uncommonly, the patient will say, "I am a size 8 on top but a 12 on bottom" or make other similar comments.

Since the medial thighs have relatively less fat, they are less frequently the focus of the patient's attention. When this area is the patient's primary concern, it is usually because of skin laxity rather than excess fat. Nevertheless, some women desire the least possible amount of fat in this area and want a relatively straight medial thigh contour. They also want to maximize the amount of space between their upper thighs.

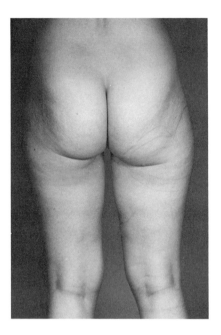 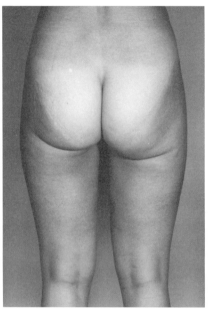

Inner thigh straightening was attained in this patient after 75 cc was removed from each upper medial thigh.

The patient with significant wrinkling and laxity of the medial thighs will sometimes place both her hands on the upper inner thigh, pull up, and eliminate every vestige of wrinkle or irregularity from knee to groin, simultaneously stating, "This is what I want!" But even the most successful thigh lift will leave some residual wrinkling, particularly in the lower third of the thigh, and the surgeon must correct any illusions to the contrary.

Significant anterior thigh fullness is usually accompanied by generalized bulkiness. Although liposuction reduces thigh bulk, the patient will be disappointed unless the surgeon educates her to the real limitations of the procedure.

A forthright discussion is essential for both patient and surgeon to select the best procedure for the patient's specific deformity, needs, and life-style. A long-term reconstructive plan may be necessary: liposuction in the immediate future and possible thigh lift later.

Informed Consent

Informed consent for liposuction of the thighs and buttocks should include all of the general issues discussed in Chapter 1 and the liposuction information letters on pp. 5-7. In my experience, secondary operations are more frequently needed for the lateral thighs than any other area. Patients are told that there is a 5% to 10% likelihood that they will have to undergo a second operation for removal of additional fat and that liposuction may result in additional irregularities.

Patients are also given complete information on the time course of resolution of swelling and bruising (see p. 70), particularly if they plan on wearing shorts or other abbreviated clothing soon after the operation.

Patients scheduled for thigh and buttock lifts require additional time to discuss the special issues related to these questions. The location, length, and permanence of scars and the potential for unfavorable results and complications are explained and described. The patient should understand that in the first few months after surgery the scar will redden and may hypertrophy, but after 6 months the redness will gradually fade, and the overall appearance will improve. Maximal improvement may take 2 years or longer. The patient also needs to be informed that scars may descend, and their final width, height, and color are unpredictable. The risk of wound dehiscence, infections, and skin necrosis should be noted as well as the possibility, however remote, of life-threatening complications such as pulmonary embolus. The inconveniences of the postoperative period, including pain and inability to sit normally for 1 to 2 weeks following medial thigh lift, should be stressed. If significant undermining is performed at surgery, the patient also needs to be prepared for return visits to the office for aspiration of seromas or hematomas.

All patients contemplating thigh and buttock lifts are given information letters specific to these operations.

INFORMATION LETTER

Thigh, Hip, and Buttock Lift

Thigh, hip, and buttock lift is a surgical procedure to tighten the skin of the outer thighs, buttocks, and hips. The operation removes elliptical segments of skin and underlying fat from the upper buttock and flank area. The remaining skin and tissues are reconstructed to achieve a tightening and smoothing effect. The operation is designed to help patients with loose, flabby skin and underlying tissues that may occur from massive weight loss, natural aging, or as a result of heredity. Although the operation is often combined with liposuction (fat removal by suction), it is primarily for skin and deep tissue tightening. As with liposuction, it is not a correction for obesity, and you should be at normal or near-normal weight before surgery.

Combined Procedures   Thigh and buttock lift may be combined with liposuction or cosmetic operations on other parts of the body.

Anesthesia   All thigh and buttock lifts require general anesthesia.

Duration of Operation   Operating time is 2½ hours.

Hospitalization   You will be admitted to the hospital the morning of surgery and discharged 1 or 2 days later.

After Surgery   You will remain in bed until the next morning. A urinary catheter may have been placed during your operation. It will be removed the next morning. Both placement and removal are painless. You will receive intravenous fluids for 24 hours after surgery.

You can expect some discomfort and pain at the incision site, but this is alleviated with medication and gradually subsides when you begin to walk. The bandage over the incision is removed the day after surgery, and you may then shower. All sutures are internal and self-dissolving.

You will find it difficult to sit for several days after the operation. Generally, by the end of the first week you are able to sit comfortably.

Physical Activity After Surgery   Patients should rest at home for 2 weeks after surgery. Walking and other activities are gradually resumed during the second week, and most people return to work at the end of 2 weeks. Strenuous sports are prohibited for 2 months.

Photographs   Photographs, which do not show the face, are taken before and several months after surgery. They aid in planning and performing the operation and become a permanent part of your patient record.

Scars   You can expect a horizontal scar in the upper buttock/flank area extending from the midline in the back to the groin area in the front. There will be scars on both sides. The scar will be positioned so that it is covered by panties or a bathing suit. You should bring a pair of panties or bathing suit of the type you normally wear (not a string bikini) to the hospital.

I make every effort to keep the scars symmetric, but perfect symmetry is not always achievable. In some patients a different type or location of scar may be necessary because of individual anatomic variation. If this is so in your case, I will inform you at the time of consultation. I will keep the scar as short and inconspicuous as possible, but this operation, of necessity, requires long scars.

The scars will be red for the first few months after surgery and gradually fade with time. Nevertheless, you should be aware that the scars are permanent, and their final width, height, and color are not totally predictable.

Diminished Sensibility As with any surgical procedure, small nerves to the skin are interrupted. Consequently, portions of your torso and your upper thighs will feel numb or have diminished feeling. Sensibility generally returns over several months, although in some cases return is incomplete.

Complications The most common complication is hematoma, or a collection of blood under the skin. This occurs infrequently but may necessitate returning to the operating room to remove the blood.

In some patients, fluid (serum) collects beneath the skin 1 or 2 weeks after surgery. If necessary, I will remove the fluid by needle aspiration in the office. This procedure is painless.

Infection or wound healing problems, including loss of skin and excessive scarring, can occur but are infrequent in my experience. Other serious or even life-threatening complications are possible.

I mention all of the above not to alarm or frighten you since, in my experience, the vast majority of patients are satisfied. I am, however, compelled to give you full information on side effects and complications no matter how remote their possibility.

Cigarette Smoking If you smoke, the likelihood of wound healing problems and other complications increases. Smokers *must stop smoking completely* at least 2 weeks prior to surgery. "Cutting down" is not enough. *Complete cessation of smoking is mandatory.*

• • •

Should you not understand any of the foregoing, or should you want more information, please ask. Occasional questions will arise after you have left the office. Feel free to call for additional information. If necessary, a second consultation can be scheduled. Find out all you need to know. I wish all patients to be fully informed.

INFORMATION LETTER

Inner Thigh Lift

Inner thigh lift is a surgical procedure to tighten the skin of the inner thighs. This operation removes elliptical segments of skin and underlying fat from the upper portions of the inner thighs. The remaining skin and tissues are reconstructed to achieve a tightening and smoothing effect. The operation is designed to help those patients who have loose, flabby skin and underlying tissues. This condition may occur from massive weight loss or natural aging or as a result of heredity. Although the operation is often combined with liposuction (fat removal by suction), it is primarily a skin and deep tissue tightening procedure. As with liposuction, it is not a correction for obesity, and you should be at normal or near-normal weight before surgery.

Combined Procedures   Inner thigh lift may be combined with liposuction or cosmetic operations on other parts of the body.

Anesthesia   Inner thigh lifts require general anesthesia.

Duration of Operation   Operating time is 2½ hours.

Hospitalization   You will be admitted to the hospital the morning of surgery and discharged 1 or 2 days after surgery.

After Surgery   You will remain in bed until the next morning. A urinary catheter, placed during your operation, is removed the morning after surgery. Both placement and removal are painless. You will receive intravenous fluids for 24 hours after surgery.

You can expect some discomfort and pain at the incision site, but this is alleviated with medication and gradually subsides when you begin to walk. The bandage over the incision is removed the day after surgery, and you may then shower. All sutures are internal and are self-dissolving.

You will find it difficult to sit for several days and sometimes weeks after the operation. For the first few days after surgery, voiding and bowel movements must be performed in a semistanding position. Generally, by the end of the first week you are able to sit comfortably.

Physical Activity After Surgery   Patients should rest at home for 2 weeks after surgery. Walking and other activities are gradually resumed during the second week, and most people return to work at the end of 2 weeks. Strenuous sports are prohibited for 2 months.

Photographs   Photographs, which do not show the face, are taken before and several months after surgery. They aid in planning and performing the operation and become a permanent part of your patient record.

Scars   You can expect a horizontal scar in the groin crease extending from the top of the pubic hair in front to the buttocks in back. The scar may in time descend to a lower level due to the ongoing forces of gravity but can usually be covered by panties or a bathing suit.

For severe deformities a portion of the scar will extend down the inner thigh. If this is so in your case, I will inform you at the time of consultation. The scars will be red for the first few months after surgery and will gradually fade with time. You should be aware, however, that they are permanent, and their final width, height, and color are not totally predictable.

Diminished Sensibility   As with any surgical procedure, small nerves to the skin are interrupted. Consequently, portions of the inner thighs will feel numb or have diminished feeling. Sensibility generally returns over several months, although in some cases return is incomplete.

Complications   Hematoma, a collection of blood under the skin, is infrequent but may necessitate returning to the operating room for removal of the blood. Infection or wound healing problems, including loss of skin, distortion of the genitalia, and excessive scarring, occur less frequently. Other serious or even life-threatening complications can occur. I mention all of the above not to alarm or frighten you since, in my experience, the vast majority of patients are satisfied. I am, however, compelled to give you full information on side effects and complications no matter how remote their possibility.

Cigarette Smoking   If you smoke, the likelihood of wound healing problems and other complications increases. Smokers must stop smoking *completely* at least 2 weeks prior to surgery. "Cutting down" is not enough. *Complete cessation of smoking is mandatory.*

• • •

Should you not understand any of the foregoing, or should you want more information, please ask. Occasional questions will arise after you have left the office. Feel free to call for additional information. If necessary, a second consultation can be scheduled. Find out all you need to know. I wish all patients to be fully informed.

LIPOSUCTION
Markings

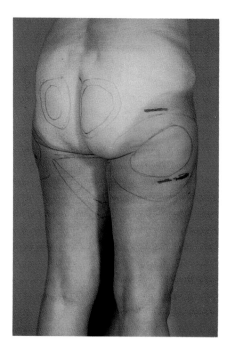 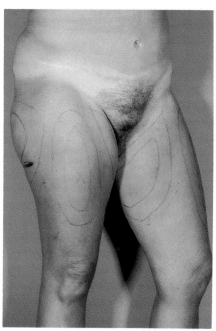

The patient stands while the lateral thigh protuberance is outlined as two or three concentric rings in the form of a rough circle. The buttock protuberance is similarly outlined. Areas to be avoided (the gluteal recess, etc.) are also marked. The exact location of access incisions is also indicated. I treat the lateral thighs through flank and gluteal crease incisions. The buttock is most accessible through an incision at the top of the natal crease and gluteal crease incision. The medial thigh bulge is outlined as a triangle with its base a line parallel to and below the groin crease and its apex pointing down the thigh. The exact size and location of the medial thigh marking depends on the size and location of the fat deposit. Most medial thigh fat excess begins several centimeters below the groin crease. Access incisions for the medial thigh are in the groin crease medial to the femoral vein and in the midthigh just below the apex of the area to be treated. The anterior thigh fullness is also marked when liposuction is planned in this area.

Operative Technique
Lateral Thighs

The lateral thighs and contiguous lower lateral buttocks are treated with the patient in the lateral decubitus position. I use Mercedes Type cannulas, 3 to 5 mm in diameter, the actual size varying with volume of aspirate, which is usually 200 to 400 cc per side. Smaller and larger volumes are not uncommon.

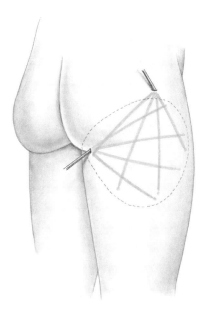

Use of gluteal crease and flank access incisions permits crisscrossing of tunnels and a smooth surface contour.

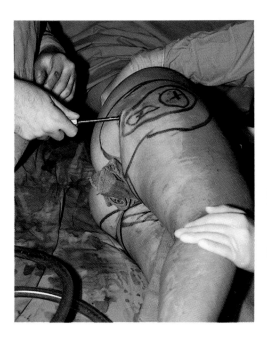
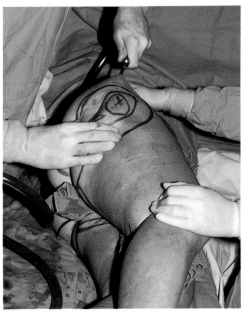

After infiltration of dilute lidocaine with epinephrine, I inspect and pinch the tissue to establish baseline appearance and feel. I then insert the cannula through the gluteal crease incision, making certain to pierce the superficial fascia with the cannula tip. I remove approximately half the planned suction volume from this incision and then inspect and pinch the tissues again to judge my progress. I also run my hand lightly over the skin surface to feel for irregularities. Additional aspirate is suctioned from the flank access incision, concentrating on areas that have a residual protuberance or feel thicker.

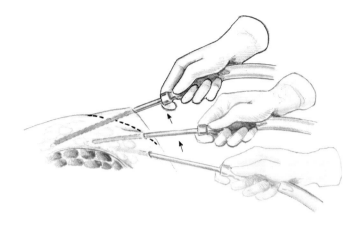

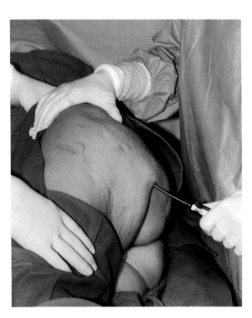

It is important to keep the tip of the cannula within the well-developed deep fat deposit in the subtrochanteric area as much as possible. When using the gluteal crease incision, the surgeon is working in a transverse direction along the convexity of the lateral thigh, and he should elevate the handle of the cannula as he thrusts forward. Elevation of the handle lowers the tip, permitting it to stay deep along the convex fascial surface. Maintenance of the cannula tip in the deep fat is technically easier from the flank access incision since there is less convexity along the length of the thigh.

The anterior border of the deep subtrochanteric fat deposit ends abruptly as the superficial fascia inserts into the zone of adherence at the iliotibial tract (see p. 344). Therefore, when treating the lateral thigh, it is particularly important to stay deep and limit suctioning as the anterior thigh is approached.

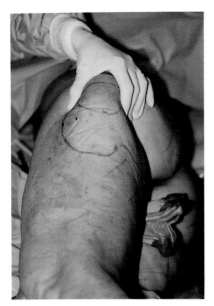 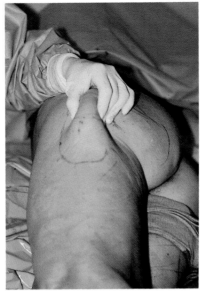 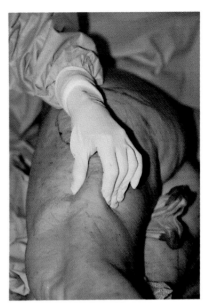

Left: The skin is pinched before suctioning. *Center:* The skin is pinched after suctioning. *Right:* A more distal area is similar in thickness to the treated proximal area.

The end point is reached when skin thickness is approximately that of adjacent skin on the lower lateral thigh. The actual thickness is usually 3 to 4 cm on pinch, but varies with each individual, depending on age, weight, body habitus, etc. The relative change from pretreatment thickness and comparison with nearby tissues is more important than absolute measured thickness.

When the second side is treated with the patient in the lateral decubitus position, it is impossible to make a synchronous visual and pinch comparison for left-to-right symmetry. Therefore it is essential to record the exact volume removed from the first side so that an identical amount can be removed from the second side (assuming preoperative symmetry). The primary criteria for judging when to stop are appearance and feel of the tissues, but matching volumes is a critical additional determinant when working with the patient in the decubitus position.

Medial Thighs

The medial thighs are treated with the patient in the frog-leg position. Because of the smaller amounts of fat in this area, cannulas that range from 2 to 4 cm in diameter are used, and volumes commonly suctioned are 50 to 100 cc per side.

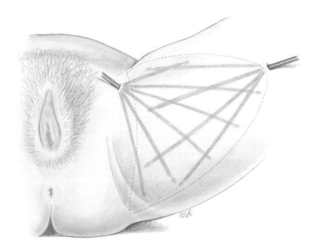

Suctioning is performed from two access incisions: one in the groin crease about 4 cm medial to the femoral pulse and a second at the lower limit of the area being treated in the proximal third of the medial thigh.

Since the femoral nerve, artery, and vein are deep to the investing fascia, they are not at risk so long as the cannula is kept superficial to the fascia lata. Nevertheless, placing the groin access incision well medial to the femoral pulse provides added safety when thrusting the cannula into the deep fat to begin suctioning. Although the saphenous vein is in the superficial fascia and thus in the field of treatment, I have never seen interruption, phlebitis, or thrombosis of this vessel.

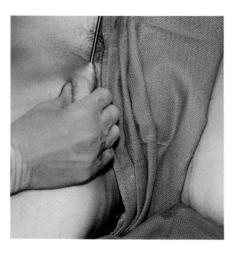 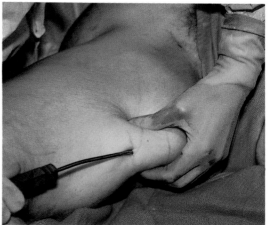

The medial thigh does not have an abundant deep layer of subcutaneous fat. However, a plane beneath the superficial fascia and above the fascia lata contains fat, and the tip of the cannula should be directed here. Reaching the correct plane in the medial thigh is facilitated by pinching the tissues adjacent to the access incision to elevate the incision away from the deep fascia (fascia lata) and stabilize the superficial tissues. The cannula can then be thrust through the incision and underlying superficial fascia to reach the deep plane without penetrating the fascia lata.

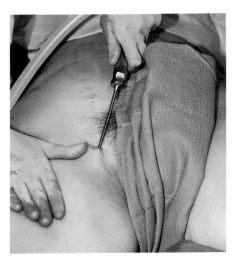 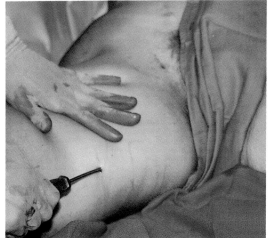

Since the fat layer is relatively thin, it is particularly important to keep the cannula tip at a deep level adjacent to the fascia lata. When the cannula is at the correct level, its movement feels unimpeded, and the skin remains smooth and undisturbed. When the cannula approaches the skin undersurface, the operator will feel a "catching" as the tip is caught by the superficial fascia. Increased dimpling and pulling of the skin will be seen as the cannula drags on the fascial connections to the skin. Once the cannula has been inserted and suctioning starts, pulling up the skin does little to help. I usually keep the hand not directing the cannula to the side so that the skin surface is visible yet the hand can still stabilize the tissues by traction. As with the other areas, about half the predicted volume is taken from each access incision.

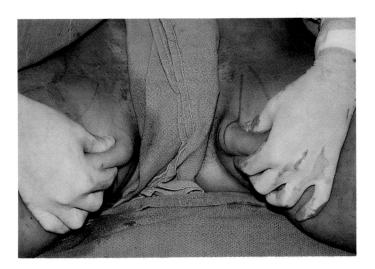

The end point is determined by the usual triad of appearance, pinch, and volume of aspirate. With the patient in the frog-leg position the two sides can be compared simultaneously. Note the difference between the treated area on the patient's right vs. the left side, which has not yet been treated. The end point on the medial thighs may be as little as 1.5 cm of pinch.

Anterior Thighs

The anterior thighs are treated with the patient supine. The fat in this area is diffusely distributed and has little localization. Conservatism is necessary to avoid creating significant contour deformities. As with the medial thighs, the fatty layer is relatively thin, dictating smaller cannulas, generally 2 to 4 mm in diameter. Volumes aspirated are in the 100 to 200 cc range.

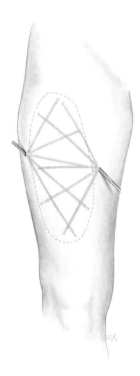

Two access incisions are placed at convenient locations. Access incisions on either side of the main anterior thigh bulk permit removal of fat in a controlled, even manner.

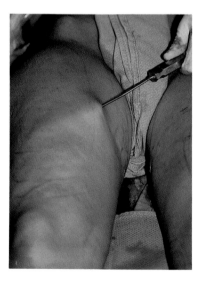
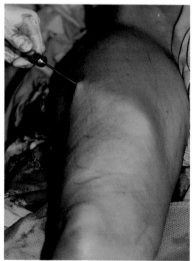

The end point is generally 3 to 4 cm of pinch, but variation is the rule, and, as with most areas, the relative difference between pre- and postoperative pinch test thickness compared to adjacent untreated areas is more important than absolute measured thickness.

Circumferential Treatment of Thighs

Circumferential treatment of the thighs is more than the sum of treatments of the various individual areas since these patients generally have diffuse fullness as well as localized excess. Therefore the entire cutaneous surface of the thigh is treated.

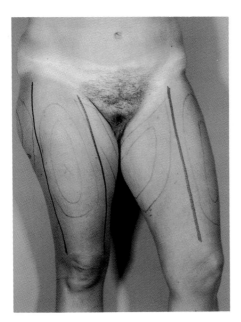 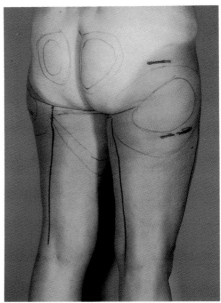

In addition to the usual markings for the anterior, medial, and lateral areas, I add vertical markings running the entire length of the thigh from groin to knee. These additional markings divide each thigh into three segments: anterior, medial, and posterolateral. Access incisions are identical to the ones for the individual areas with additional incisions added as necessary.

Initially, I suction from one segment until I am satisfied with the shape and feel of that area. The volume is recorded, and I proceed to the next segment, also recording the volume. Equal volumes are removed from symmetric segments on the right and left. This method ensures that no area will be left untreated. The quantitative recording of volumes removed from each segment also facilitates achieving a symmetric result.

Buttocks

The buttocks, especially the upper buttocks (steatopygia), are treated by rolling the patient slightly more prone from the lateral decubitus position. Careful sculpting to retain roundness dictates the use of somewhat smaller cannulas than in the lateral thigh. I most frequently use Mercedes Type cannulas ranging in size from 3 to 5 mm in diameter. Volumes suctioned are usually in the 100 to 250 cc range.

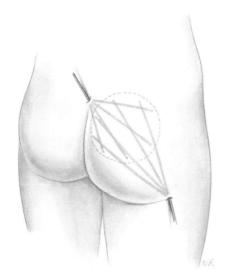

One access incision at the top of the natal crease permits treatment of both buttocks. A second incision for each side is made in the gluteal crease. The subcutaneous fat is abundant, and there is usually a well-defined deep subcutaneous fat layer, permitting the operator to keep the cannula in the deep fat without difficulty.

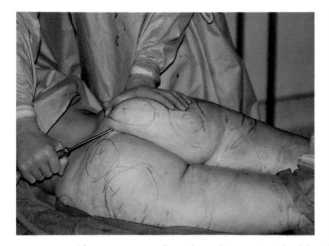 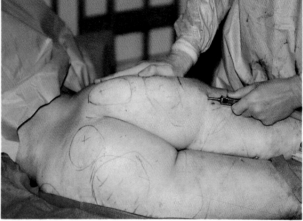

The surgeon normally works on the opposite side of the table from that shown here. This position was taken so as not to block the camera's view of the buttocks.

Half of the predicted volume is removed from the natal crease access incision and half from a secondary incision in the gluteal crease. Continual pinching, feeling for irregularities, and inspection of shape are used to judge the end point. As in the lateral thighs, pinch comparison with an adjacent area is helpful. Comparing left and right volumes also aids in achieving symmetry.

Problems to be avoided are uneven or overaggressive resection producing a flat or hollowed buttock. In particular, resection in the lower medial buttock should be avoided. The goal is overall reduction with selective removal from the most protuberant areas to produce a smaller but still rounded buttock.

Postoperative Care and Recovery

Most patients wear compressive garments immediately after surgery. The surgeon or hospital may stock a supply of these and give them to the patient. If not, the patient should be told in advance what garment to purchase so that she may bring it with her to surgery. I prefer a strong stretch garment with side closures for ease of fitting the unconscious patient (see p. 67). The patient should have two garments so that she can wear one while the other is being washed.

Patients having only one or two areas treated do not require garments. Instead the areas will be covered in the operating room after surgery with a ¼-inch thick layer of self-adhering foam sponge (see p. 67).

Patients are told to allow a week for full resumption of daily activities but are also told that most patients are up and about in 72 hours. Similarly, patients are warned that it takes 3 to 4 weeks for full return to vigorous sports but that most patients resume light conditioning regimens at the end of a week. Patients must also be informed that in the first few hours after surgery pain may be severe enough to require narcotics but that the necessity for any pain medication after the first postoperative day is uncommon. They should also be alerted to the possibility of late momentary pain over the treated area on vigorous motion. This pain, which may occur as late as 2 to 3 months after surgery, is probably due to sudden stretching as the muscle and investing fascia are moved through an increased range of motion.

Results
Thighs

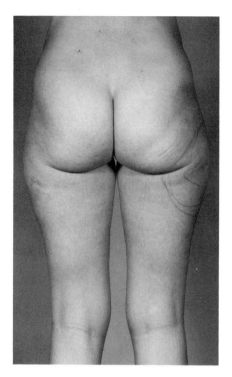 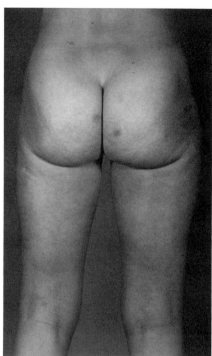

This 30-year-old woman's 120 pounds was distributed on a 5-foot 4-inch frame. Although the subtrochanteric area was of normal size and proportion, she sought fashion's ideal of a perfectly smooth, unbroken curve from iliac crest to below the greater trochanter. Her skin was relatively taut. Removing 350 cc of fat from each lateral thigh and 50 cc from each medial thigh fulfilled her goals. She is shown 2 years after surgery.

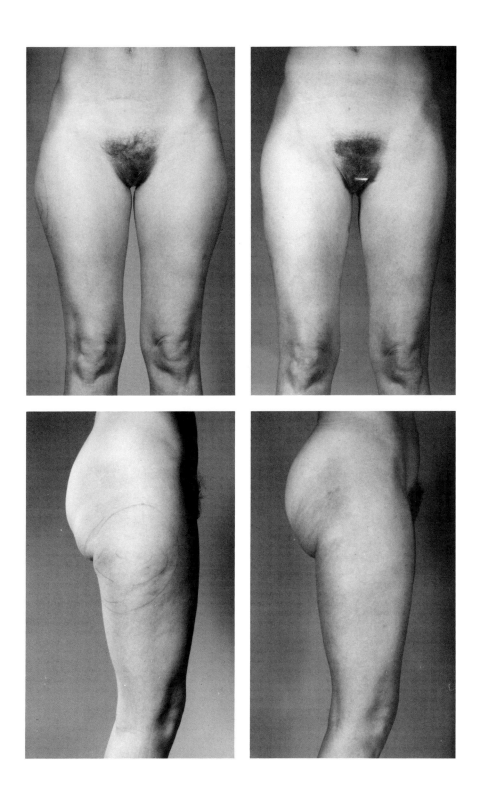

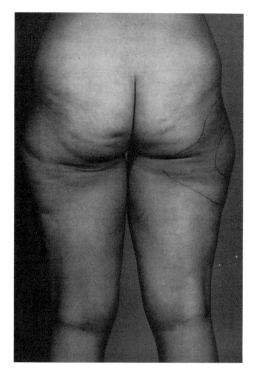 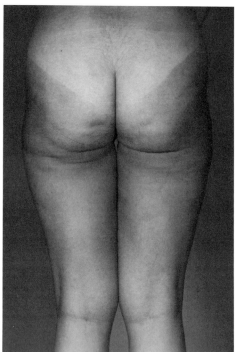

This 22-year-old, 5-foot 6-inch woman had gone from 210 to 145 pounds by dieting; her weight remained stable for more than a year. Her skin was lax and irregular. Lifting up her skin and subcutaneous tissues during the physical examination (see p. 357) eliminated most of her lateral thigh fullness and smoothed her medial thigh skin. I suggested lateral and medial thigh lifts, but she was unwilling to accept the associated scarring and opted for liposuction only. She is shown 1 year after aspiration of 400 cc from each lateral thigh and 75 cc from each medial thigh. I also performed simultaneous mastopexy. Her postoperative result was surprisingly good. Nevertheless, the looseness of her inner thigh skin still troubled her, and she subsequently underwent medial thigh lift. She did not return for photographs after the second procedure.

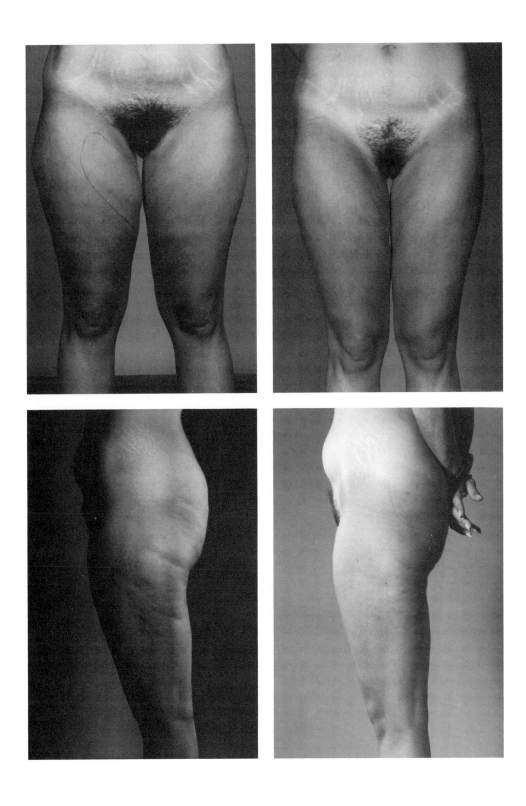

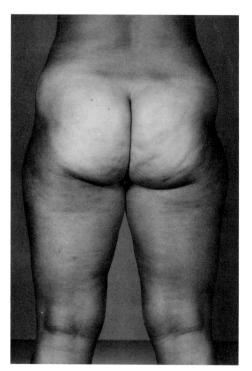 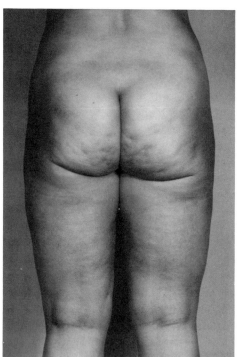

This 45-year-old woman sought overall reduction in contour and skin tightening. At 5 feet 3 inches and 135 pounds she was moderately overweight. Although she had localized fat excess in the lateral and medial thighs, diffuse fullness was also present. The skin was reasonably elastic and tight but rippling was pronounced.

A thigh lift was not indicated since her skin was not loose, and lifting up the skin during physical examination did not change contour. I explained to her that liposuction would reduce her contour but not make her skin perfectly smooth. She is shown 2 years after removal of 500 cc from each lateral thigh, 100 cc from each medial thigh, and 100 cc from each anterior thigh. The hips and medial knees were also treated. She was pleased with her reduced contour and eventually became more accepting of her residual skin irregularities.

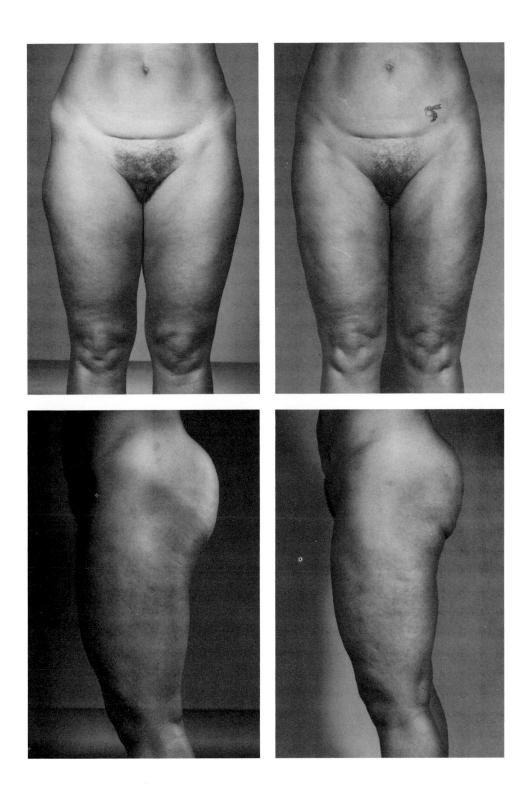

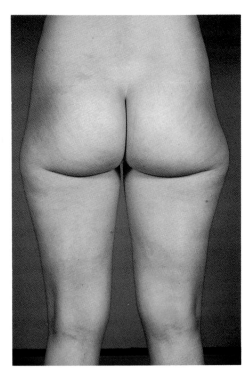 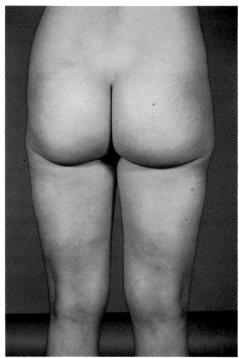

The most notable results are achieved when excess fat is well localized. This rather petite woman (5 feet 3 inches, 108 pounds, dress size 3 on top, 5 on bottom) had small but very sharply localized excess fat. I was able to achieve a striking change in contour by removing less than 150 cc of aspirate from each lateral thigh. Postoperatively, her weight remained constant, and she was able to fit in a size 3 bottom as well as top.

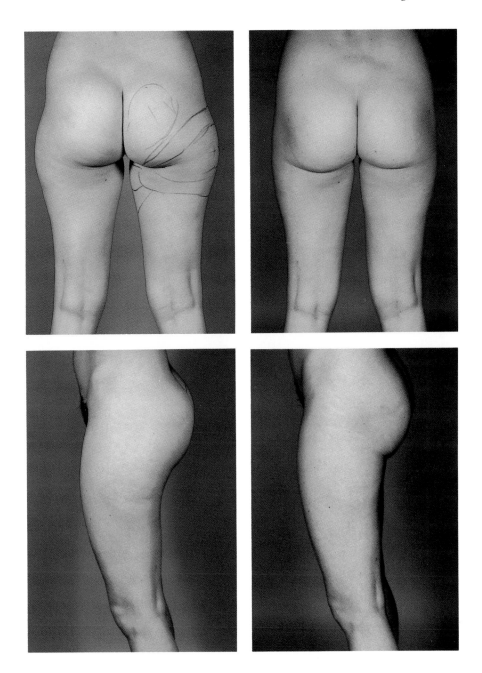

Although this 31-year-old woman carried only 100 pounds on a 5-foot 2-inch frame, she was troubled by disproportionate buttock and thigh fullness. Removal of 75 cc from each upper buttock eliminated her steatopygia. I also removed 75 cc from each inner medial thigh and 350 cc from each outer lateral thigh. Six months later I removed an additional 150 cc from the left lateral thigh and 100 cc from the right lateral thigh. She is shown before any surgery and 6 months after her secondary procedure. This patient illustrates two important points: removal of relatively small amounts of upper buttock fat can reduce contour yet preserve roundness, and treatment of the lateral thighs may require two operations for maximum reduction without depressions or other surface irregularities.

Buttocks

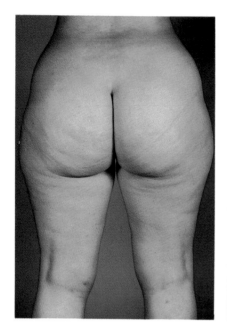 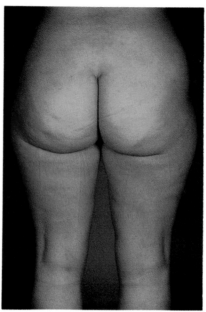 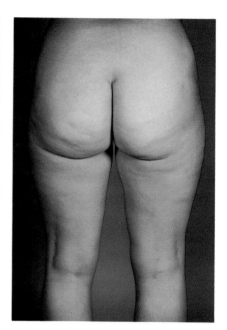

This full-figured woman (5 feet 3 inches, 140 pounds, dress size 12) had pronounced localization of excess fat in her lateral thighs. I removed 425 cc from the left and 475 cc from the right outer thigh in one operation and 350 cc from the left and 450 cc from the right at a second operation 8 months later for a total of 775 cc from the left and 875 cc from the right outer thigh. I also treated her anterior thighs, medial thighs, buttocks, hips, and knees. By the time the last photograph was taken, she had lost 10 pounds by dieting and wore a size 8 dress. The dramatic change in contour could not have been realized with weight loss alone. Localization of fat permitted an outstanding result in the subtrochanteric area.

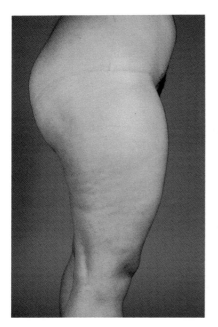 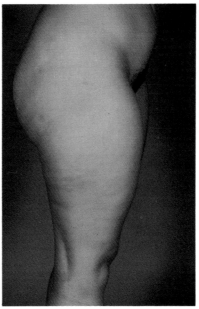 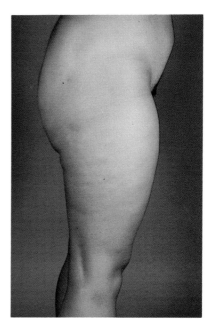

The lateral views show the particularly well–localized upper buttock excess fat. She exhibited true steatopygia, and, for her, the upper buttocks were an area of particular concern. Although the buttocks were quite large, I wanted to be certain that a normal, rounded posterior contour would be retained. Staged removal of 175 cc per side at the first operation and 100 cc per side at the second surgery gave her the smaller appearance she desired. Despite loss of bulk, she exhibits a softly convex buttock slope.

MEDIAL THIGH LIFT

Medial thigh lift with a scar confined to the groin permits lifting and tightening of the upper third of the thigh. It does not address circumferential laxity and massive amounts of loose skin. These conditions require a vertically oriented excision extending variable distances down the medial aspect of the thigh to the knee or below.

Markings

With the patient standing and feet about 12 inches apart, I estimate medial thigh excess by lifting and pinching the medial thigh skin up to the groin crease. The lower limit of the medial thigh excess is marked. The remainder of the marking can be done after the patient is anesthetized. The patient is then placed in the frog-leg position, and I pinch the skin again to be certain that the estimated lower limit of medial thigh skin excess can still be brought to the groin crease. If the previously marked point will not reach to the groin, I adjust it to a more cephalad location.

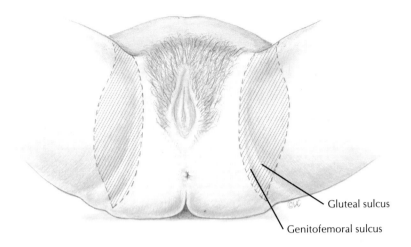

Gluteal sulcus

Genitofemoral sulcus

I then mark the upper limb of a planned elliptical excision in or slightly above the genitofemoral sulcus and groin crease. The central portion of this line should be as cephalad as possible without impinging on the labia. The anterior portion runs parallel and superior to the inguinal crease, ending at the lateralmost extent of the pubic hairline. The direction of this line can be varied to create a narrow or wide escutcheon, the former giving a more youthful appearance,[48] but sometimes requiring a transverse extension to take out extra skin. The posterior portion of the upper limb is marked above the gluteal crease and genitofemoral sulcus. The posterior limb should not be visible on the standing patient viewed from behind.

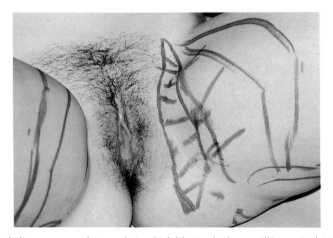

Arrows indicate cephalic movement of tissues during thigh lift. Hatched area will be excised. More distal markings indicate areas to be suctioned.

Once the superior limit of planned excision is marked, lines are drawn from the previously marked inferior point of skin excess to connect to the anterior and posterior limits of the groin crease marking. These markings define the area of planned elliptical excision. The width of the ellipse has ranged up to 7 cm.

Operative Technique

After anesthesia is established, a Foley catheter is inserted, and the patient remains in the frog-leg position.

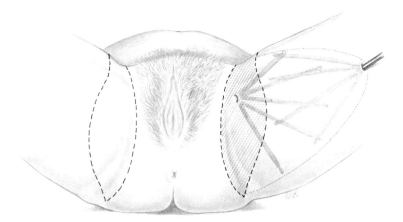

If there is excess fat, the medial thighs are suctioned through access incisions. The superior access incision will be included in the final excision.

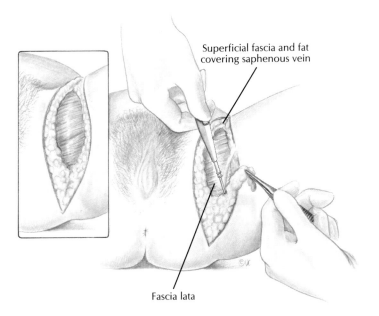

Superficial fascia and fat covering saphenous vein

Fascia lata

After suctioning is completed, the previously marked ellipses are excised. The depth of excision is to the fascia lata in the midportion of the ellipse, exposing the strong fascia along the ischiopubic ramus. The anterior portion of the excision is through the superficial fascia so that the saphenous vein and groin lymphatics are left undisturbed. The posterior portion of the excision also comes through the superficial fascia, the exact depth of excision depending on individual circumstances. No undermining is carried out.

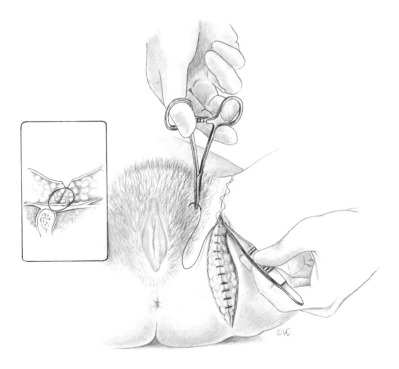

The midportion of the lower flap is advanced in a superior direction, and the deep portion of the superficial fascia is sutured to the deep fascia along the ischiopubic ramus using 2-0 Neurolon interrupted sutures. The fascia along the ischiopubic ramus is composed of elements of the fascia lata as well as the investing fascia of the pelvic diaphragm and a thickened band of Colles' fascia. Joining these fascial elements produces a thick, strong anchor for the lower flap, taking all tension off of the skin closure and preventing any possible pulling on the labia. The remainder of the deep tissue is closed with interrupted chromic sutures to the subdermal level. Dog ears are removed at the anterior or posterior extremities of the excision as necessary.

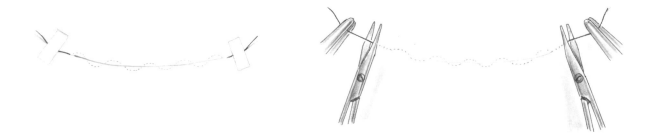

Final skin closure is accomplished with running intracuticular 3-0 poly-dioxanone sutures (PDS), which are not tied beneath the skin but are brought out through the skin and taped to the skin surface. The ends will be cut and allowed to retract beneath the skin a few days after surgery.

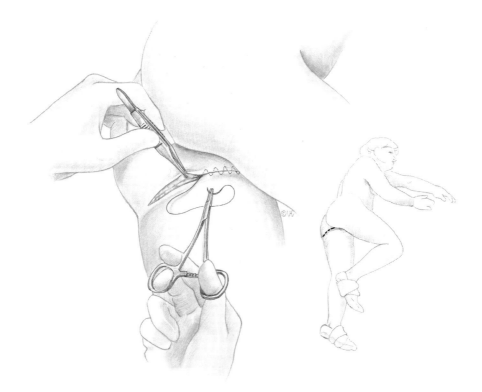

Exposure for the posterior portion of the incision is facilitated by turning the patient to the lateral decubitus position.

Postoperative Care and Recovery

No dressings or drains are needed. The patient ambulates the morning after surgery with the help of two staff members. The bed is locked in position before moving the patient so it cannot roll. The staff assists the patient to lie prone at the edge of her bed. The patient pushes her upper body up to a 45-degree angle off the bed with the help of one assistant. As one assistant helps the patient maintain her upper body off of the bed, the second assists the patient in sliding her feet and legs off the edge of the bed to the floor. Syncopal episodes are not uncommon, and staff should be prepared to return the patient to bed quickly. Once the patient is able to stand, graduated ambulation is begun.

The patient is able to leave the hospital on the first or second postoperative day. Voiding and defecation are performed from a semistanding position until the patient is able to sit comfortably (usually sometime during the second week after surgery). Most patients are able to engage in sedentary activities 2 weeks after surgery, although prolonged sitting may cause discomfort for some time thereafter. At 2 weeks the patient can gradually increase levels of exercise, but vigorous sports are not permitted for 2 months.

Results

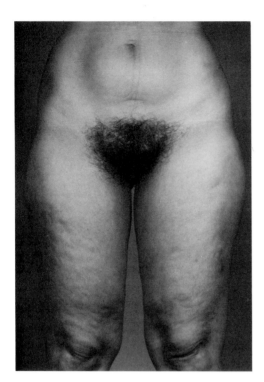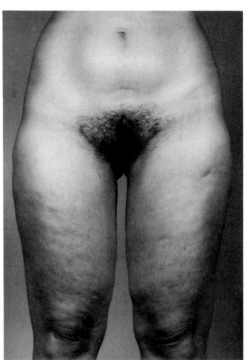

This 40-year-old patient was desperately unhappy over the appearance of her thighs. Her overall bulkiness was superimposed on excessive localized fat in the lateral and medial thighs. Her problem was compounded by her lax, rippled skin. She particularly disliked the loose skin in her upper medial thighs. Although the quality of her skin and overall bulkiness precluded an outstanding result, I believed liposuction of the upper and medial thighs should be supplemented by a medial thigh lift for maximal smoothing and tightening of the medial thigh area. I considered her result mediocre; however, her expressions of gratitude were touching, and she stated 9 months after surgery that she felt confident enough to wear a bathing suit in public for the first time in her adult life.

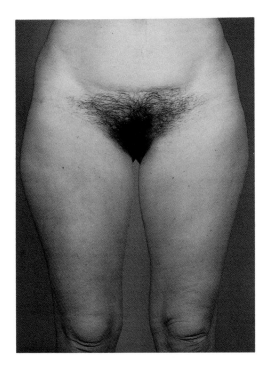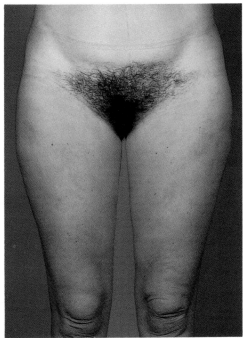

This 49-year-old, 5-foot 6-inch, 130-pound woman requested reduction of fullness in her hips, thighs, and knees. Her medial thigh skin was only moderately lax, but she wished this area to be as tight and smooth as possible and was willing to accept the associated scarring. I combined liposuction of the medial thighs, lateral thighs, hips, and knees with medial thigh lift as described previously. She is shown before and 8 months after surgery. The smooth, straight contour of the upper inner thigh is attributable to medial thigh lift.

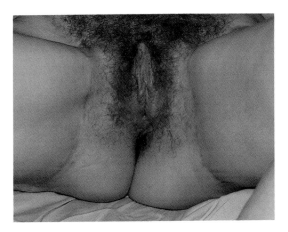

The medial thigh lift scar is inconspicuous with the patient in the standing position, even when she is disrobed. Although these scars may become hyperpigmented in the crural area, they can still remain relatively thin and well positioned, as in this 45-year-old woman 2 years after surgery.

LATERAL THIGH AND BUTTOCK LIFT

Problems with excessive scarring and contour depressions prompted attempts to treat buttock and lateral thigh laxity by other means.[26,29,30] Since liposuction permits removal of subtrochanteric fat, the design for a lateral thigh and buttock lift incision need not allow for direct removal of subtrochanteric fat. Therefore the incision can be removed from the buttock and placed in the flank area.

The transverse flank/thigh/buttock lift[30] has several advantages over a diagonal elliptical excision on the buttock. The excision is made in the hip/flank area, which usually has tissue excess, whereas the Pitanguy excision is performed over the gluteal recess, requiring careful sculpting to retain sufficient tissues to prevent exaggeration of the gluteal depression. The design of the hip/flank excision permits the soft tissues to be pulled up over the buttock without destroying the normal anatomy of the gluteal crease. The transverse excision avoids separation of the dominant inferior and superior gluteal artery blood supply from portions of the lower flap. Finally, the transverse excision is technically easier to execute and produces less postoperative disability than the Pitanguy excision.

If lateral thigh lift is the only procedure to be done, preparations for blood transfusion are usually not necessary, but if simultaneous suction of large volumes is carried out, the patient donates autologous blood well before surgery. Decisions about blood transfusion, of course, have to be individualized for each patient.

Markings

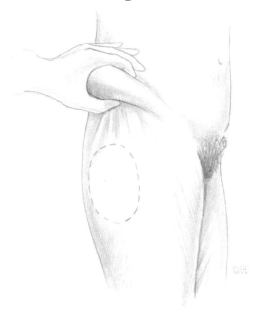

Skin laxity above and below the scar line is estimated by pinching and pulling up the skin. If there is excess fat in the subtrochanteric area, it is marked while the flank tissues are elevated to simulate the final position of the fat excess and to reduce the component of the protuberance due to gravity.

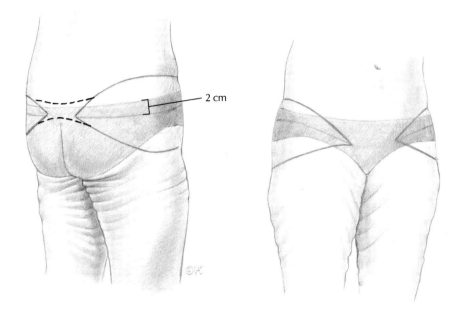

Markings for skin excision are made with the patient standing with feet 12 inches apart. The patient's normal underwear or semi-bikini bathing suit outline is marked first. A transverse line 2 cm below and parallel to the top of the bathing suit line is drawn from near the natal crease to the anterior groin area. This line represents the line of closure of the excision and the eventual scar position. As the line comes anterior, it is directed to a more inferior position to approach the groin.

Long ellipses are drawn from near the posterior midline to the groin. If there is sufficient posterior excess, the left and right excisions can be joined at the posterior midline. The maximal width of excision in my experience has ranged up to 18 cm. Symmetry of planned excisions should be verified by measuring right and left widths of excision and by using a tape measure fixed to the midline and swung from side to side. Underlying skeletal asymmetries will preclude exact soft tissue symmetry, but planned excisions should be as symmetric as possible.

Operative Technique

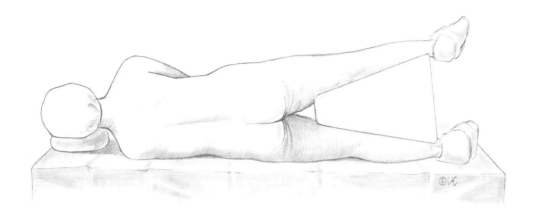

The patient is induced and intubated while lying on a position maintenance device (Vac-Pac; Olympic Medical, Seattle, Wash.) After anesthesia is established, a Foley catheter is inserted, and the patient is turned to the lateral decubitus position. A wedge is placed between the knees and ankles to maintain hip abduction. The Vac-Pac is evacuated of air, creating firm and protective support. Adhesive strapping helps to maintain the lateral decubitus position (strapping and Vac-Pac not shown above).

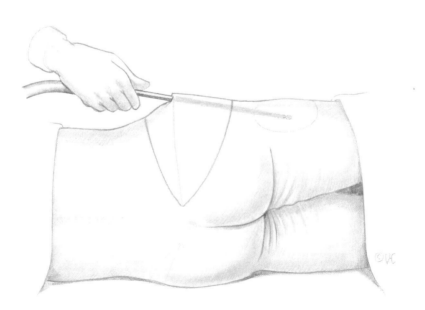

After the patient is prepped and draped, the operative area is infiltrated with dilute lidocaine with epinephrine, and the subtrochanteric area is suctioned to remove excess fat if necessary.

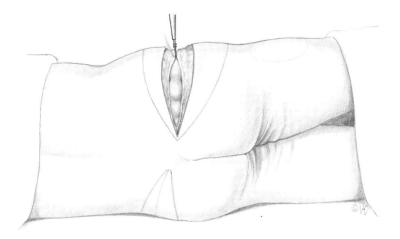

The line of the scar is then incised through the skin and superficial fascia. The deep limit of incision over the buttock and flank is the plane between the superficial and deep fat. The incision is deepened over the anterior abdomen to the external oblique fascia.

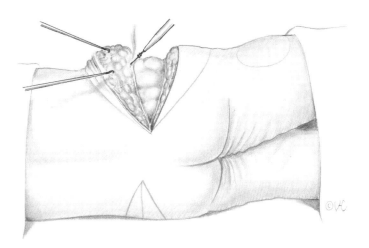

The superior flap is undermined as far as the planned upper limit of excision.

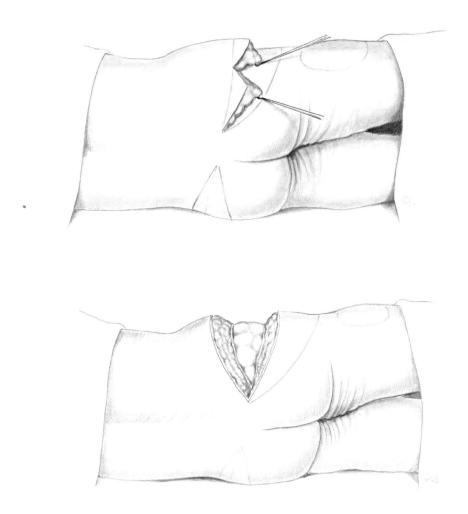

The flap is then grasped and pulled down to ascertain how much can be excised. No more should be removed than can be easily pulled down over the scar line. The flap is divided vertically at its midpoint and temporarily fixed to the lower flap. Excess anterior and posterior segments of the flap are then excised.

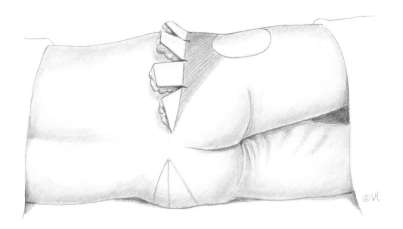

The inferior flap is undermined slightly beyond the planned limit of resection but no further than the superior edge of the subtrochanteric fat deposit. This undermining frees connections to the deep fascia so that thigh and buttock tissues can be advanced. Undermining should be limited to the minimal amount necessary. The presence of postoperative seromas or hematomas is directly related to the extent of undermining. The flap is advanced, divided into segments, and held in place with towel clips while excess skin and subcutaneous tissues are excised.

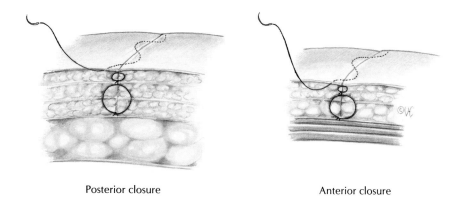

Posterior closure   Anterior closure

Interrupted 0 Mersilene is used to close the superficial fascial system, interrupted 2-0 PDS to close the subdermal level, and running intracuticular 3-0 PDS to close the skin. When closing the anterior portion of the wound, the deep sutures should include the external oblique muscle fascia to fix the closure to the deep fascia. After the first side is completed, the patient is turned to the opposite lateral decubitus position for treatment of the opposite side.

Postoperative Care and Recovery

The postoperative care and recovery are similar to that for medial thigh lift except that the patient has less postoperative discomfort, and recovery is somewhat quicker. Patients may lie in any comfortable position. For the first 3 to 4 days a pillow is kept between the knees to maintain hip abduction. Most patients resume normal activities 10 days after surgery.

Results

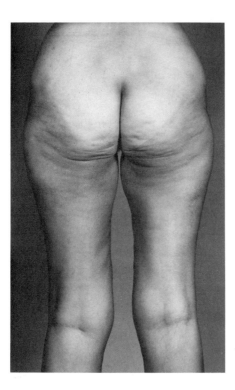 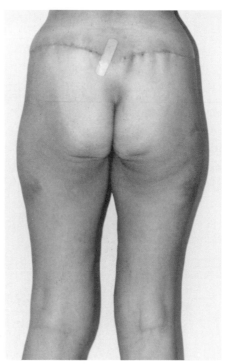

This 44-year-old woman was dissatisfied with the appearance of her thighs and buttocks. The skin and underlying tissues were lax, and the pinch test revealed little subcutaneous fat. Pulling up the hip and flank tissues reduced the lateral thigh bulges. I performed a transverse thigh, buttock, and flank lift, removing an 18 cm ellipse from each side and suctioning 100 cc from each lateral thigh and 50 cc from each medial thigh. The patient is seen before and 3 weeks after surgery. Although some of the smoothing effect of the skin is due to postoperative edema, there will be a long-lasting improvement in shape and surface contour. The patient did not return for further photographs.

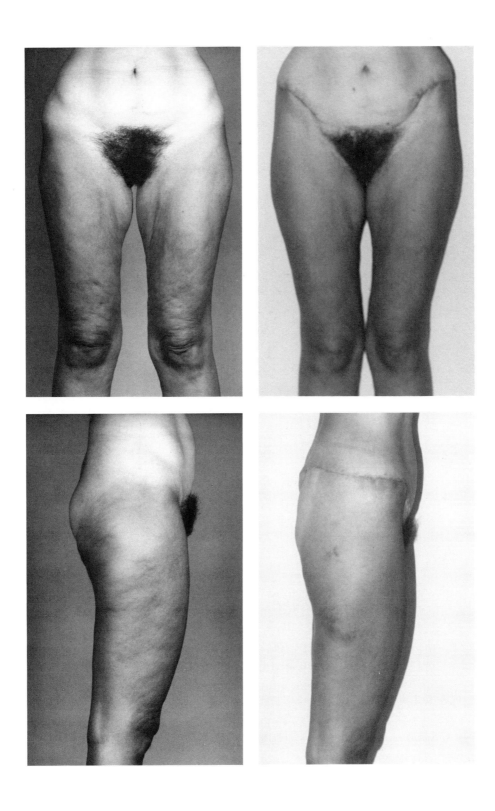

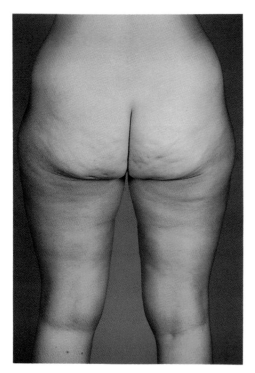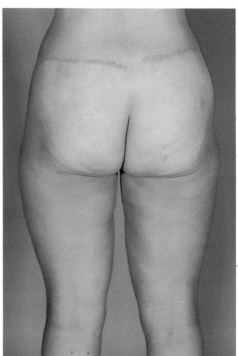

At 5 feet 7 inches this 135-pound woman was thin except for hip and thigh fullness. She was a size 6 on top and a size 10 on bottom. The pinch test documented excess subcutaneous fat of the thighs and hips. In addition, the skin was lax with fine and coarse wrinkling over the thighs, hips, and buttocks.

I suctioned 350 cc from each lateral thigh, 200 cc from each hip, and 100 cc from each anterior thigh and medial thigh. Although liposuction slightly reduced all areas, the patient was displeased because the skin was still rippled and the disproportion was still pronounced. Six months after liposuction I performed a transverse thigh/buttock/flank lift, removing 14 cm ellipses from each side. The patient is shown before liposuction and 7 months after transverse lift. Her skin is smoother, contour is reduced, and top/bottom disproportion is less despite a weight gain of 7 pounds.

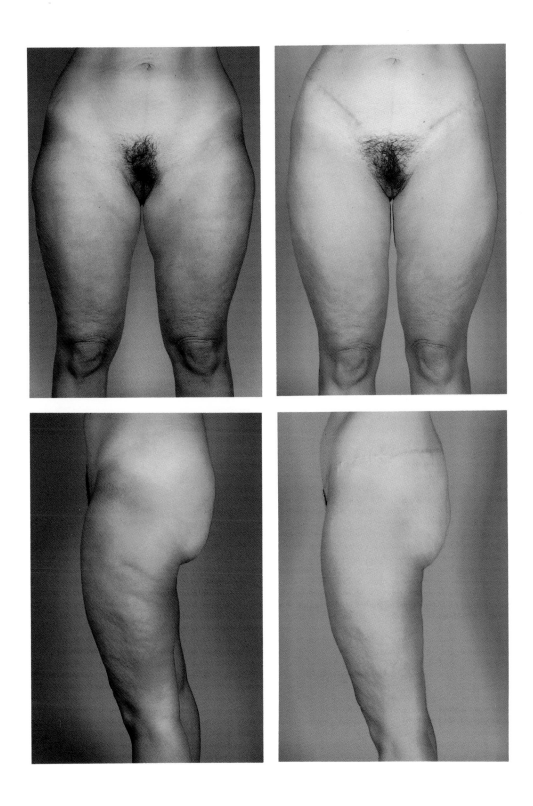

COMBINED MEDIAL AND LATERAL THIGH LIFT

The lateral flank/buttock/thigh lift can be combined with medial thigh lift to produce a near circumferential lift with one continuous scar on each side. When the procedures are combined, autologous blood should be available. The operation begins with the patient in the supine frog-leg position for resection and closure of the medial thigh. The patient is then turned successively into the left and right lateral decubitus positions for completion of flank/buttock/lateral thigh excision and closure.

GLUTEAL CREASE EXCISION

Minor degrees of buttock ptosis may be corrected with simple elliptical skin excision on the axis of the gluteal crease. A modest amount of fat may also be removed. Ideally, the scar is confined to the gluteal crease, but most patients require lateral extension of the scar beyond the actual crease. The operation may be done under local anesthesia as an outpatient. Aside from inability to sit for 1 to 2 weeks, disability is less than for medial or lateral thigh lifts.

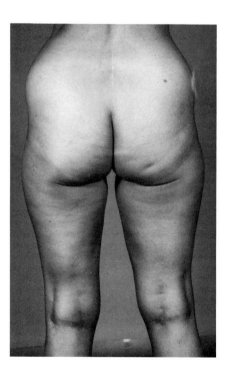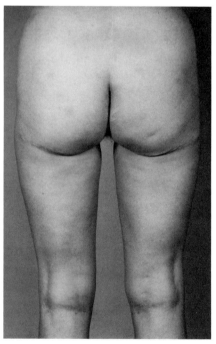

This 40-year-old woman was 128 pounds and 5 feet 6 inches tall. She complained of excessive fullness of her thighs and what she described as "a sagging rear end." I performed liposuction of the hips, lateral thighs, medial thighs, and medial knees and excised a 5 cm wide wedge of skin and subcutaneous tissue from each buttock crease. She is shown before and 2 years after surgery. The patient was satisfied with her overall reduction in contour but was particularly pleased with the subtle change in shape at the buttock–upper thigh junction.

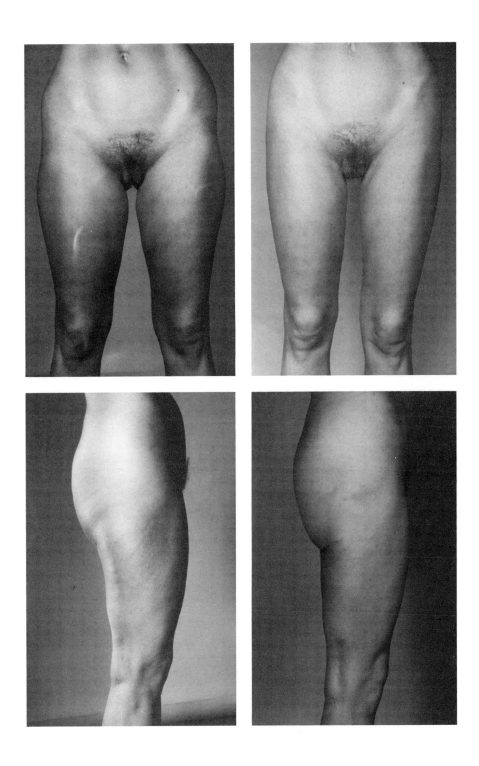

COMPLICATIONS AND UNAESTHETIC RESULTS
Liposuction

Major medical complications are discussed on pp. 464-466. Unaesthetic results such as surface irregularities, depressions, asymmetries, and hyperpigmentation occur in the thighs and buttocks, as in other areas. These problems are minimized by adhering to the basic precepts of liposuction technique outlined in Chapter 3: use of small cannulas for small volumes of fat, keeping the cannulas in the deep central fat, cross-tunneling, and conservatism in resection. Certain problems peculiar to the thighs and buttocks can be avoided by attention to the unique features and requirements of this anatomic area.

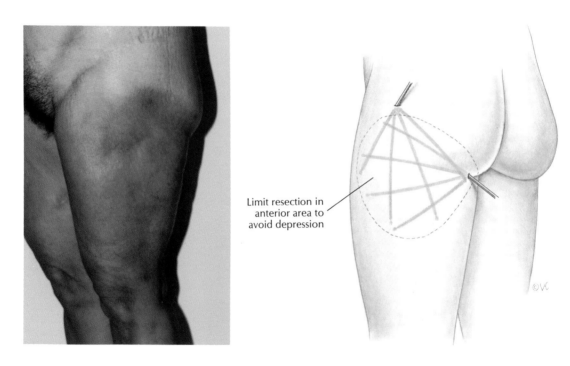

Limit resection in anterior area to avoid depression

In the lateral thigh the deep subtrochanteric fat deposit ends abruptly at the iliotibial tract. Thus depressions and overresections are most common on the anterolateral aspect of the thigh just beyond the iliotibial tract. This problem is avoided by limiting resection in the anterior area.

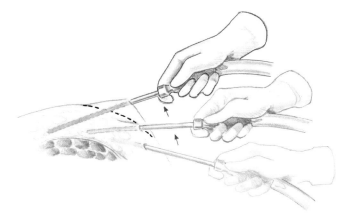

It is also important to maintain the tip of the cannula in the deep fat along the convexity of the lateral thigh by elevating the hand as the cannula is thrust forward.

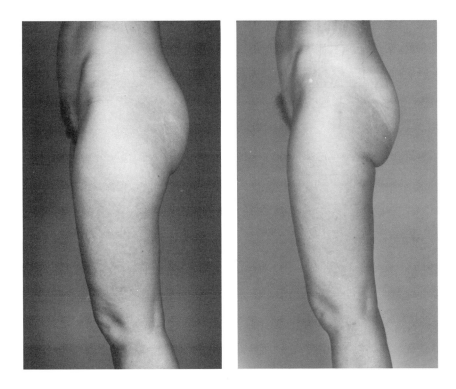

Overresection in the lower lateral buttock and posterolateral thigh adjacent to the buttock crease can exaggerate buttock ptosis and produce an unpleasant appearance from the side when the buttock hangs over the thigh. Aggressive attempts to create or lengthen a gluteal crease will have the same effect. This can be avoided by preoperative marking of this area to limit the volume of resection.

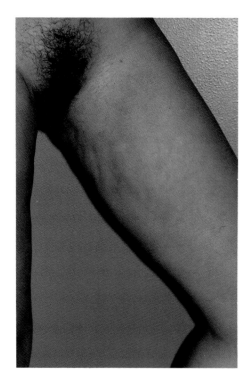 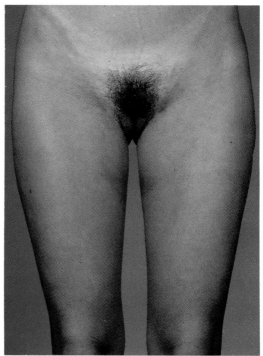

The medial thighs are more subject to postoperative surface irregularities and hyperpigmentation because of the relatively small amount of fat in this area. The key to avoiding these problems is gentleness in handling of tissues and conservatism in resection. Surface depressions such as those on the left may sometimes be ameliorated by using ultra-fine cannulas for removal of small amounts of fat from the raised areas. The problem is never entirely eliminated, however, and is best avoided rather than treated. Although topical hydroquinones are used to treat hyperpigmentation, efficacy is limited. The darkness tends to fade with time, but some residual pigmentation may persist. In the patient on the right the pigmentation was present for 18 months after surgery. She did not return for further follow-up, and I assume the discoloration is permanent.

The upper buttocks are subject to unattractive flattening if excessive volume is removed. Removal of fat in this area should be conservative and incremental to maintain a normal, rounded appearance. Aspiration of small amounts of fat can produce a satisfactory contour reduction.

Thigh and Buttock Lift
Scars

The most frequent complication following thigh and buttock lift involves scars. The lateral scars will predictably redden and hypertrophy in the first few months after surgery. By about 6 to 8 months this phase has peaked and there is gradual deflorescence. Persistent hyperemia or florid hypertrophy may be associated with overresection and excessive tension, but such scars sometimes have no known antecedents.

If incisions are placed too low, the scars will be visible on the medial thigh below underwear or shorts. The medial scars can also spread and descend spontaneously, eventually becoming visible. Placing the scars above the genitofemoral crease and anchoring the lower flap to the investing fascia over the ischiopubic ramus makes descent of the scars less likely but is no guarantee of stability. Groin scars have a tendency to become hyperpigmented.

Scars may be asymmetric because of inaccurate preoperative measurements or because of improper preoperative marking. Unequal surgical excisions result. Checking and rechecking the markings for symmetry prior to starting surgery is an important step in prevention. Equal segments of tissue should be removed from right and left sides.

Correction of scars may require revisional surgery, which should not be done until at least a year after the original operation. The patient's postoperative complaints about cicatricial problems are frequently inversely related to the amount of time the surgeon took in the preoperative consultation to explain the permanent nature and unpredictability of scarring.

Hematomas and Seromas

Early expanding hematomas are infrequent, but if there has been undermining of flaps, collections of bloody fluid or serum beneath the flap are common in the first 2 weeks. The more extensive the undermining, the more likely repeat aspirations will be necessary. The fluid reaccumulations gradually get smaller with weekly or more frequent aspirations and eventually resorb completely. Using drains does not prevent seromas or hematomas.

Wound Problems

Medial thigh wound dehiscence in the early postoperative period is usually secondary to the patient sitting too soon or straining at stool. Repair must be done under general anesthesia. Both patients and nursing staff must be instructed repeatedly that medial thigh lift patients not sit until 1 week after surgery.

Wound infections are rare and are usually associated with poor preoperative hygiene in the medial thigh area or unrecognized hematoma. Treatment consists of rest and appropriate antibiotic therapy after culture. If there is an abscess or suspected abscess, the wound should be opened to facilitate drainage. The wound can be closed at a later date when the infection has subsided or can be permitted to heal by secondary intention.

Small necrotic areas at the edge of the wound usually require no treatment. They will separate spontaneously as the underlying area epithelializes. Major necrosis is rare in the absence of infection or unrecognized hematoma. Conservative debridement will usually permit complete healing by secondary intention, and it is best to avoid a skin graft if at all possible.

Vulvar Problems

Too much tension on the medial thigh lift closure can result in vulvar eversion, drying, and pain. If the problem is temporary, it can be treated with estrogen-containing lubricating ointments. If the problem is severe and permanent, reoperation to release the tight scar with Z-plasty[20] or a skin graft is required. It is best prevented by avoiding excess tension on the medial closure and by anchoring the inferior flap to the deep fascia.

Contour Deformities

Uneven resection, overresection, and underresection can all cause contour deformity and asymmetry. Careful preoperative marking is the best prevention. If the deformity is an error relating to underresection, it may be correctable by a second operation. If too much has been resected, the error may not be retrievable.

Lymphocele

Lymphocele has been reported following thigh lift.[49] It is prevented by preserving the deep fat over the saphenous vein and femoral triangle.

Neuropathy

Traction injuries to the brachial plexus or upper extremity peripheral nerve compression can cause transient or permanent neuropathies. Preventing hyperabduction at the shoulder and using protective padding and positioning will minimize the occurrence of these injuries.

================================ REFERENCES ================================

1. Posse RP. Cirurgia esthetica. Cited in Pitanguy I. Aesthetic plastic surgery of the upper and lower limbs. Aesthetic Plast Surg 4:363–372, 1980.
2. Lewis JR. The thigh lift. J Int Coll Surg 27:330–334, 1957.
3. Lewis JR. Correction of ptosis of the thighs: The thigh lift. Plast Reconstr Surg 37:494–498, 1966.
4. Lewis JR. Atlas of Aesthetic Plastic Surgery. Boston: Little, Brown, 1973, pp 271–276.
5. Farina R, Baroudi R, Golcman B, de Castro O. Lipodistrofia pelvi-crural tipo calcas de montaria. O Hospital 57:135–140, 1960.
6. Farina R, Baroudi R, Golcman B, de Castro O. Riding-trousers like type of pelvi-crural lipodystrophy (trochanteric lipomatosis). Br J Plast Surg 13:174–178, 1960.
7. Pitanguy I. "Lipodistrofia trocanteriana." Rev Bras Chir 7:69–74, 1964.
8. Pitanguy I. Trochanteric lipodystrophy. Plast Reconstr Surg 34:280–286, 1964.
9. Pitanguy I. Technique for trunk and thigh reductions. In Hueston J, ed. Transactions of the Fifth International Congress of Plastic Surgeons. Melbourne: Butterworths, 1971, pp 1204–1210.
10. Pitanguy I. Aesthetic plastic surgery of the upper and lower limbs. Aesthetic Plast Surg 4:363–372, 1980.
11. Pitanguy I. Aesthetic Plastic Surgery of Head and Body. New York: Springer-Verlag, 1981, pp 129–153.
12. Hoffman S, Simon BE. Experiences with the Pitanguy method of correction of trochanteric lipodystrophy. Plast Reconstr Surg 55:551–558, 1975.
13. Delerm A, Cirotteau Y. Plastie cruro-femoro-fessière ou circum fessière. Ann Chir Plast 18:31–36, 1973.
14. Agris J. Use of dermal-fat suspension flaps for thigh and buttock lifts. Plast Reconstr Surg 59:817–822, 1977.
15. Guerrerosantos J. Secondary thigh-buttock lift. In Ely JF, ed. Transactions of the Seventh International Congress of Plastic and Reconstructive Surgery. São Paulo: Cartgraf, 1979, pp 650–651.
16. Teimourian B, Adham MN. Anterior periosteal dermal suspension with suction curettage for lateral thigh lipectomy. Aesthetic Plast Surg 6:207–209, 1982.
17. Grazer FM, Klingbeil JR. Body image: A surgical perspective. St. Louis: CV Mosby, 1980, pp 238–356.
18. Shaer WD. Gluteal and thigh reduction: Reclassification, critical review, and improved technique for primary correction. Aesthetic Plast Surg 8:165–172, 1984.
19. Aston SJ. Buttocks and thighs. In Rees TD, ed. Aesthetic Plastic Surgery. Philadelphia: WB Saunders, 1980, pp 1039–1066.
20. Regnault P, Daniel R. Aesthetic Plastic Surgery: Principles and Techniques. Boston: Little, Brown, 1984, pp 655–678.
21. Planas J. The "crural meloplasty" for lifting of the thighs. Clin Plast Surg 2:495–503, 1975.
22. Schultz RC, Feinberg LA. Medial thigh lift. Ann Plast Surg 2:404–410, 1979.
23. Vilain R, Dardour JC, Bzowski A. Use of dermal-fat flaps in treating abdominal scars in abdominoplasty and in subtrochanteric lipectomy. Plast Reconstr Surg 60:876–881, 1977.
24. Lockwood TE. Fascial anchoring technique in medial thigh lifts. Plast Reconstr Surg 82:299–304, 1988.
25. Hodgkinson DJ. Medial thighplasty, prevention of scar migration, and labial flattening. Aesthetic Plast Surg 13:111–114, 1989.

26. Baroudi R. Body contour surgery. Clin Plast Surg 16:263–277, 1989.

27. Baroudi R. Flankplasty. In Hetter GP, ed. Lipoplasty: The Theory and Practice of Blunt Suction Lipectomy. Boston: Little, Brown, 1990, pp 399–416.

28. Baroudi R, Moraes M. Philosophy, technical principles, selection, and indication in body contouring surgery. Aesthetic Plast Surg 15:1–18, 1991.

29. Lockwood TE. Superficial fascial system (SFS) of the trunk and extremities: A new concept. Plast Reconstr Surg 87:1009–1018, 1991.

30. Lockwood TE. Transverse flank, thigh, buttock lift with superficial fascial suspension. Plast Reconstr Surg 87:1019–1027, 1991.

31. Schrudde J. Lipektomie und Lipexehaerese im Bereich der unteren Extremitäten. Langenbecks Arch Chir 345:127–131, 1977.

32. Schrudde J. Lipexeresis as a means of eliminating local adiposity. Aesthetic Plast Surg 4:215–226, 1980.

33. Fischer A, Fischer GM. Revised techniques for cellulitis fat. Reduction in riding britches deformity. Bull Int Cosmetic Surg, vol 2, No. 4, 1977. Cited in Illouz Y-G. The origin of lipoplasty. In Hetter GP, ed. Lipoplasty: The Theory and Practice of Blunt Suction Lipectomy, 2nd ed. Boston: Little, Brown, 1990.

34. Kesselring UK, Meyer R. A suction curette for removal of excessive local deposits of subcutaneous fat [letter]. Plast Reconstr Surg 62:305, 1978.

35. Illouz Y-G. Une nouvelle technique pour les lipodystrophies localisées. Rev Chir Esth Franc 6:3, 1980.

36. Illouz, Y-G. Réflexions après 4 ans et demi d'expérience et 800 cas de ma technique de lipolyse. Rev Chir Esth Franc 6:24, 1981.

37. Illouz Y-G. Body contouring by lipolysis: A 5-year experience with over 3000 cases. Plast Reconstr Surg 72:591–597, 1983.

38. Teimourian B, Fisher JB. Suction curettage to remove excess fat for body contouring. Plast Reconstr Surg 68:50–58, 1981.

39. Fournier PF, Otteni FM. Lipodissection in body sculpturing: The dry procedure. Plast Reconstr Surg 72:598–609, 1983.

40. Kesselring UK. Regional fat aspiration for body contouring. Plast Reconstr Surg 72:610–619, 1983.

41. Courtiss, EH. Suction lipectomy: A retrospective analysis of 100 patients. Plast Reconstr Surg 73:780–794, 1984.

42. Teimourian B. Suction Lipectomy and Body Sculpturing. St. Louis: CV Mosby, 1987, pp 339–494.

43. Illouz Y-G, Dardour JC. Combined procedures: The thighs and buttocks. In Illouz Y-G, de Villers YT. Body Sculpturing by Lipoplasty. New York: Churchill Livingstone, 1989, pp 340–352.

44. Illouz Y-G, de Villers YT. Body Sculpturing by Lipoplasty. New York: Churchill Livingstone, 1989, pp 29–38.

45. Manchot C. The Cutaneous Arteries of the Human Body. Leipzig: FCW Vogel, 1889. (First English edition translated by Morain WD, Ristic J. New York: Springer-Verlag, 1983.)

46. Salmon M. Arteries of the Skin. Paris: Masson & Cie, 1936. (First English edition edited by Taylor GI, Tempest MN. Translated by Hueston P, Cuthbertson A, Tempest MN. New York: Churchill Livingstone, 1988.)

47. Lewis CM. Dissatisfaction among women with "thunder thighs" undergoing closed aspirative lipoplasty. Aesthetic Plast Surg 11:187–191, 1987.

48. Loeb R. Narrowing of the mons pubis during thigh lifts. Ann Plast Surg 2:290–297, 1979.

49. Leitner DW, Sherwood RC. Inguinal lymphocele as a complication of thighplasty. Plast Reconstr Surg 72:878–881, 1983.

────────── SUGGESTED READINGS ──────────

Baroudi R. Thigh-lift and buttock-lift. In Courtiss EH, ed. Aesthetic Surgery: Trouble, How to Avoid It and How to Treat It. St. Louis: CV Mosby, 1978, pp 223-231.

Baroudi R, Carvalho CGS. Lifting of the inner third of the thigh; an analysis of immediate and mediate results. Cir Plast Iber Lat Am 7:275, 1981. (Abstracted in Plast Reconstr Surg 74:160, 1984.)

Clarkson P. Lipodystrophies. Plast Reconstr Surg 37:499-503, 1966.

Ducourtioux J-L. Technique et indications des dermolipectomies crurales. Ann Chir Plast 17:204-211, 1972.

Franco T. Aesthetic surgery of the upper and lower limbs. Aesthetic Plast Surg 4:245-256, 1980.

Guerrerosantos J. Secondary hip-buttock-thigh plasty. Clin Plast Surg 11:491-503, 1984.

Ichida M, Kamiishi H, Shioya N. Aesthetic surgery of the trunk and extremities in the Japanese. Ann Plast Surg 5:31-39, 1980.

Lewis JR. Surgery of the hips, buttocks, and thighs. In Goldwyn RM, ed. Long-Term Results in Plastic and Reconstructive Surgery. Boston: Little, Brown, 1980, pp 774-789.

Lockwood TE. Medial thighplasty. In Hetter GP, ed. Lipoplasty: The Theory and Practice of Blunt Suction Lipectomy. Boston: Little, Brown, 1990, pp 375-383.

Muhlbauer W. Radical abdominoplasty including body shaping: Representative cases. Aesthetic Plast Surg 13:105-110, 1989.

Regnault P, Baroudi R, Carvalho C. Correction of lower limb lipodystrophy. Aesthetic Plast Surg 3:233-249, 1979.

Regnault P, Daniel R. Secondary thigh, buttock deformities after classical techniques. Clin Plast Surg 11:505-516, 1984.

Rosenthal SG. Trochanteric lipectomy: A new approach. Plast Reconstr Surg 69:356-358, 1982.

Vilain R. Surgical correction of steatomeries. Clin Plast Surg 2:467-470, 1975.

Vilain R, Dardour JC. Aesthetic surgery of the medial thigh. Ann Plast Surg 3:176-183, 1986.

Vogt PA. Lateral thighplasty. In Hetter GP, ed. Lipoplasty: The Theory and Practice of Blunt Suction Lipectomy. Boston: Little, Brown, 1990, pp 383-397.

Zook EG. The massive weight loss patient. Clin Plast Surg 2:457-466, 1975.

Chapter 12

KNEES, CALVES, AND ANKLES

The knee-calf-ankle complex constitutes a highly visible and important aesthetic unit. While hips and thighs can be camouflaged by ample dresses and skirts, only slacks can hide the legs. Consequently, successful treatment of this area gives the patient an emotional and social gain that exceeds the sometimes subtle visual changes.

HISTORY

As early as the 1920s, surgeons attempted to reduce bulky legs by removing fat with curettes. The procedure fell into disrepute following an operation in which Dujarrier, a French physician, injured a major vessel while using a curette to remove fat from the legs of a dancer. The operation eventuated in amputation.[1]

Fat curetting of calves and ankles was not revived until 1964 when Schrudde of Cologne operated on his first patient. Although some of Schrudde's results were excellent, he reported skin necrosis in 4 of 15 patients, two of whom required skin grafts. To avoid necrosis he recommended treating the lower leg in two stages, medial and lateral.[2,3] Pfulg[4] also reported a case of skin necrosis at the ankle.

Understandably, early practitioners of liposuction were reluctant to treat the leg. Kesselring[5] confined his treatment exclusively to the trochanteric region, whereas Courtiss[6] treated the knees but not distal areas. Other surgeons treated calves and ankles but not as frequently as knees.[7-11]

HISTORICAL REVIEW OF LIPOSUCTION PROCEDURES ON CALVES AND ANKLES VS. KNEES FROM 1981 TO 1988			
Authors	No. of Operations or Patients	% Involving Calves and Ankles	% Involving Knees
Teimourian and Fisher, 1981[7]	54	2	16
Illouz, 1983[8]	1326	12	39
Pitman and Teimourian, 1985[9]	1249	2	12
Ersek et al., 1986[10]	101	3	22
Hetter, 1988[11]	1078	4	34

By 1987 treatment of calves and ankles was becoming more frequent,[12] but not until 1989 and 1990 did surgeons report large numbers of cases.[13-16] Most expressed faint enthusiasm for liposuction of the calves and ankles, cautioning against "limited success"[14] and "not always dramatic" results.[15] In a survey of his Japanese patient population, Wanatabe[17] reported a low level of satisfaction with treatment of the calves and ankles as compared to other areas.

Notwithstanding others' limited enthusiasm for treating calves and ankles, my personal experience has been gratifying. I find results in this area compare favorably to those elsewhere and can be outstanding. Patient satisfaction is high.

AESTHETIC AND ANATOMIC CONSIDERATIONS

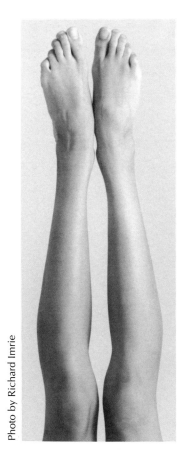

Photo by Richard Imrie

Attractive legs are characterized by a gradual tapering from strong thighs to delicate ankles. Although slight fullness at the knees is a normal anatomic feature, most women regard their knees as unattractive and wish to eliminate any bulge in this area. Thin calves and elegant ankles are universally desired.

Fullness at the knees reflects the underlying skeletal bulging of the femoral condyles, the patella, and the tibial plateau. The quadriceps femoris adds bulk above the patella, and the gracilis, sartorius, and hamstrings fill out the medial contour. A well-localized subcutaneous fat collection overlies the medial muscle group, softening contour but also adding bulk.

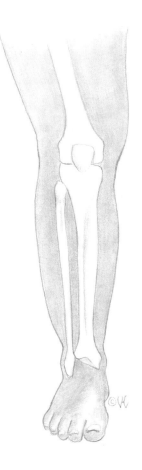

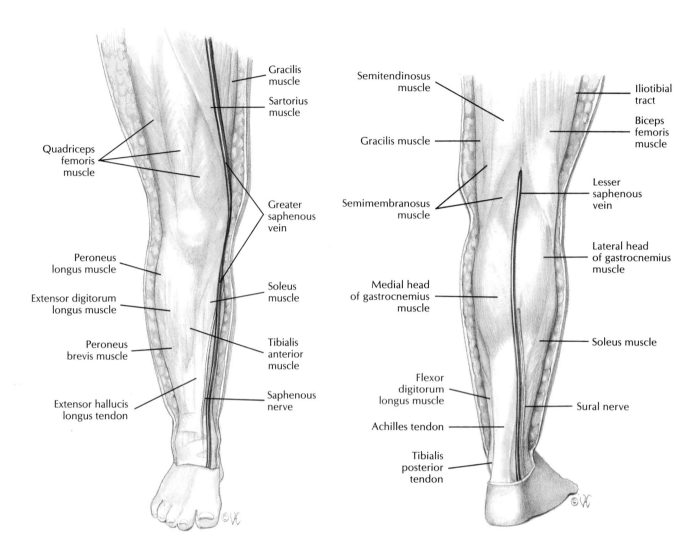

The lower extremity narrows at the distal border of the medial knee fat collection, which is also the locus of insertion of the thigh musculature. The silhouette fills out again in midcalf to accommodate the medial and lateral heads of the gastrocnemius. The soleus adds bulk, particularly in the distal half of the leg. The leg narrows at the ankle as the soleus and gastrocnemius insert into the Achilles tendon. A wide distal soleus or excessive fullness of the peroneus brevis and flexor digitorum longus can obliterate the graceful taper from calf to ankle.

All major arteries and nerves run beneath the investing fascia. The greater and lesser saphenous veins, accompanied, respectively, by the saphenous and sural nerves, run along the investing fascia in the superficial fat.

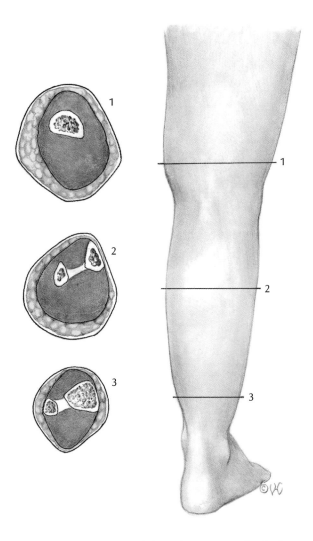

Although basic contour is dictated by the musculoskeleton, the subcutaneous fat plays an important additional role in defining overall shape. The top cross section shows a well-defined and localized fat collection at the medial knee. The center cross section illustrates the more diffuse and circumferential distribution of fat in the midleg. Note the relative paucity of fat over the anterior tibia. At this level the fat also softens the abrupt contour change caused by the gastrocnemius muscle belly entering its tendon of insertion. The bottom cross section shows that fat distribution at the ankle remains diffuse and circumferential, but localized excess can create lateral and medial fullness.

PATIENT TYPES AND TREATMENT OPTIONS

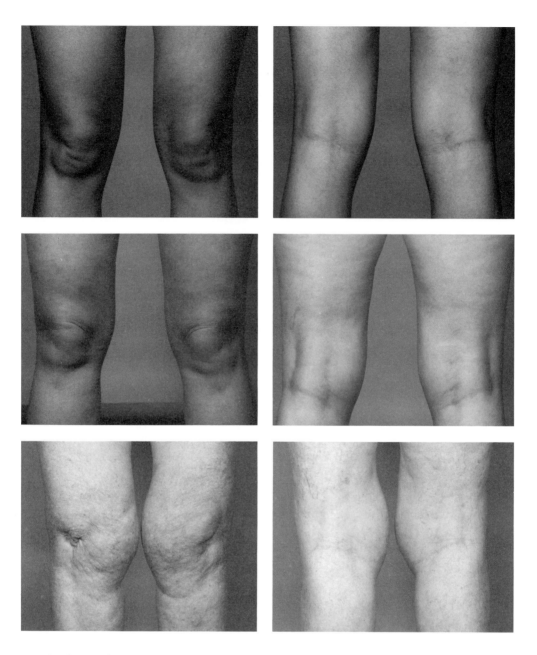

At the knee the most common correctable deformity is bulging in the area of the medial femoral condyle. A variety of patients request correction of medial knee bulges. Even a small and natural-looking fullness (top) may be unwanted. Disproportionate bulkiness is never desirable (center and bottom). Treatment by liposuction is straightforward and effective.

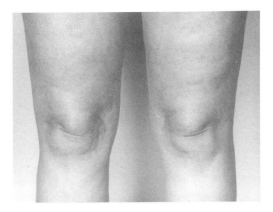

Patients may also complain of anterior fullness near the patella, but this problem is usually accompanied by skin laxity and is not easily remedied with liposuction.

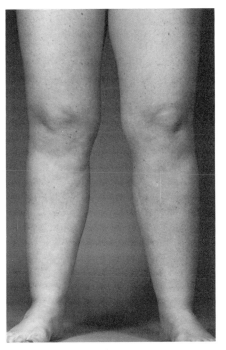 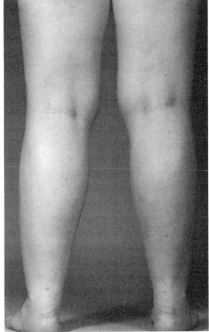

The entire leg may be bulky below the knee. This fullness may be caused by excessive fat and/or musculoskeletal hypertrophy. The pinch test determines to what degree subcutaneous fat is involved. When excess fat contributes to the thickness, it can be treated by circumferential liposuction.

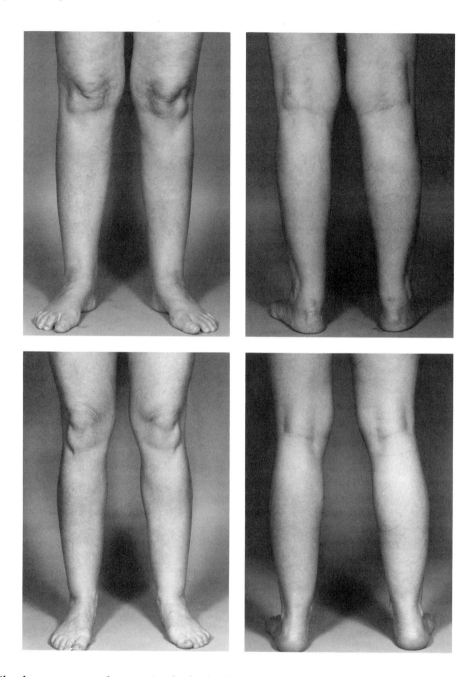

The leg may not be particularly bulky, but it may lack pleasing shape and proportion as a result of localized excess fat. The surplus fat may occur either in the calves or ankles but is most commonly seen on either side of the Achilles tendon. Side-to-side fullness at the ankle can also be muscular in origin. Again, the pinch test will differentiate the two.

Liposuction of the localized areas of excess fat can dramatically improve contour. Fullness in the anteroposterior dimension, however, is always determined by the distance between the anterior tibia and posterior surface of the Achilles tendon. Since there is sparse fat over both of these structures, suction does not change the anteroposterior dimension at the ankle.

PATIENT EVALUATION AND COUNSELING
Physical Examination

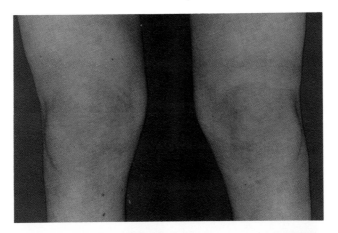

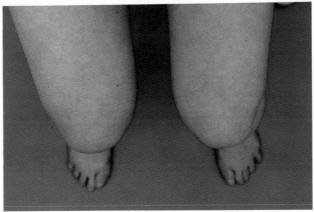

Patients are examined while standing (top), a position in which the medial knee fat bulge is more obvious. When the knee is flexed to 90 degrees, as when sitting (bottom), most small and moderate fat protrusions disappear, and the inner knee appears to have a rather straight outline. If the patient is unable to visualize the planned reduction in medial knee bulk, it is helpful to have her sit with knees flexed to 90 degrees so that the future improvement becomes evident.

Of course, if the surgeon removes enough fat so that the inner contour is completely straight when the knee is extended, there will be a pronounced concavity when the patient sits, a point worth remembering during surgery to prevent overresection.

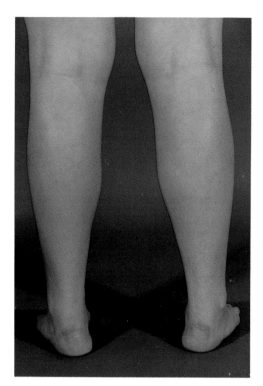 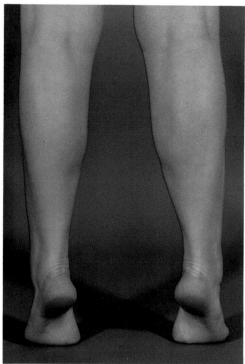

The calves and ankles are examined with the patient standing flat-footed and then again with the patient on her toes to delineate the mass and location of the medial and lateral heads of the gastrocnemius. The distal end of the gastrocnemius is an important landmark in determining leg contour and will influence how the surgeon sculpts the fat to obtain the most pleasing shape.

The presence of varicosities, pitting edema, and any asymmetries are noted. Mild varicosities do not preclude liposuction, and these patients are not subject to increased postoperative morbidity.

It is not uncommon for one leg to be larger than the other. Although this is usually a benign condition, the patient should be questioned for a past history of phlebitis or deep vein thrombosis. Complaints of severe swelling, either intermittent or continuous, should also prompt the surgeon to investigate the venous and/or lymphatic systems prior to liposuction. Swelling due to lymphatic insufficiency may be ameliorated by liposuction (see pp. 458-459).

If the patient has severe varicosities and vein stripping is planned, it should precede liposuction by 3 months. Sclerosing solutions to treat mild varicosities should not be injected for 3 weeks before a liposuction procedure. Active phlebitis is an absolute contraindication to surgery.

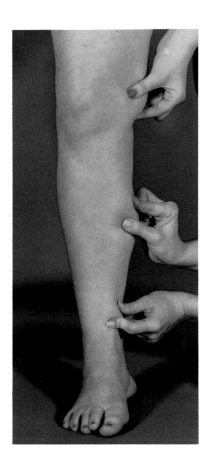

The pinch test should be performed with the patient standing, placing most of her weight on the opposite leg. As with all areas, no absolute guidelines exist, but a pinch test of 3 to 4 cm at the medial knee, 2 cm at the calf, and 1.5 cm at the ankle generally indicates a favorable candidate.

Defining Patient Goals

Patients who seek treatment of the medial knees are usually quite concrete in their requests and realistic in their expectations—they want flattening and reduction of the localized bulge. Since this is a straightforward and attainable goal, little discussion is required. If the patient also wants prepatellar fullness and wrinkling addressed, the limitations of liposuction in this area must be made clear.

The patient may be quite unrealistic in her desires concerning the calves and ankles. She frequently wants surgery to give her the legs and ankles of a high fashion model but does not voice this to the surgeon. Her inner wishes form a hidden agenda never openly expressed. The surgeon must be alert to the patient's unconscious desires and gently but firmly explain the limitations of liposuction while encouraging her to reap the real benefits of surgery—a delicate task.

Most patients, if properly educated before surgery, are grateful for even subtle improvements and pleased with modest results. Simply making legs smaller is an acceptable goal for surgeon and patient. As the surgeon gains experience, he will find he can also satisfy the patient's desire for better shape.

Patients with massive accumulation of fat in the medial knees may seek liposuction to eliminate the irritation from the friction of the knees rubbing together while walking. Overweight patients with massive fat accumulation around the knee may also request suction to reduce bulk prior to orthopedic procedures. In these cases liposuction is performed at least 6 weeks prior to orthopedic surgery.

Informed Consent

The surgeon should discuss several issues unique to the treatment of the knees, calves, and ankles in addition to the standard informed consent topics for liposuction procedures.

If only the knees are being treated, the patient should expect that the recovery period will be considerably shorter than for other areas of the body. Except for participating in sports, most of these patients resume full activity in 48 hours.

When calves and ankles are treated, recovery will be more prolonged than for most other areas. Patients may return to work in a week, but still have some discomfort for an additional week. Patients who have calf and ankle liposuction can also expect intermittent ankle swelling for up to 3 months, although swelling is much less after 6 weeks. Patients also need to be told they must wear strong, heavy support stockings for 4 to 6 weeks and occasionally longer.

Irregularities in surface texture are more common in the calves and ankles than elsewhere since the fat layer is relatively thin. The irregularities are more frequently palpable than visible. Hyperpigmentation also occurs more frequently in this area because of the thinness of the fat layer and the dependent position.

LIPOSUCTION OF THE KNEES

Liposuction of the knees involves volume reduction in a small, well-circumscribed area. Treatment is straightforward, and although overresection and contour irregularities can occur here as elsewhere, results are usually excellent.

Markings

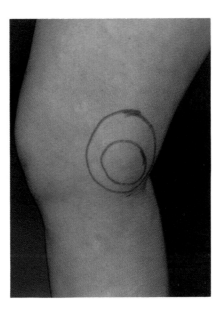

The surgeon kneels in front of the patient while she rotates her foot outward and flexes slightly at the knee. This position accentuates the bulge of the medial knee and puts the area in front of the surgeon for easy marking. The access incision is marked in the posteromedial knee crease adjacent to the area to be treated. I routinely use only one access incision to treat the medial knee, one of the few areas for which this is possible.

Operative Technique

The knees are easily treated with the patient under local anesthesia. General or regional anesthesia is used if the knees are treated in conjunction with the calves and ankles.

The knees are treated most conveniently with the patient in the frog-leg position. If calves and ankles are also to be suctioned, the patient is placed in the lateral decubitus position.

Volumes removed range from 25 to 200 cc, the average being 50 to 100 cc. Cannula size is most commonly 3.0 or 3.7 mm in diameter but may be larger or smaller depending on volume of fat.

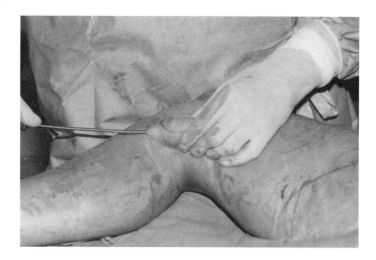

With the patient in the frog-leg position a stab incision is made in the posterolateral knee crease. Exposure is improved by pulling the access incision to a more anterior position. The surgeon grasps the medial knee tissues, slides the access incision toward the front of the knee, and inserts the cannula into the deep level of the superficial fascia and subcutaneous fat. The cannula is directed away from the popliteal fossa.

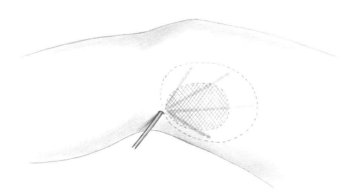

The cannula is moved through the fat in a series of tunnels radiating from the single access incision. Although tunnels extend to the outer perimeter of the treated area, most of the suctioning and therefore most of the fat removal occurs in the lower central portion (cross-hatching). Excessive suction outside of this area will result in postoperative contour depressions.

Contour and side-to-side symmetry are checked by placing the legs in the extended position and comparing the two sides. The visual end point is a flattened contour with the knees extended.

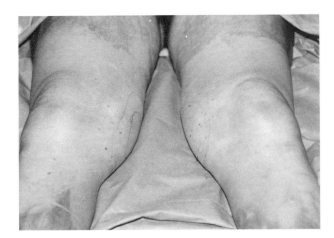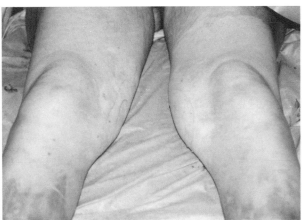

In this patient, left and right medial knee contours are near identical prior to suctioning. After the right knee is suctioned, the contour on that side is reduced in comparison to the left knee.

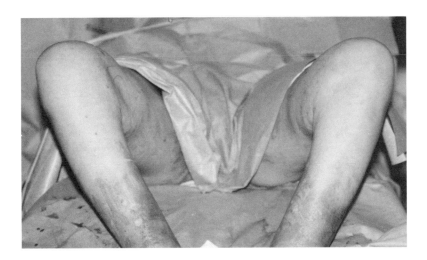

With the patient in the frog-leg position the right knee shows a concavity after aspiration not seen when the knee is extended.

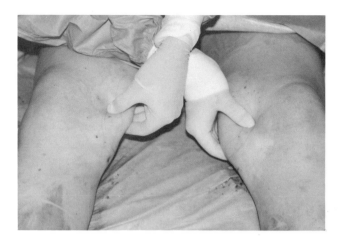

Gentle pinching and rolling of the skin also help determine the end point, usually 1 or 2 cm of pinch thickness. The left knee has not yet been treated.

Postoperative Care and Recovery

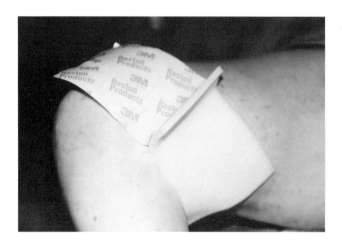

The wound is closed with one or two staples, and a self-adherent ¼-inch thick foam sponge (Reston) is firmly placed over the medial half of the knee.

If only the knees have been treated, recovery is more rapid than after liposuction of any other body area. The patient is instructed to rest in bed with feet and knees elevated for 24 hours. She may resume all nonsports-related activities the day after surgery and full sports activities in 1 week. The sponge and staples are removed 2 days after surgery.

Bruising and swelling are usually much less than in other areas treated. Ecchymosis usually resolves in 2 weeks, and 90% of swelling resolves by 6 weeks.

Results

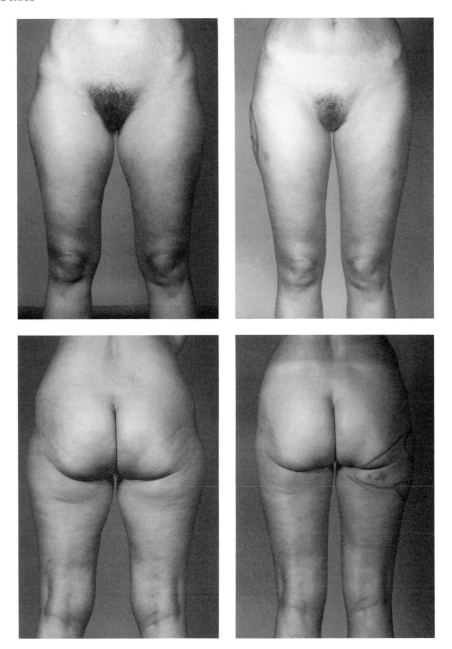

This 32-year-old, 5-foot 5-inch, 124-pound woman requested reduction in the size of her thighs and hips. At the initial consultation I suggested treatment of her medial knees as well as the thighs and hips. Women seeking thigh and hip reduction are sometimes not focused on the inner knees, but treatment of this area adds very little time to the surgery and the results are almost always gratifying to the patient. She is shown 6 months after aspiration of 50 cc from each medial knee as well as liposuction of the thighs and hips. The right lateral thigh is marked in the postoperative view because the patient desired secondary liposuction of this area.

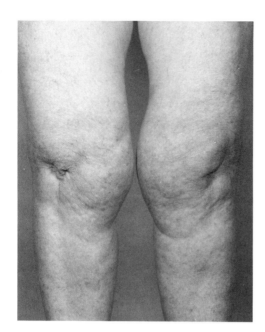 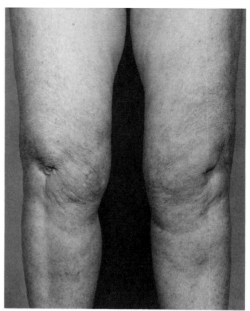

This 53-year-old woman consulted me initially for facial rejuvenation. Almost in passing, she asked if something could be done to improve the appearance of her knees. Liposuction of the knees was performed along with face, neck, and brow lift and four-lid blepharoplasty. She is shown before and 13 months after aspiration of 200 cc from each knee.

Additional examples of knee liposuction are shown on pp. 436-443.

LIPOSUCTION OF THE CALVES AND ANKLES

Treatment of the calves and ankles usually requires circumferential reduction of the entire lower leg subcutaneous mass as well as localized fat removal to form the desirable contours dictated by the musculoskeletal framework. The subcutaneous fat in this area is relatively sparse, leaving little margin for error. Even small irregularities may be noticeable after swelling has subsided. The surgeon should gain experience in more forgiving areas before treating the calves and ankles.

Prior to surgery the patient is fitted for an elastic support stocking (Sigvaris graduated compression garment; Ganzoni & Cie AG, St. Gallen, Switzerland, and Branford, Conn.). These garments are the type worn for severe venous insufficiency or lymphedema and exert a pressure of 30 to 40 mm Hg. Use of department store garments or the typical hospital-supplied antiembolism stockings will not be sufficient to prevent postoperative edema. The patient needs to be informed prior to surgery that continuous wearing of this garment is critical to smooth and rapid recovery from surgery. In my experience, the most frequent cause of persistent and recurring edema has been the patient's failure to wear strong support hose on a continuous basis.

Markings

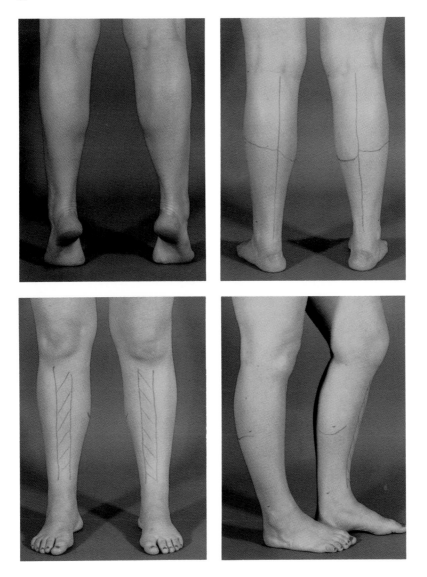

The calf is marked by having the patient stand on her toes facing away from the kneeling surgeon. This position emphasizes the shape of the gastrocnemius and permits the surgeon to accurately mark the lower borders of this muscle. Areas of special interest to the patient or areas that require special attention (e.g., medial and lateral to the Achilles tendon above the malleoli) are marked at this time. A vertical line is drawn down the midline of the posterior leg. The pretibial area is marked with vertical lines on either side of the anterior tibia since there is generally little fat in the pretibial area and suction is rarely necessary. By marking the vertical midline and the anterior tibia, the surgeon divides the leg into medial and lateral halves. The leg is further divided into upper and lower segments by the markings at the lower border of the gastrocnemius. Thus the leg is divided into four roughly equal quadrants. Three access incisions (upper, lower, and middle) are marked along both medial and lateral sides of each leg.

Operative Technique

Patients are treated under general or spinal anesthesia. The six access incisions allow for total coverage of the leg using 15 to 20 cm long cannulas. If longer cannulas (30 cm) are used, the middle access incisions may be eliminated. I find, however, that the shorter cannulas permit greater control and precision. Since the incisions are only 3 to 4 mm in length, the additional scars are inconsequential.

Suction volumes range from 200 to 800 cc for each calf and ankle. Cannulas range in diameter from 2.4 to 3.7 mm, with the 3.0 cannula being used most often. Use of the finer cannulas makes the operation slower and more tedious, but this relative disadvantage is more than offset by the smoother results and minimal irregularities made possible by the finer instruments.

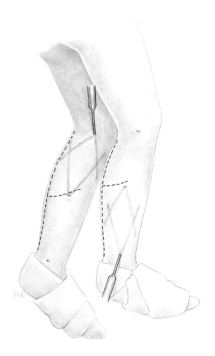

The patient is placed in the left lateral decubitus position initially. The upper and middle access incisions are used for the calves and the middle and lower access incisions for the ankles to create crisscross mesh tunneling. It is easy to overresect around the access incisions, and the operator should direct the tip of the cannula away from the incisions as much as possible.

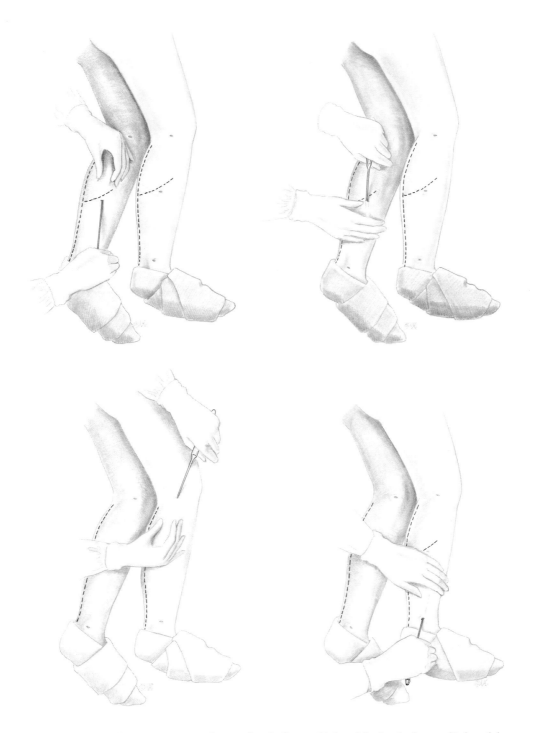

Fat is suctioned in sequence from the left medial calf, the left medial ankle, the right lateral calf, and the right lateral ankle. The volume aspirated from each quadrant is recorded accurately. Special attention is paid to areas requiring extra definition. Depending on the patient, these may include the lower border of the gastrocnemius, the areas on either side of the Achilles tendon, and the fullness over the bellies of the gastrocnemius.

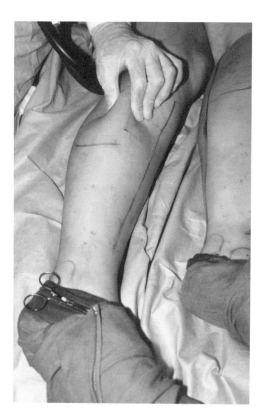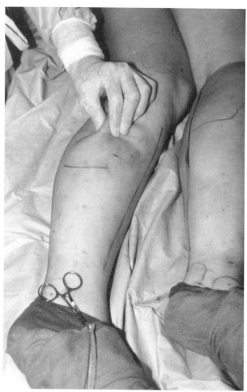

The end point of suctioning in each area is judged by gently squeezing and rolling the skin between the fingers to determine the relative thickness of tissues. Note the pinch thickness of the medial calf before and after suction in the patient shown above. Light palpation while rubbing the fingers over the surface of the skin will detect residual excess fat that can be removed with extra fine cannulas. The end point differs for each patient, but certain principles apply. Palpable skin thickness should be less and contour should be visibly reduced. Enough residual fat should remain to provide smooth subcutaneous cover. In this area, particularly, "less is best." Secondary liposuction can improve an underresection, but overresections are irretrievable.

When treatment of the left medial calf and ankle and the right lateral calf and ankle have been completed, the patient is turned 180 degrees to the right lateral decubitus position. The identical procedure is carried out on the right medial calf and ankle and the left lateral calf and ankle. Again, the surgeon's aesthetic judgment is key to determining the proper thickness and smoothness of the subcutaneous tissues. In operating on the second side, however, he must also match volumes with the opposite leg, removing the identical volume from the right medial calf as removed from the left medial calf and the identical volume from the right medial ankle as from the left medial ankle (assuming the legs are of equal volume prior to surgery).

Segmenting each leg into four quadrants and removing identical volumes from each area gives the surgeon an added measure of control in achieving symmetry. A simple chart kept in the operating room ensures equality of volumes.

	Left	Right
MEDIAL CALF	125	125
MEDIAL ANKLE	100	100
LATERAL CALF	125	125
LATERAL ANKLE	100	100

Postoperative Care and Recovery

After the wound is closed, patients are placed in custom-fitted support hose (Sigvaris), which they must wear for 3 to 6 weeks. Most of these patients stay overnight in the hospital and are kept on strict bed rest with feet elevated until the morning, at which time staples are removed from the wounds, fresh garments are put on, and the patients are discharged. If patients are treated on an ambulatory basis, they remain in bed at home with feet elevated for 48 hours and then return to the office for follow-up.

Patients wear the stockings continuously (even while sleeping). They are instructed to place blocks under the front of their beds to elevate the legs a few degrees. Alternatively, they may use pillows. Garments may be removed for showering, but the stockings fit quite snugly and are difficult to take on and off, particularly in the immediate postoperative period when swelling and tenderness are maximal. Use of a silk undersock facilitates removal and replacement. After 3 weeks patients no longer wear stockings at night but do wear them for at least another week during the day. By the end of the fourth week patients remove the garments during the day on a trial basis. If swelling returns, they continue to wear the garments until they are able to remove them without recurrence of swelling. Most patients discard the garments altogether between the fourth and sixth week.

Patients undergoing calf and ankle liposuction require longer to recover than those having liposuction of the thighs or torso. They generally refrain from even sedentary activities for a full week and are warned against sitting for more than an hour at a time when they do return to work, usually 1 week after surgery. They will experience some discomfort in walking for 2 weeks. Sports generally cannot be resumed for 4 weeks since running may be painful.

Results

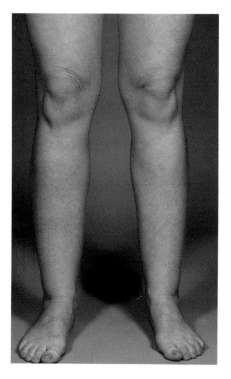 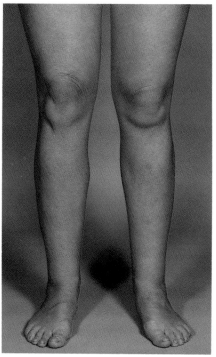

This 35-year-old, 5-foot 3-inch, 135-pound woman was displeased with the shape of her calves and ankles. She felt they did not taper enough and were excessively full. I treated her calves and ankles circumferentially, aspirating 300 cc from each leg to produce an overall size reduction. Removal of fat from the areas proximal to the lateral and medial malleoli narrowed the ankles in the anterior and posterior views. I also aspirated 50 cc from each medial knee.

Photographs 6 months after surgery show a subtle improvement. Removal of a small additional volume from the right calf over the medial gastrocnemius would further improve her appearance, but she did not desire additional surgery.

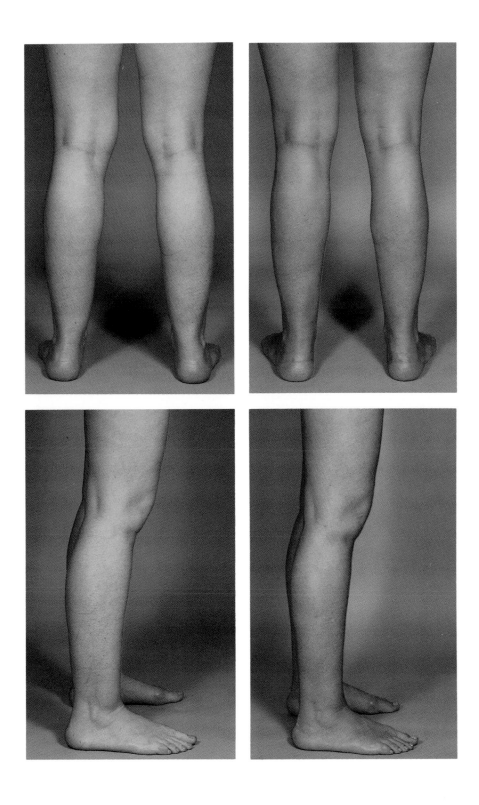

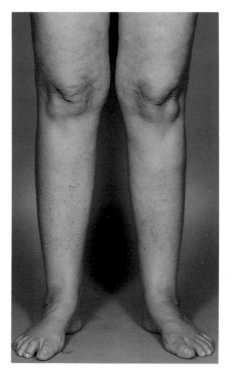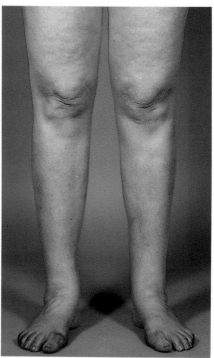

This 50-year-old, 5-foot 5-inch, 135-pound woman complained that her ankles had thickened in the past few years, during which time she had gained 15 pounds. Mild venous insufficiency was manifest as ankle swelling and a reticular vascular pattern on her skin. I recommended liposuction of the calves and ankles and medial knees. The patient requested treatment of the prepatellar region as well, but skin laxity precluded effective treatment of this area.

She is shown before and 6 months after aspiration of 425 cc from each calf and ankle and 75 cc from each medial knee. The quality of her result is diminished by faint skin irregularities seen on the posterior view and by asymmetry of resection in the medial ankle. The patient was unaware of the irregularities since they were only evident in the stark light used for these photographs. She did, however, complain of the ankle asymmetry, which I corrected by secondary aspiration of 50 cc from the left medial ankle.

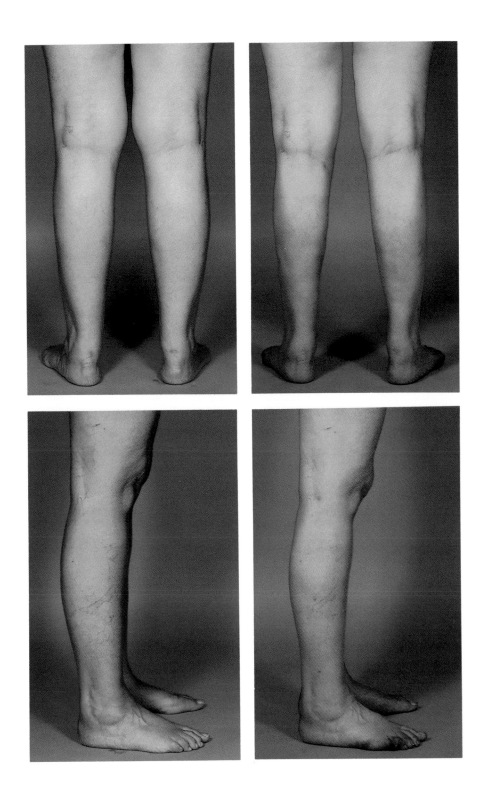

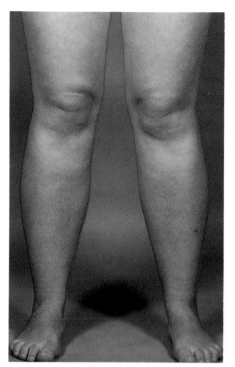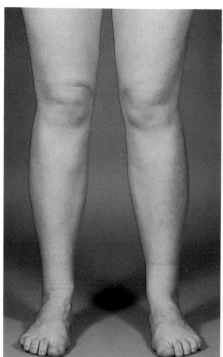

Having had large calves since she was a "baby," this 23-year-old, 5-foot 9-inch, 164-pound woman requested reduction of this area. I performed circumferential liposuction, removing 600 cc from each calf and ankle and 50 cc from each medial knee. She is shown before and 6 months after surgery, by which time she had also lost 25 pounds through diet and increased exercise. Her calf circumference was reduced from 17½ to 14½ inches. Although surgery contributed to this patient's striking contour improvement, her weight loss was instrumental in improving her result. Most patients do not lose weight following liposuction, but a few are inspired to change their eating habits and actively participate in their therapy, a happy event for all!

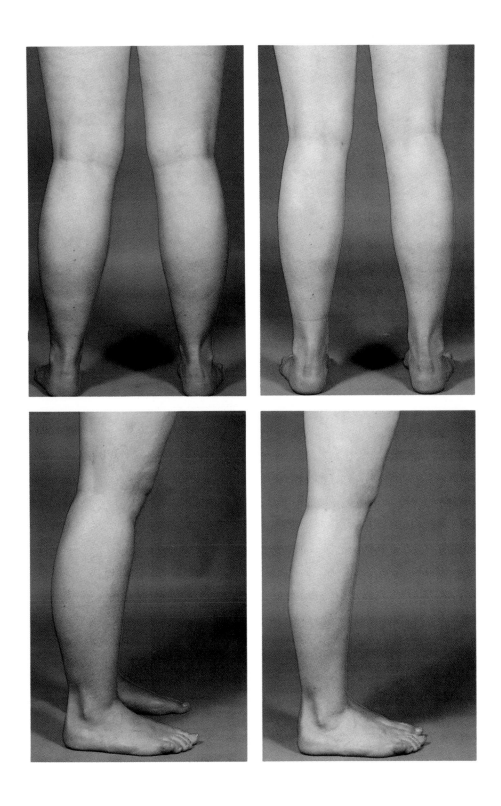

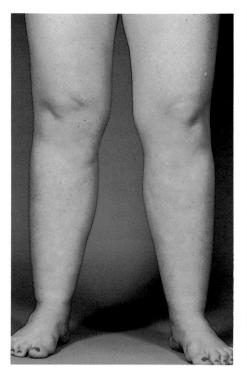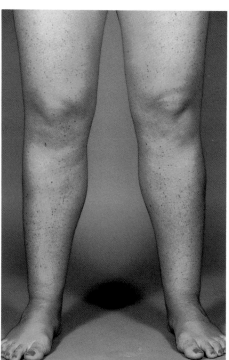

This 25-year-old, 5-foot 1-inch, 125-pound woman complained of heavy legs and painful, swollen ankles. Her father's legs were of similar shape. She took diuretics periodically with partial relief. She is shown before and 6 months after circumferential liposuction to remove 700 cc from each calf and ankle and aspiration of 100 cc from each medial knee. Her weight was unchanged. The dramatic contour reduction was gratifying to both patient and surgeon. The patient was particularly pleased to fit into over-the-calf boots. She no longer had ankle pain and stopped taking diuretics.

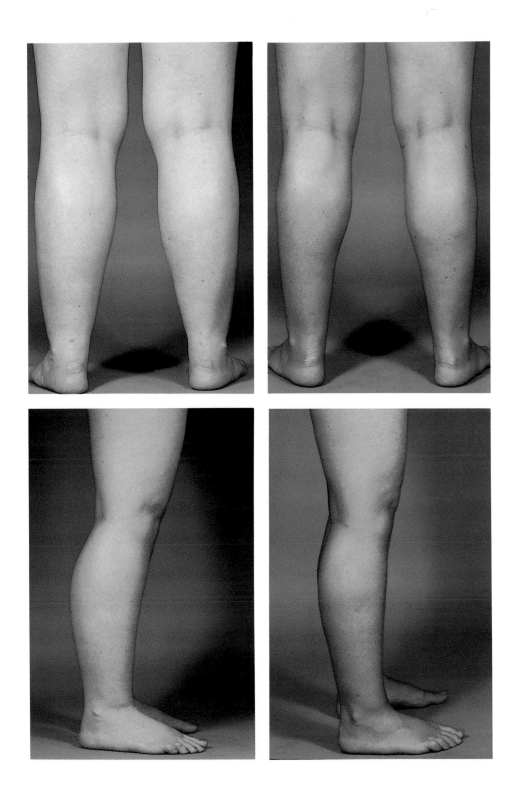

COMPLICATIONS AND UNAESTHETIC RESULTS
Knees

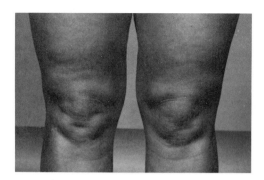 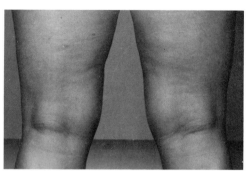

Left-to-right asymmetry may occur following liposuction of the knees, but this problem is uncommon if the surgeon is meticulous in removing equal volumes from both sides. Overresection of the area just above the medial knee protuberance on the lower thigh results in a more or less noticeable indentation in the area above the medial knee. This problem is avoided by keeping the cannula confined to the area adjacent to the medial femoral condyle. Secondary surgery, if necessary, is usually to remove more volume or to correct minor side-to-side asymmetries.

Calves and Ankles

Irregularity of the skin surface is the most common complication. Although this waviness is more frequently palpable than visible, it sometimes may be seen, particularly in harsh side lighting. A visible depression may be created by overresection, especially at the site of the middle access incisions. Irregularities and depressions are avoided by using ultra-fine cannulas and resecting conservatively. Given the relatively thin layer of fat in this area, some slight irregularities are almost unavoidable and patients should be informed of this in advance. Hyperpigmentation can also occur because the thinness of the subcutaneous fat layer makes the dermis more susceptible to injury. Again, fine cannulas, gentleness of technique, and conservative resections will minimize this problem. Significant swelling beyond 6 weeks may occasionally occur, but is preventable if the patient is assiduous in wearing strong support hose.

REFERENCES

1. Otteni F, Fournier PF. A history and comparison of suction techniques until their debut in North America. In Hetter GP. Lipoplasty: The Theory and Practice of Blunt Suction Lipectomy. Boston: Little, Brown, 1990, p 23.

2. Schrudde J. Lipexeresis as a means of eliminating local adiposity. Aesthetic Plast Surg 4:215-226, 1980.

3. Schrudde J. Suction curettage for body contouring. Clin Plast Surg 11:445-456, 1984.

4. Pfulg ME. Complications of suction for lipectomy [letter]. Plast Reconstr Surg 69: 562, 1982.

5. Kesselring UK. Suction curettage to remove excess fat for body contouring [letter]. Plast Reconstr Surg 69:572, 1982.

6. Courtiss EH. Suction lipectomy: A retrospective analysis of 100 patients. Plast Reconstr Surg 73:780-794, 1984.

7. Teimourian B, Fisher JB. Suction curettage to remove excess fat for body contouring. Plast Reconstr Surg 68:50-58, 1981.

8. Illouz Y-G. Body contouring by lipolysis: A 5-year experience with over 3,000 cases. Plast Reconstr Surg 72:591-597, 1983.

9. Pitman GH, Teimourian B. Suction lipectomy: Complications and results by survey. Plast Reconstr Surg 76:65-69, 1985.

10. Ersek RA, Zambrano J, Surak GS, Denton DR. Suction assisted lipectomy for correction of 202 figure faults in 101 patients: Indications, limitations, and applications. Plast Reconstr Surg 78:615-624, 1986.

11. Hetter GP. Closed suction lipoplasty in 1078 patients: Illouz told the truth. Aesthetic Plast Surg 12:183-185, 1988.

12. Teimourian B. Suction Lipectomy and Body Sculpturing. St. Louis: CV Mosby, 1987, pp 495-542.

13. Pitman GH. Liposuction of the knees, calves and ankles. Presented at the Annual Meeting of the Northeast Society of Plastic Surgeons. Lake George, N.Y.: October 7, 1990.

14. Reed LS. Lipoplasty of the calves and ankle. Clin Plast Surg 16:365-368, 1989.

15. Mladick RA. Lipoplasty of the calves and ankles. Plast Reconstr Surg 86:84-93, 1990.

16. Wanatabe K. Discussion of Mladick RA: Lipoplasty of the calves and ankles. Plast Reconstr Surg 86:94-96, 1990.

17. Wanatabe K. Circumferential liposuction of calves and ankles. Aesthetic Plast Surg 14:259-269, 1990.

Chapter 13

ODDS AND ENDS

LIPOMAS, FLAP DEBULKING, LYMPHEDEMA, FAT REINJECTION, AND ADDITIONAL COMPLICATIONS

"Odds and Ends" deals with topics that do not fall within the anatomic organization of the table of contents but are nonetheless worthy of consideration. These procedures range from the commonplace to the controversial and include excision of lipomas, flap debulking, amelioration of lymphedema, and reinjection of autologous fat.

Liposuction offers indisputable advantages in treating lipomas. With the use of aspiration this most common of soft tissue tumors can be removed through a small incision. Because minimal dissection is required, recovery is more rapid even for very large lipomas.

Flap debulking using liposuction permits precise contour reduction without jeopardizing blood supply. Suction can also be used in conjunction with scar revision along the flap periphery and excision of redundant skin.

Liposuction is beneficial for the palliation of lymphedema. Although the effects are sometimes temporary, the procedure itself is simple and safe. Cutaneous scarring is inconspicuous compared to other methods of surgical bulk reduction.

The fourth application, reinjection of autologous fat, offers the seductive potential of providing a readily available soft tissue fill. Unfortunately, long-term results have been disappointing.

General observations and recommendations concerning each of these subjects are supplemented by case reports. A brief discussion of complications not covered in earlier chapters concludes "Odds and Ends."

LIPOMAS

Lipomas constitute 80% of all benign soft tissue tumors. They occur most frequently on the torso and extremities but can be found anywhere in the subcutaneous fat as well as other tissues throughout the body. Tumors occur at all ages but are seen most commonly in the fourth decade of life. Although they are generally only a few centimeters in diameter, they can become massive.

Grossly, lipomas appear as bright yellow fat separated by fibrous trabeculae. Microscopically, most are indistinguishable from normal fat. About 2% contain increased fibrous elements and are designated fibrolipomas. Another 10% have increased vascular elements and are termed angiolipomas. Angiolipomas are usually close to the undersurface of the skin and may be painful.

Multiple lipomas occur in about 5% of patients and are associated with three conditions. *Familial multiple lipomatosis* is a common inherited disease that usually becomes manifest in patients in their thirties. It is characterized by multiple, usually painless lipomas of the torso and extremities. *Madelung's disease* is marked by large, painless, coalescent lipomas around the neck, shoulders, and upper arms and is seen most commonly in middle-aged men. *Dercum's disease* occurs in overweight, menopausal women and consists of symmetric, painful, circumscribed fatty deposits.

In contrast to lipomas, liposarcomas are rare. Although they are the most common soft tissue malignancy, only about 1600 cases occur each year in the United States. They can appear anywhere in the body but have a predilection for the upper thigh and retroperitoneum. They do not arise from lipomas.

Patients with lipomas commonly present with one or more subcutaneous tumors. A history of slow growth is not uncommon. The tumors have usually been present for more than a year and sometimes longer than 10 years.

On physical examination the tumors are usually soft and movable. Occasionally they are quite firm. Most are in the subcutaneous space, but they can lie beneath the investing fascia in an inter- or intramuscular location. Since lipomas occur almost anywhere in the body, the surgeon cannot assume they are subcutaneous.

The differential diagnosis includes sebaceous cysts, dermoids, and other tumors of epithelial appendages and the subcutaneous space.

For tumors less than 6 cm in diameter, treatment is usually dictated by the history and physical examination. For larger tumors (>10 cm), CT scans or MRI can confirm the diagnosis and pinpoint the anatomic location. If the diagnosis remains in doubt, preliminary incisional biopsy with microscopic evaluation of permanent fixed sections will usually establish an unequivocal diagnosis prior to treatment. Frozen sections of fatty tumors are difficult to interpret.

Liposuction has improved our ability to treat patients with these common tumors. Many of these masses can be removed through small incisions with reduced scarring. Multiple lipomas can be removed through a single incision. The use of liposuction for removal of larger tumors has also shortened recovery.

It is impossible to anticipate which lipomas will be amenable to liposuction. I tell the patient that I will make a small initial incision to establish by visual inspection that the tumor is fat. If not and if it is small, I will perform an excisional biopsy. If the tumor is hard or large or if the diagnosis is otherwise in doubt, I perform an incisional biopsy and defer treatment until the diagnosis is established by microscopic examination.

When gross inspection establishes that the tumor is fat, it is aspirated through the original incision and a secondary incision if necessary. The tumor should be stabilized with the left hand while the right hand repeatedly drives the tip of the cannula into the central portion of the mass. There is usually a gradual reduction of contour as the tumor is aspirated. The surgeon should continually inspect the area, pinch up the tissues for thickness, and run his hands over the skin to check for smoothness of resection.

If the tumor is very fibrous, complete aspiration will not be possible, and the subcutaneous mass persists. For these patients, the incision is enlarged just enough to insert a curved Stevens scissors, which is gently spread to divide fibrous bands. The fragmented fat is extruded from the incision by gently squeezing and milking the tissues. If necessary, a mosquito hemostat is used to pull out fibro-fatty elements. No matter how large the tumor, a 2 cm incision will usually suffice. Obviously, this method of extraction can only be used if the surgeon is absolutely certain the tumor is indeed a benign lipoma confined to the subcutaneous space.

Case Reports

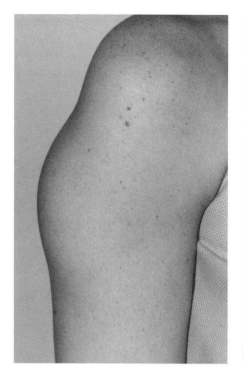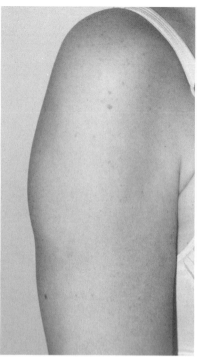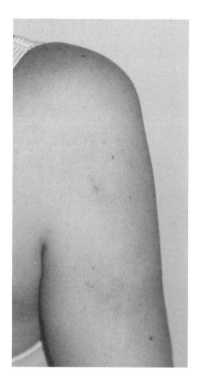

This 41-year-old woman had a 4-year history of a slow-growing mass of the upper right arm. A small lipoma had been surgically excised from her back 5 years ago, and she was troubled by the scar. Her brother and mother had both had lipomas removed. Examination showed a 9.5 cm soft, movable mass overlying the lower portion of the right deltoid muscle. Under local anesthesia a preliminary incision was made directly over the superior pole of the mass to verify the fatty nature of the tumor. An additional access incision was made in the posterior axillary crease, and 2.4 and 3.0 mm Mercedes Type cannulas were used to extract 150 cc of fatty tissue. She is shown before and 3 months following surgery. The posterior view shows the scar.

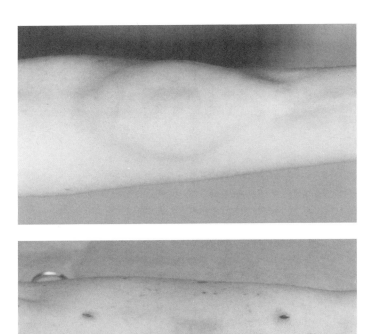

A slow-growing mass in the left forearm of this 41-year-old woman had been present for more than 10 years. Examination revealed a soft, movable, 13 × 8.5 cm tumor of the flexor surface of the left midforearm. With the patient under local anesthesia, a 1.5 cm incision was made over the proximal pole of the mass to visually confirm the diagnosis. Liposuction through this incision and an additional access incision at the lower pole of the mass evacuated only a portion of the tumor. Therefore both incisions were enlarged and the remaining tumor removed by milking out fragments and extracting residual fat and fibrous tissue with a mosquito hemostat. All dissection was kept superficial to the investing fascia. The patient is shown before and immediately after surgery. The linear dark area between the two access incisions is a small hematoma from injection of the local anesthetic. The tumor had not recurred at follow-up 1 year later.

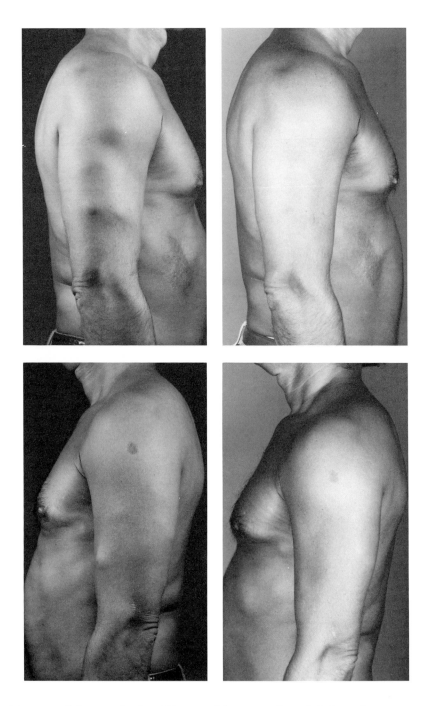

This 45-year-old man had a 25-year history of multiple subcutaneous tumors of the torso and extremities. Three of the tumors had been removed by conventional surgery that left unsightly scars. His mother had had a large lipoma of the face. Multiple, nodular, movable masses of the soft tissues of the trunk and extremities were found on examination. Most of the tumors were soft, but some were firm. The largest measured 4 cm in diameter. With the patient under general anesthesia, small incisions were

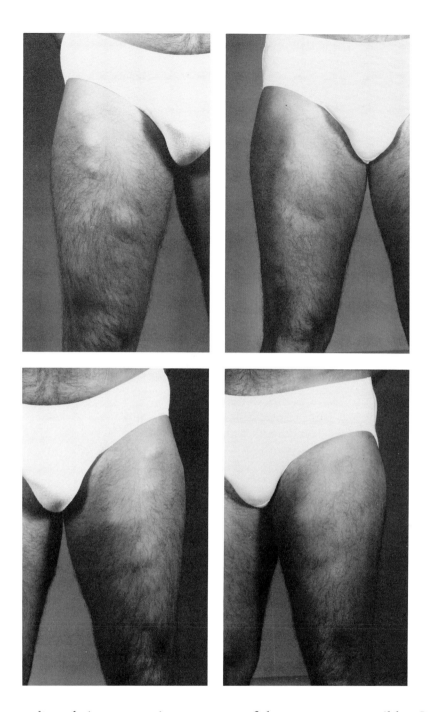

made at selected sites to suction as many of the tumors as possible. Generally one incision permitted access to four to eight separate tumors. Those that persisted were excised through 1 cm incisions directly over the tumor. Liposuction permitted treatment with minimal scarring. The patient is shown before and 6 months following surgery. The postoperative photographs are somewhat overexposed compared to the postoperative views, but the change in contour and minimal scarring are evident.

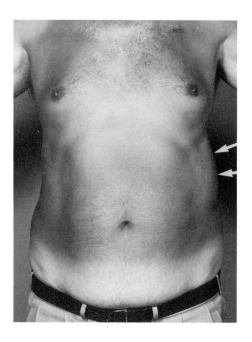

This 60-year-old man had a a 12 × 14 cm mass on his left anterolateral chest wall. The mass had been gradually growing for 2 years. In addition, he had a 10- to 15-year history of two smaller growths in the posterior cervical and occipital areas. His maternal grandmother had had multiple fatty tumors. Examination showed a compressible, rounded mass of the soft tissues overlying the left anterior axillary line just caudal to the rib cage. I could not tell if the mass was subcutaneous or deep. There were, in addition, 6 and 2.5 cm tumors in the hair-bearing skin of the posterior cervical and occipital areas.

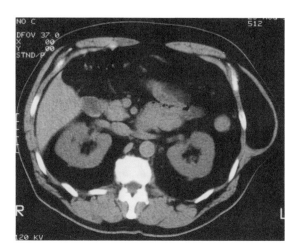

Because of the large size of the thoracic tumor and my uncertainty as to its precise anatomic location, I obtained a preoperative CT scan. The scan revealed a mass with the radiodensity of fat deep to the serratus anterior muscle. The patient's operation, performed under general anesthesia, consisted of direct surgical excision of all tumors. The serratus anterior muscle was split in the direction of its fibers for access to the thoracic lipoma. Liposuction was not used. He was back at work 4 days after surgery.

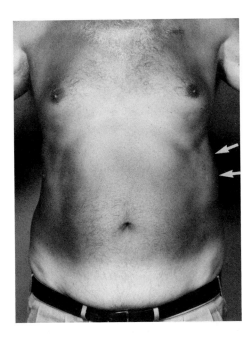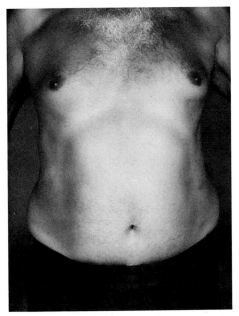

The patient is shown before (arrows point to lipoma) and 9 months after surgery. In the postoperative view the anterior portion of the scar is visible in the flank area.

See pp. 140-141 for treatment of lipomas of the submental area.

FLAP DEBULKING

Transfer of large flaps for reconstructive procedures frequently results in oversized, bulky, and unaesthetic tissue masses. In the past, secondary flap contouring was performed in stages to preserve flap blood supply. Liposuction, however, permits rapid, efficient contouring of the entire flap in one stage with preservation of the blood supply. Since the flap does not have to be totally elevated and blood supply is preserved, there is minimal swelling and more rapid recovery. Secondary liposuction for contouring can theoretically be performed as early as 3 weeks after surgery or as soon as the recipient site blood supply is established through the base of the flap. I prefer to wait 3 months or longer to permit complete resolution of swelling. Once the flap has been debulked, a portion of the redundant skin can be excised.

Case Reports

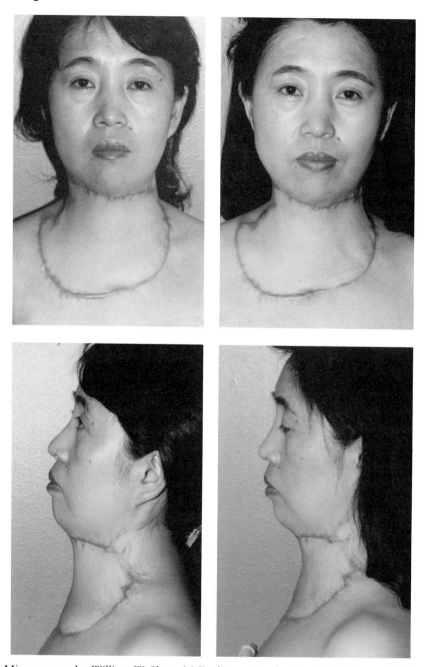

Microsurgery by William W. Shaw, M.D.; liposuction by Gerald H. Pitman, M.D.

This 20-year-old woman had a severe anterior cervical skin contracture from a thermal burn as a child. She was treated with release of the scar contracture and placement of a large microvascular groin flap. Six months postoperatively the bulky flap was reduced by liposuction of 100 cc. Simultaneously a Z-plasty was performed along one edge of the scar. She is shown 6 months after placement of the free flap on the left and 6 months after liposuction on the right.

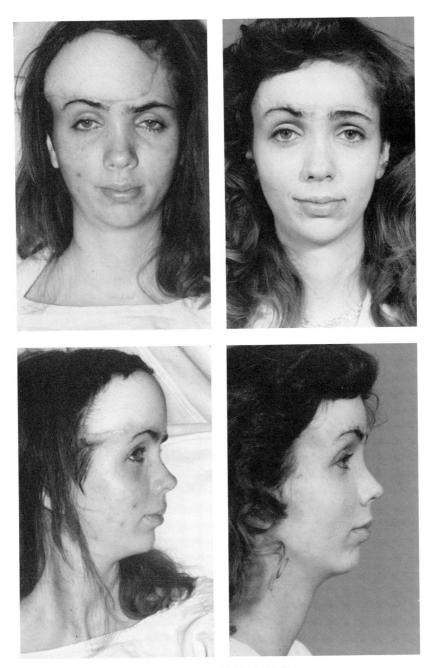

Courtesy Foad Nahai, M.D.

This 25-year-old woman underwent excision of a dermatofibrosarcoma of the forehead and frontal bone in a combined neurosurgery and plastic surgery procedure. The cranial defect was repaired with an acrylic plate. Soft tissue cover was accomplished with a free flap based on the superficial inferior epigastric artery (SIEA). Two months later the excessive bulk of the flap was thinned by liposuction. The patient is shown 10 months after flap reconstruction on the left and 5 months after liposuction on the right.

LYMPHEDEMA

The primary treatment for lymphedema is medical. Complex decongestive physiotherapy, as suggested by Clodius, will improve almost all lymphedematous conditions, and surgery is indicated only for those patients whose disease progresses despite medical therapy. Surgery is palliative not curative, and results may be temporary.

Surgical procedures fall into two categories: those designed to increase lymph drainage and those that reduce the load for lymphatic clearance. Theoretically, procedures to increase lymph drainage (transposed flaps, lymphovenous anastomoses) should be performed early in the disease before distal lymphatics are obscured. Procedures that reduce the load for lymphatic clearance include direct excision of subcutaneous tissue and, more recently, liposuction.

Debulking by directly removing the subcutaneous tissue and a portion of the skin permits the surgically reduced skin envelope to serve as a compression device. This debulking is more effective than liposuction, albeit at the cost of increased morbidity and cutaneous scarring. Liposuction produces negligible morbidity and minimal cutaneous scars. Its major limitation is that no skin is excised, and thus reduction of the skin envelope depends on the ability of the skin to shrink to the reduced volume. Continuous wearing of a compressive garment following surgery is an integral component of liposuction therapy.

Hygiene of the integument should be optimized prior to liposuction. This may involve a course of intense physiotherapy and use of antibiotics to control bacterial and/or fungal infections. Limb circumferences should be measured at 10 cm intervals. Water displacement volumetric measurements also help compare pre- and postoperative limb size.

Liposuction is performed under general anesthesia using the technique outlined for treatment of the calf and ankle on pp. 432-435. Tourniquets are not necessary. Aspirate removed is generally more watery and less bloody than in patients without lymphedema.

Postoperative care differs in several respects from that following cosmetic liposuction of the calves and ankles. An elastic garment is not placed on the patient immediately after surgery. Instead, the extremity is wrapped with strips of Reston foam sponge as an inner layer supplemented by an elastic bandage. The patient is kept on bed rest with feet elevated for 48 hours, after which the initial dressings are removed and measurements taken for a custom compression garment. The patient is redressed with foam sponge and elastic bandages until the garment is ready. Ambulation is not begun until the patient can wear the garment. Continuous wearing of the compression garment is critical to maintaining the result. As swelling continues to recede during the first weeks following surgery, the patient is remeasured, and if necessary, a new smaller garment is purchased for continued wear.

Results are initially impressive, but recurrences and reoperation are not uncommon. Nevertheless, the procedure is simple, causes minimal associated cutaneous scars, and there has been no significant morbidity.

To date the procedure has been used only in patients with early stages of lymphedema who have good skin elasticity and limited tissue fibrosis. Although I have not tried this procedure on patients with severe fibrosis, it seems only logical that the tissues in patients with late disease would be less easily aspirated.

Case Report

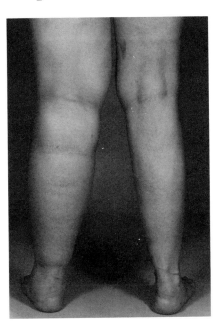 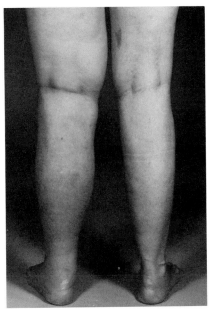

This 45-year-old woman underwent resection of an undifferentiated soft tissue malignancy of the left groin and left radical lymph node dissection followed by postoperative radiotherapy. She developed persistent lymphedema, which initially was successfully managed conservatively. Despite intensive therapy the swelling became worse, and the patient had to give up playing tennis. Three years following her cancer surgery I performed circumferential liposuction of the lower extremity, removing 1800 cc from the ankle to midthigh. A few days after surgery the patient was placed in a custom compression garment, which she wore diligently. She was able to resume playing tennis. Six months following liposuction surgery she noted an increase in the circumference of her leg. Although the contour was still improved at 1 year, I performed a secondary procedure. I also suctioned the right knee. She is shown before and 1 year after her second liposuction. She maintained the incremental improvement obtained by the secondary procedure at 2-year follow-up.

FAT REINJECTION

Autologous fat grafting was first reported in the late nineteenth century.[1] Peer[2,3] investigated the behavior of free fat grafts in humans prior to World War II, and in 1950 he reported that approximately 50% of grafted adipocytes survived. Stimulated by Peer, plastic surgeons attempted fat grafts for multiple indications, including breast augmentation. When prosthetic breast implants became readily available in the 1960s, interest in fat transplantation waned. With the popularization of liposuction in the 1980s, however, plastic surgeons expressed a renewed interest in fat grafting. Fat was used initially for restoration of volume deformity resulting from liposuction, but eventually plastic surgeons began to use it as a convenient filler material. It has been used to fill depressions and lines on the face and has recently been touted as a remedy for cellulite (see Chapter 5, p. 105).

Several plastic surgeons have reported successful reinjection of fat[4-9] or transplantation of small "pearls" of fat.[10] Others have expressed skepticism,[11] reported negative results,[12] or retracted previous favorable reports.[13,14]

Bircoll[15] described breast augmentation using autologous fat reinjection, but the presence of calcifications in the breasts of injected patients makes this technique unacceptable.

It is not surprising that injection of aspirated fat does not give uniformly consistent results. Successful grafting of any tissue requires a few basic prerequisites: a favorable recipient bed, meticulous hemostasis, atraumatic handling of the graft, adequate immobilization, and maximal contact of graft and recipient site. Most of these requirements are not met during fat reinjection.

My personal experience with reinjection of aspirated fat began in 1985, and I have used a wide variety of techniques involving washing, centrifugation, and filtering of the fat to rid it of water, oil, and blood. I have injected fat into multiple recipient sites on the face and the body in amounts ranging from a few cubic centimeters up to 150 cc. It has not been helpful for correction of fine lines and scars. Occasional patients have benefited in the short term by improvement of contour depressions, but results have been inconsistent and unpredictable.

Despite my disenchantment with fat recycling, a good alternative is not available. We do not have a reliable, safe, injectable, nonallergenic filler. Moreover, *occasional* patients do benefit from fat reinjection. Therefore I use the technique in selected patients. Most frequently these are patients undergoing liposuction who request that their aspirated fat be used to fill various contour defects. My best results have been in nonscarred areas requiring relatively small volumes to increase bulk. More than one treatment is always required.

Techniques for collection and injection of large volumes of fat for the torso and extremities are described in Chapter 5. Smaller volumes for the face are most conveniently collected using a 3 to 5 ml Luer-Lok syringe with an 18-gauge needle.

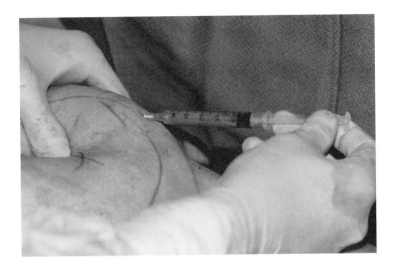

The fat is simply aspirated from the anesthetized tissues of the abdomen, thigh, or buttock. An important technical point, particularly in a patient with small fat deposits, is to fully distend the tissues with dilute local solution. As many syringes as necessary are filled with fat.

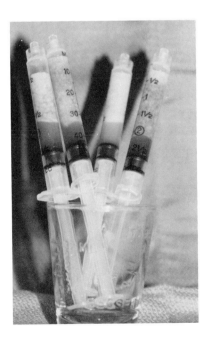

The syringes are then set aside in an upright position for a few minutes to permit separation of fat from water and oil.

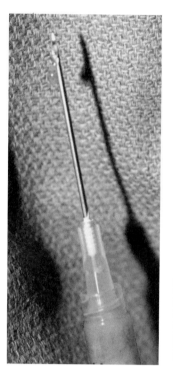 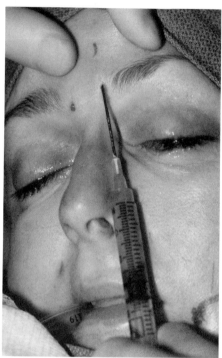

The supernatant oil is ejected prior to injecting the fat into the defect. I use nerve block anesthesia for the recipient site supplemented, when necessary, with infiltration of small amounts of local anesthetic. I generally overcorrect by 50% and repeat the treatment in 6 weeks. Most results do not persist beyond 6 months. Occasional patients have more long-lasting benefits.

Case Reports

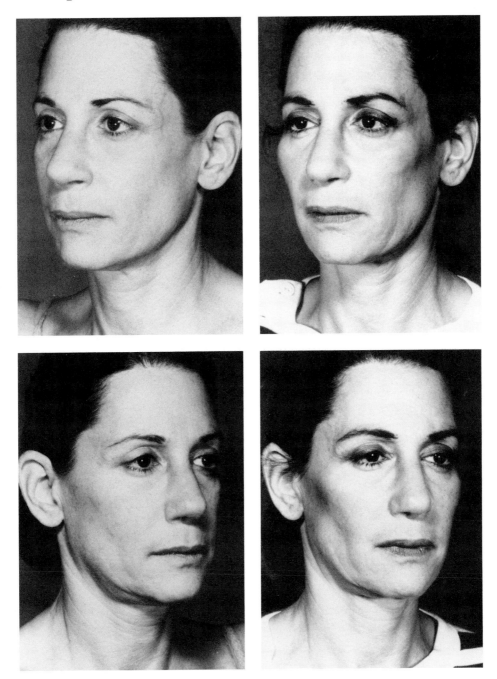

This 42-year-old woman requested malar augmentation. I injected 5 cc of fat into each malar eminence and repeated the injection at 6 weeks and 6 months. She is shown 1 year following the last injection. The improvement has been maintained for longer than 2 years. This patient is atypical; generally results do not last beyond 6 months.

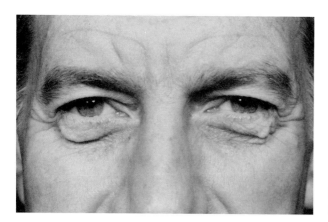 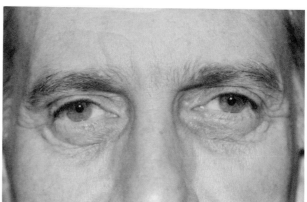

This 48-year-old man had fat grafted to his glabellar creases. Initially he demonstrated dramatic improvement, but by 3 months all beneficial effects had receded.

■   ■   ■

Plastic surgeons continue to search for a nonallergenic, injectable soft tissue filler that is both safe and reliable. A substance meeting all of these requirements does not exist. Autologous fat is readily available, meets some of these requirements, and has been used extensively. But what some have heralded as a panacea has not fulfilled its promise.

ADDITIONAL COMPLICATIONS

Most complications were discussed in Chapters 3, 4, and 6 to 12, the latter chapters describing detailed operative treatment by anatomic area. Chapters 3 and 6 to 12 also dealt with prevention and management of unaesthetic results. In this concluding section additional complications not specific to a particular anatomic area and those not previously considered are discussed. Although some of the material may overlap earlier chapters, the serious nature of these complications justifies repetition.

It is reassuring that liposuction alone rarely results in a serious complication.[1-4] It is particularly noteworthy that liposuction is a safer operation than abdominoplasty or other procedures involving dermatolipectomy.[2] Nevertheless, as with any surgery, serious complications are always a potential threat.

Deaths

Teimourian and Roger's 1989 survey reported two deaths in 75,591 "major" liposuction procedures (they left it to the respondents to define what was major and minor).[2] One mortality was attributed to pulmonary thromboembolism and the other to fat embolism.

Case reports of deaths in the literature have almost always involved patients who had procedures in addition to liposuction (usually abdominoplasty).[5-7] But mortalities have occurred in patients who had liposuction only.[7]

The case histories of mortalities frequently share common elements:
- An overweight patient
- Large-volume liposuction combined with another procedure (usually abdominoplasty)
- Inappropriate fluid and blood replacement (too much or too little)
- Pulmonary decompensation
- Sepsis

Stringent patient selection, limiting the scope of surgical procedures in accordance with the abilities and experience of the surgical team, and appropriate fluid management can reduce the already low mortality rate associated with liposuction.

Deep Venous Thrombosis and Pulmonary Thromboembolism

Deep venous thrombosis was the single most frequent serious complication reported by Teimourian and Rogers,[2] occurring in 33.1/100,000 (0.03%) of operations. The incidence of pulmonary embolism was considerably less, 11.9/100,000 (0.01%). On the other hand, large personal series of pure liposuction procedures have been reported without pulmonary embolism.[3,4]

Obesity predisposes to pulmonary embolism and is probably the most prevalent risk factor in the population of patients seeking liposuction. Other causes include disorders of clotting, cancer, advanced age, sepsis, immobilization, dehydration with venous stasis, and prior thromboembolism.[8]

Prevention of thromboembolism was discussed on pp. 303-304. Grazer and Mathews[4] have advocated intravenous alcohol, but no controlled trials have validated its efficacy. Low-dose heparin will reduce the incidence of thromboembolism[8-10] but predisposes to bleeding.[11]

My approach to this important problem is to refuse liposuction to patients at high risk for pulmonary thromboembolism. All my patients are well hydrated during surgery and mobilized rapidly after surgery. No thromboembolic complications have occurred in my personal practice.

Fat Embolism and Fat Embolism Syndrome

The fat embolism syndrome, consisting of respiratory failure, fever, petechiae, and changes in sensorium, occurs infrequently after long-bone fractures or other major trauma. The postmortem presence of pulmonary fat emboli has led to the belief that breakdown of fat in the lungs leads to increased pulmonary capillary permeability, leakage of fluid into the interstitium, and respiratory failure; but it has not been documented that fat embolization is the cause rather than an associated finding.[12-14]

Fat embolization probably occurs in every liposuction patient. Respiratory decompensation occurs rarely. In a small clinical investigation, Hunstad and Withers[15] were able to demonstrate free fat in the blood of all patients undergoing liposuction of more than 900 cc. In a parallel laboratory study they found free fat in the blood of all pigs undergoing liposuction but could find no evidence of fat pulmonary embolism in multiple lung biopsies.

Pulmonary fat embolism syndrome was reported only twice in the more than 75,000 operations surveyed by Teimourian and Rogers.[2] Even that low incidence may reflect overreporting since the few reports in the literature do not withstand critical analysis. The cases either are respiratory failure not proved to be caused by pulmonary fat embolism,[16-18] involve patients who underwent abdominoplasty and other procedures, [6,16-18] or are clearly respiratory distress secondary to inappropriate fluid management.[18]

Treatment of the liposuction patient in respiratory distress should include medical consultation, identification of the underlying cause (rarely, if ever, fat embolization), vigorous treatment of fluid imbalance, and respiratory support ranging from supplemental oxygen to endotracheal intubation with controlled ventilation. Early recognition and prompt intervention will permit a happy resolution in most of these uncommon cases.

Infection

Infections are seen infrequently. Dillerud[3] reported 1 in 2009 cases, and I have yet to see a clinical infection in my personal practice. Most of my patients do not receive prophylactic antibiotics. I believe strict surgical asepsis and avoidance of a hypovolemic or shock state are important determinants of a negligible infection rate.

Alexander et al.[7] reported the case of a 36-year-old woman who developed a fatal streptococcal soft tissue infection and septicemia following liposuction alone. She had had a hypotensive episode during a 3000 cc extraction. Although she was able to go home after volume replacement and treatment with corticosteroids, 48 hours later she was readmitted in a moribund state. Despite heroic measures, including surgical debridement, she never recovered.

Hematoma

Hematoma also occurs uncommonly. If hematomas of the body are small, stable, and do not cause pressure symptoms, they will resorb, and drainage is unnecessary. A large, expanding hematoma should be evacuated. Although drainage is imperfect because of the loculated cavity, it is better to relieve pressure and permit egress of blood. The bleeding generally stops spontaneously. Most of these hematomas are secondary to inadvertent injury to the deep muscle fascia, although Teimourian[5] reported an injury to the femoral vein due to misdirection of the cannula. Keeping the cannula in the central fat will minimize hematoma formation.

Seroma

Seromas were frequent when sharp cannulas were used, but they are seen only rarely with blunt cannulas.

Skin Irritation

Occasional patients are allergic to the latex garments and develop skin rashes. More commonly, use of an adhesive-backed dressing can irritate the skin.

▪   ▪   ▪

Overall, the reported incidence of major complications associated with liposuction is 0.1% compared to a rate of 2.0% for abdominoplasty and 0.9% for other dermolipectomies.[2] Liposuction is safe when patients are selectively screened for surgery, surgical technique is precise, and attention is directed to appropriate fluid management.

─────────────── SUGGESTED READINGS ───────────────

Lipomas

Adair FE, Pack GT, Farrior JH. Lipomas. Am J Cancer 16:1104-1120, 1932.
Allen PW. Tumors and Proliferation of Adipose Tissue. New York: Masson Publishing, 1981.
Armoid HL, Odom RB, James WD. Andrews' Diseases of the Skin. Philadelphia: WB Saunders, 1990, pp 734-736.
Comings DE, Glenchur H. Benign symmetric lipomatosis. JAMA 203:305, 1968.
Enzinger FM, Weiss SW. Soft Tissue Tumors. St. Louis: CV Mosby, 1983.
Krizek TJ, Feinstein RF. Tumors of soft tissue. In Jurkiewicz MJ, Krizek TJ, Mathes SJ, Ariyan S, eds. Plastic Surgery: Principles and Practice. St. Louis: CV Mosby, 1990, pp 1307-1310.
Leffell DJ, Braverman IM. Familial multiple lipomatosis. Report of a case and a review of the literature. J Am Acad Dermatol 15:275-279, 1986.
Miee JM. The soft tissues. In Coulson WF, ed. Surgical Pathology, vol 2, 2nd ed. Philadelphia: JB Lippincott, 1988, pp 1230-1232, 1290-1299.
Rosai J. Ackerman's Surgical Pathology, 6th ed. St. Louis: CV Mosby, 1981.

Flap Debulking

Baird W, Nahai F. The use of lipoplasty in contouring and debulking of flaps. Clin Plast Surg 16:395-399, 1989.

Hallock GG. Liposuction for debulking free flaps. J Reconstr Microsurg 2:235-238, 1986.

Stallings J. The defatting of flaps by lipoplasty. In Hetter GP, ed. Lipoplasty: The Theory and Practice of Blunt Suction Lipectomy, 2nd ed. Boston: Little, Brown, 1990, pp 417-430.

Lymphedema

Clodius L. Lymphedema. In McCarthy JG, ed. Plastic Surgery. Philadelphia: WB Saunders, 1990, pp 4093-4120.

Louton RB, Terranova WA. The use of suction curettage as adjunct to the management of lymphedema. Ann Plast Surg 22:354-357, 1989.

Miller TA. Surgical management of lymphedema of the extremity. Plast Reconstr Surg 56:633-641, 1975.

Nava VM, Lawrence WT. Liposuction on a lymphedematous arm. Ann Plast Surg 21:366-368, 1988.

O'Brien BM, Khazanchi RK, Kumar PA, Dvir E, Pederson WC. Liposuction in the treatment of lymphoedema: A preliminary report. Br J Plast Surg 42:530-533, 1989.

Sando WC, Nahai F. Suction lipectomy in the management of limb lymphedema. Clin Plast Surg 16:369-373, 1989.

REFERENCES

Fat Reinjection

1. Billings E Jr, May JW Jr. Historical review and present status of free fat graft autotransplantation in plastic and reconstructive surgery. Plast Reconstr Surg 83:368-381, 1989.

2. Peer LA. Loss of weight and volume in human fat grafts. With postulation of a "cell survival theory." Plast Reconstr Surg 5:217-230, 1950.

3. Peer LA. The neglected "free fat graft." Its behavior and clinical use. Am J Surg 92:40-47, 1956.

4. Chajchir A, Benzaquen I. Fat-grafting injection for soft tissue augmentation. Plast Reconstr Surg 84:921-934, 1989.

5. Horl HW, Feller AM, Biemer E. Technique for liposuction fat reimplantation and long-term volume evaluation by magnetic resonance imaging. Ann Plast Surg 26: 248-258, 1991.

6. Illouz Y-G. The fat cell "graft": A new technique to fill depressions. Plast Reconstr Surg 78:122-123, 1986.

7. Moscona R, Ullman MD, Har-Hashi Y, Hirscowitz B. Case report: Free-fat injections for the correction of hemifacial atrophy. Plast Reconstr Surg 84:501-507, 1989.

8. Matsudo PK, Toledo LS. Experience of injected fat grafting. Aesthetic Plast Surg 12:35-38, 1988.

9. Teimourian B. Repair of soft-tissue contour deficit by means of semi-liquid fat graft [letter]. Plast Reconstr Surg 78:123-124, 1986.

10. Ellenbogen R. Free autogenous pearl fat grafts in the face: A preliminary report of a rediscovered technique. Ann Plast Surg 16:179-194, 1986.

11. Fredericks S. Discussion of Chajchir A, Benzaquen I. Fat-grafting injection for soft tissue augmentation. Plast Reconstr Surg 84:935, 1989.

12. Ersek RA. Transplantation of purified autologous fat: A 3-year follow-up is disappointing. Plast Reconstr Surg 87:219-229, 1991.

13. Ellenbogen R. Invited commentary. Ann Plast Surg 24:297, 1990.

14. Ellenbogen R. Autologous fat injection [letter]. Plast Reconstr Surg 88:543, 1991.

15. Bircoll M. Cosmetic breast augmentation using autologous fat and liposuction techniques. Plast Reconstr Surg 79:267-271, 1987.

Additional Complications

1. Pitman GH, Teimourian B. Suction lipectomy: Complications and results by survey. Plast Reconstr Surg 76:65-69, 1985.
2. Teimourian B, Rogers WB. A national survey of complications associated with suction lipectomy: A comparative study. Plast Reconstr Surg 84:628-631, 1989.
3. Dillerud E. Suction lipoplasty: A report on complications, undesired results, and patient satisfaction based on 3511 procedures. Plast Reconstr Surg 88:239-246, 1991.
4. Mathews WA, Grazer FM. Operative management. In Grazer FM. Atlas of Suction Assisted Lipectomy in Body Contouring. New York: Churchill Livingstone, 1992, pp 82-92.
5. Teimourian B. Suction Lipectomy and Body Sculpturing. St. Louis: CV Mosby, 1987.
6. Christman KD. Death following suction lipectomy and abdominoplasty [letter]. Plast Reconstr Surg 78:428, 1986.
7. Alexander JM, Takeda D, Sanders G, Goldberg G. Fatal necrotizing fasciitis following suction-assisted lipectomy. Ann Plast Surg 20:562-565, 1988.
8. Roberts HR, Adel S, Bernstein EF. Prevention of venous thrombosis and pulmonary embolism: Consensus conference. JAMA 256:744-749, 1986.
9. Kakkar VV, Field ES, Nicolaides AN, Flute PT, Wessler S, Yin ET. Low doses of heparin in prevention of deep-vein thrombosis. Lancet 2:669-671, 1971.
10. Kakkar VV, Corrigan T, Spindler J, Flossard DP, Flute PT, Crellin RQ, Wessler S. Efficacy of low doses of heparin in prevention of deep-vein thrombosis after major surgery. Lancet 2:101-106, 1972.
11. Pachter HL, Riles TS. Low dose heparin: Bleeding and wound complications in the surgical patient. Ann Surg 186:669-674, 1977.
12. Bowe RC, Brown RC. Lung injury and prospects for therapy. In Vincent JL, ed. Update in Intensive Care and Emergency Medicine. New York: Springer-Verlag, 1987, pp 109.
13. Chan KM, Tham KT, Chow YW, Leung PC. Posttraumatic fat embolism: Its clinical and subclinical presentation. J Trauma 24:45-49, 1984.
14. Fabian TC, Hoots AV, Stanford DS, et al. Fat embolism syndrome: Prospective evaluation in 92 fracture patients. Crit Care Med 18:42-46, 1990.
15. Hunstad JP, Withers JP. Pulmonary fat embolism: Does it occur following suction assisted lipectomy. Presented at the Fifty-Sixth Annual Scientific Meeting of the American Society of Plastic and Reconstructive Surgeons. Atlanta: November 13, 1987.
16. Abbes M, Borergean Y. Fat embolism after dermolipectomy and liposuction [letter]. Plast Reconstr Surg 84:546, 1989.
17. Laub D Jr, Laub D Sr. Fat embolism syndrome after liposuction. A case report and review of the literature. Ann Plast Surg 25:48-52, 1990.
18. Ross RM, Johnson GW. Fat embolism after liposuction. Chest 93:1294-1295, 1988.

Credits

Chapter 1

p 13 (top), after Mladick RA. The big six: Six important tips for a better result in lipoplasty. Clin Plast Surg 16:249-262, 1989.

p 27, from Pitman GH. Suction lipectomy of the face and body: Precision and refinement. In Riley WB Jr, ed. Plastic Surgery Educational Foundation Instructional Courses, vol 1. St. Louis: CV Mosby, 1988, p 80.

Chapter 2

p 39, courtesy Grams Medical, Costa Mesa, Calif.

p 40, courtesy M.D. Engineering Company, Hayward, Calif.

p 42, courtesy Wells-Johnson Company, Tucson, Ariz.

Chapter 3

p 46, from Pitman GH. Suction lipectomy of the face and body: Precision and refinement. In Riley WB Jr, ed. Plastic Surgery Educational Foundation Instructional Courses, vol 1. St. Louis: CV Mosby, 1988, p 82.

p 53, courtesy M.D. Engineering Company, Hayward, Calif.

p 67, courtesy Caromed International, Inc., Raleigh, N.C.

p 68, courtesy Augustine Medical, Inc., Eden Prairie, Minn.

Chapter 4

pp 74, 77, 78, 79, from Pitman GH, Holzer J. Safe suction: Fluid replacement and blood loss parameters. Perspect Plast Surg 5(1):79-89, 1991.

Chapter 5

pp 92 (bottom), 97 (top), courtesy Wells-Johnson Company, Tucson, Ariz.

pp 101, 102, from Nürnberger F, Müller G. So-called cellulite: An invented disease. J Dermatol Surg Oncol 4:221-229, 1978 (copyright 1978 by Elsevier Science Publishing Co., Inc.).

p 105 (bottom), after Grazer FM. Cellulite lysing. Aesthetic Surg 11:11, 1991.

p 107, from Pitman GH. Suction lipectomy of the face and body: Precision and refinement. In Riley WB Jr, ed. Plastic Surgery Educational Foundation Instructional Courses, vol 1. St. Louis: CV Mosby, 1988, pp 80, 93.

Chapter 6

p 114, from Marino H, Galeano EJ, Gandolfo EA. Plastic correction of double chin: Importance of the position of the hyoid bone. Plast Reconstr Surg 31:45-50, 1963.

p 117 (right), after Pernkopf E. Atlas of Topographical and Applied Human Anatomy, vol 1. Philadelphia: WB Saunders, 1963, p 225.

p 127, from Pitman GH. Face and neck contouring by fat removal. In Courtiss EH, ed. Male Aesthetic Surgery. St. Louis: Mosby–Year Book, 1991, p 309.

p 134 (bottom), from Pitman GH. Suction lipectomy of the face and body: Precision and refinement. In Riley WB Jr, ed. Plastic Surgery Educational Foundation Instructional Courses, vol 1. St. Louis: CV Mosby, 1988, p 96.

p 141 (lower left), from Pitman GH. Face and neck contouring by fat removal. In Courtiss EH, ed. Male Aesthetic Surgery. St. Louis: Mosby–Year Book, 1991, p. 141.

Chapter 7

p 174, after Guerrerosantos J. Arm-lift. In Courtiss EH, ed. Aesthetic Surgery: Trouble, How to Avoid It and How to Treat It. St. Louis: CV Mosby, 1978, pp 232-246, and Guerrerosantos J. Brachioplasty. Aesthetic Plast Surg 3:1-44, 1979.

p 192 (top), after Grazer FM. Body contouring. In McCarthy JG, ed. Plastic Surgery. Philadelphia: WB Saunders, 1990.

Chapter 8

p 206, courtesy Caromed International, Inc., Raleigh, N.C.

Chapter 9

p 277, courtesy Caromed International, Inc., Raleigh, N.C.

Chapter 10

p 319, after Lockwood TE. Superficial fascial system (SFS) of the trunk and extremities: A new concept. Plast Reconstr Surg 87:1009-1018, 1991.

p 333 (bottom), from Pitman GH. Suction lipectomy of the face and body: Precision and refinement. In Riley WB Jr, ed. Plastic Surgery Educational Foundation Instructional Courses, vol 1. St. Louis: CV Mosby, 1988, p 89.

Chapter 11

p 345, modified from Lockwood TE. Superficial fascial system (SFS) of the trunk and extremities: A new concept. Plast Reconstr Surg 87:1009-1018, 1981.

pp 346, 347, after Manchot C. The Cutaneous Arteries of the Human Body. Leipzig: FCW Vogel, 1889. (First English edition translated by Morain WD, Ristic J. New York: Springer-Verlag, 1983.)

p 351 (lower right), from Pitman GH. Suction lipectomy of the face and body: Precision and refinement. In Riley WB Jr, ed. Plastic Surgery Educational Foundation Instructional Courses, vol 1. St. Louis: CV Mosby, 1988, p 93.

Chapter 12

pp 419 (bottom), 442, 443 (top), from Pitman GH. Suction lipectomy of the face and body: Precision and refinement. In Riley WB Jr, ed. Plastic Surgery Educational Foundation Instructional Courses, vol 1. St. Louis: CV Mosby, 1988, p 91.

Index